Recent Advances and Future Directions in Trauma Care

Guest Editor

JEREMY W. CANNON, MD, SM

SURGICAL CLINICS OF NORTH AMERICA

www.surgical.theclinics.com

Consulting Editor
RONALD F. MARTIN, MD

August   2012 • Volume 92 • Number 4

SAUNDERS an imprint of ELSEVIER, Inc.

W.B. SAUNDERS COMPANY

A Division of Elsevier Inc.

1600 John F. Kennedy Blvd., Suite 1800, Philadelphia, PA 19103-2899

http://www.surgical.theclinics.com

SURGICAL CLINICS OF NORTH AMERICA Volume 92, Number 4
August 2012 ISSN 0039–6109, ISBN-13: 978-1-4557-4964-5

Editor: John Vassallo, j.vassallo@elsevier.com

Developmental Editor: Teia Stone

Surgical Clinics of North America (ISSN 0039–6109) is published bimonthly by Elsevier Inc., 360 Park Avenue South, New York, NY 10010-1710. Months of publication are February, April, June, August, October, and December. Business and Editorial Offices: 1600 John F. Kennedy Blvd., Suite 1800, Philadelphia, PA 19103-2899. Periodicals postage paid at New York, NY and additional mailing offices. Subscription prices are $339.00 per year for US individuals, $575.00 per year for US institutions, $166.00 per year for US students and residents, $415.00 per year for Canadian individuals, $714.00 per year for Canadian institutions, $468.00 for international individuals, $714.00 per year for international institutions and $229.00 per year for Canadian and foreign students/residents. To receive student/resident rate, orders must be accompanied by name of affiliated institution, date of term, and the *signature* of program/residency coordinator on institution letterhead. Orders will be billed at individual rate until proof of status is received. Foreign air speed delivery is included in all *Clinics* subscription prices. All prices are subject to change without notice. POSTMASTER: Send address changes to *Surgical Clinics*, Elsevier Health Sciences Division, Subscription Customer Service, 3251 Riverport Lane, Maryland Heights, MO 63043. **Customer Service (orders, claims, online, change of address): Telephone: 1-800-654-2452 (U.S. and Canada); 314-447-8871 (outside U.S. and Canada). Fax: 314-447-8029. E-mail: journalscustomerservice-usa@elsevier.com (for print support); journalsonline support-usa@elsevier.com (for online support).**

Reprints. For copies of 100 or more, of articles in this publication, please contact the Commercial Reprints Department, Elsevier Inc., 360 Park Avenue South, New York, New York 10010-1710. Tel. (212) 633-3812, Fax: (212) 462-1935, e-mail: reprints@elsevier.com.

The Surgical Clinics of North America is also published in Spanish by McGraw-Hill Interamericana Editores S.A., P.O. Box 5-237 06500 Mexico D.F. Mexico; and in Portuguese by Interlivros Edicoes Ltda., Rua Comandante Coelho 1085, CEP 21250, Rio de Janeiro, Brazil; and in Greek by Paschalidis Medical Publications, Athens Greece.

The Surgical Clinics of North America is covered in *MEDLINE/PubMed (Index Medicus)*, *EMBASE/Excerpta Medica, Current Contents/Clinical Medicine, Current Contents/Life Sciences, Science Citation Index*, and *ISI/BIOMED*.

Printed and bound by CPI Group (UK) Ltd, Croydon, CR0 4YY

Transferred to Digital Print 2012

Contributors

CONSULTING EDITOR

RONALD F. MARTIN, MD
Staff Surgeon, Department of Surgery, Marshfield Clinic, Marshfield, Wisconsin; Clinical
Associate Professor, University of Wisconsin School of Medicine and Public Health,
Madison, Wisconsin; Colonel, Medical Corps, United States Army Reserve

GUEST EDITOR

LtCOL JEREMY W. CANNON, MD, SM
US Air Force, Norman M. Rich Department of Surgery, Bethesda, Maryland; Division
of Trauma and Acute Care Surgery, San Antonio Military Medical Center, Fort Sam
Houston, Texas

AUTHORS

COL EDWARD D. ARRINGTON, MD, FACS
Colonel, US Army; Department of Orthopedic Surgery, Madigan Army Medical Center,
Tacoma, Washington

JEFFREY BAILEY, MD
US Army Institute of Surgical Research, Joint Trauma System, Fort Sam Houston, Texas

ALEC C. BEEKLEY, MD, FACP
Associate Professor of Surgery, Thomas Jefferson University, Philadelphia, Pennsylvania

COL LORNE H. BLACKBOURNE, MD, FACS
Commander, US Army Institute of Surgical Research, Fort Sam Houston, Texas

LAURA R. BROSCH, RN, PhD
Office of Research Protections, Headquarters, United States Army Medical Research and
Materiel Command, Fort Detrick, Maryland

COL LEOPOLDO C. CANCIO, MD, FACS
Medical Corps, US Army, US Army Institute of Surgical Research, Fort Sam Houston,
Texas

LtCOL JEREMY W. CANNON, MD, SM
US Air Force, Norman M. Rich Department of Surgery, Bethesda, Maryland; Division
of Trauma and Acute Care Surgery, San Antonio Military Medical Center, Fort Sam
Houston, Texas

JOHN CHOVANES, DO
Department of Surgery, Cooper University Hospital, Camden, New Jersey

KEVIN K. CHUNG, MD
Lieutenant Colonel, US Army, Clinical Division, US Army Institute of Surgical Research, Fort Sam Houston, San Antonio, Texas

MITCHELL JAY COHEN, MD, FACS
Department of Surgery, San Francisco General Hospital, University of California, San Francisco, San Francisco, California

MARIANNE V. CUSICK, MD, MSPH
Resident, Department of Surgery, University of Alabama at Birmingham, Birmingham, Alabama

MICHAEL DECUYPERE, MD, PhD
Neurosurgery Resident, Department of Neurosurgery, University of Tennessee Health Science Center, Memphis, Tennessee

Lt COL JOSEPH J. DUBOSE, MD, FACS
US Air Force; Division of Trauma, Acute Care Surgery and Surgical Critical Care, R Adams Cowley Shock Trauma Center, University of Maryland, Baltimore, Maryland

JOHN B. HOLCOMB, MD
Professor of Surgery, Center for Translational Injury Research, Department of Surgery, University of Texas Health Science Center, Houston, Texas

DAVID HOYT, MD
Executive Director, American College of Surgeons, Chicago, Illinois

JOSEPH R. HSU, MD
Lieutenant Colonel, US Army; Department of Orthopedic Surgery and Rehabilitation, San Antonio Military Medical Center, Fort Sam Houston, Texas

EDWARD KELLY, MD
Assistant Professor of Surgery, Director of Acute Care Surgery Fellowship, Division of Trauma, Burn, and Surgical Critical Care, Harvard Medical School, Brigham and Women's Hospital, Boston, Massachusetts

JEFFREY D. KERBY, MD, PhD
Professor of Surgery, Section of Trauma, Burns, and Surgical Critical Care, Department of Surgery; Director, Alabama Resuscitation Center, University of Alabama at Birmingham, Birmingham, Alabama

MANSOOR KHAN, MBBS(Lond), MRCS(Eng), FRCS(GenSurg)
Surgeon Lieutenant Commander, Royal Navy; Division of Trauma, Acute Care Surgery and Surgical Critical Care, R Adams Cowley Shock Trauma Center, University of Maryland, Baltimore, Maryland

DAVID R. KING, MD
Major, US Army Reserve, Division of Trauma, Emergency Surgery and Surgical Critical Care, Massachusetts General Hospital and Harvard Medical School, Boston, Massachusetts

JOSEPH M. KLAUSNER, MD, FACS
Professor of Surgery, Chairman, Division of Surgery, Tel-Aviv Medical Center, Sackler Faculty of Medicine, Tel-Aviv University, Tel-Aviv, Israel

PAUL KLIMO Jr, MD, MPH
Assistant Professor of Neurosurgery, Department of Neurosurgery, University of Tennessee Health Science Center; Semmes-Murphey Neurologic and Spine Institute; LeBonheur Children's Hospital, Memphis, Tennessee

MAJ JONATHAN B. LUNDY, MD, FACS
Medical Corps, US Army, US Army Institute of Surgical Research, Fort Sam Houston, Texas

JONATHAN J. MORRISON, MB, ChB, MRCS
The Academic Department of Military Surgery and Trauma, Royal Centre for Defence Medicine, Birmingham, United Kingdom; US Army Institute of Surgical Research, Fort Sam Houston, Texas

ALAN MURDOCK, MD
US Air Force Medical Service and University of Pittsburgh, Pittsburgh, Pennsylvania

TIMOTHY C. NUNEZ, MD
Division of Trauma and Acute Care Surgery, San Antonio Military Medical Center, Fort Sam Houston, Texas

JEREMY G. PERKINS, MD
Associate Professor of Medicine, Hematology-Oncology Service, Uniformed Services University of the Health Sciences, Walter Reed National Military Medical Center, Bethesda, Maryland

TODD E. RASMUSSEN, MD, FACS
US Army Institute of Surgical Research, Fort Sam Houston, Texas; US Air Force Medical Service, 59th Medical Deployment Wing, Science and Technology Section, Lackland Air Force Base, Texas; The Norman M. Rich Department of Surgery, The Uniformed Services University of the Health Sciences, Bethesda, Maryland

SELWYN O. ROGERS Jr, MD, MPH
Associate Professor of Surgery, Chief, Division of Trauma, Burn, and Surgical Critical Care, Harvard Medical School, Brigham and Women's Hospital, Boston, Massachusetts

ROBERT M. RUSH Jr, MD, FACS
Colonel, US Army; Chief, Department of Surgery, Madigan, Army Medical Center, Tacoma, Washington

COL ROBERT L. SHERIDAN, MD, FACS
Medical Corps, US Army Reserve, Burn Surgery Service, Shriners Hospital for Children; Massachusetts General Hospital, Surgical Critical Care, Boston VA Healthcare System, Boston, Massachusetts

DROR SOFFER, MD
Director, Associate Professor of Surgery, Division of Surgery, The Yitzhak Rabin Trauma Center, Tel-Aviv Medical Center, Sackler Faculty of Medicine, Tel-Aviv University, Tel-Aviv, Israel

SCOTT TREXLER, MD
Department of Surgery, San Antonio Military Medical Center, Fort Sam Houston, Texas

CHARLES E. WADE, PhD
Professor of Surgery, Center for Translational Injury Research, Department of Surgery, University of Texas Medical School, Houston, Texas

KELLY L. WARFIELD, PhD
Integrated Biotherapeutics, Inc, Gaithersburg, Maryland

Lt COL DAVID ZONIES, MD, MPH, FACS, USAF, MC
Director, Department of Trauma and Critical Care, Landstuhl Regional Medical Center,
Landstuhl; Director, 86th MDS Acute Lung Rescue Team, Ramstein Air Base, Germany

Contents

> Prehospital care of the trauma patient is continuing to evolve; however, the principles of airway maintenance, hemorrhage control, and appropriate resuscitative maneuvers remain central to the role of the emergency medical care provider. Recent changes in the regulations for research in emergency settings will allow randomized trials to proceed to test new devices, drugs, and resuscitative strategies in the prehospital environment. The creation of prehospital research networks will provide the appropriate infrastructure to greatly facilitate the development of new protocols and the execution of large-scale randomized trials with the potential to change current prehospital practice.

> Trauma resulting in hemorrhage from vascular disruption within the torso is a challenging scenario, with a propensity to be lethal in the first hour following trauma. The term noncompressible torso hemorrhage (NCTH) was only recently coined as part of contemporary studies describing the epidemiology of wounding during the wars in Afghanistan and Iraq. This article provides a contemporary review of NCTH, including a unifying definition to promote future study as well as a description of resuscitative and operative management strategies to be used in this setting, and sets a course for research to improve mortality following this vexing injury pattern.

> The philosophy of damage control surgery has developed tremendously over the past 10 years. It has expanded outside the original boundaries of the abdomen and has been applied to all aspects of trauma care, ranging from resuscitation to limb-threatening vascular injuries. In recent years, the US military has taken the concept to a new level by initiating a damage

control approach at the point of injury and continuing it through a transcontinental health care system. This article highlights many recent advances in damage control surgery and discusses proper patient selection and the risks associated with this management strategy.

During the past decade there has been a profound change in the understanding of postinjury coagulation. Concurrently, new data suggest that a resuscitative strategy to minimize large volumes of crystalloid while recreating whole is associated with reduced morbidity and mortality. This article outlines the history of resuscitation and transfusion practices in trauma, the changing understanding of coagulation and inflammation, and clinical data driving changes in resuscitative conduct. Finally, the current state of the science suggests future basic science and clinical investigation that will drive changes in transfusion and resuscitation in severely injured military personnel and civilian patients.

Optimal care of critically ill trauma patients remains a challenge within modern medical systems. During the past decade, emerging technologies and organizational improvements have greatly advanced the care of these patients. The effective implementation of best practice initiatives has led to measurable improvement in outcomes while also reducing health care costs. Continued advances in the implementation of these initiatives and ICU organization are required, however, to insure that optimal care is provided to this unique patient population.

Care of critically injured patients has evolved over the 50 years since Shoemaker established one of the first trauma units at Cook County Hospital in 1962. Modern trauma intensive care units offer a high nurse-to-patient ratio, physicians and midlevel providers who manage the patients, and technologically advanced monitors and therapeutic devices designed to optimize the care of patients. This article describes advances that have transformed trauma critical care, including bedside ultrasonography, novel patient monitoring techniques, extracorporeal support, and negative pressure dressings. It also discusses how to evaluate the safety and efficacy of future advances in trauma critical care.

Long-range critical care aeromedical evacuation has significantly contributed to the unprecedented survival during recent military operations. With advances in critical care, patients with increased injury severity and overall complexity are routinely evacuated while resuscitation is ongoing. Additional specialty teams now provide advanced pulmonary rescue therapies for the most critically ill patients. As part of the continuum of trauma care, an overseas fixed facility provides follow-on emergency surgical critical care to optimize patient outcomes before final evacuation to the continental United States.

Traumatic brain injury (TBI) involves significant damage of the brain parenchyma, and is the leading cause of morbidity and mortality after trauma. It is thus essential for all physicians involved in acute care medicine and surgery to have a thorough understanding of TBI. Management of the patient with TBI is a rapidly advancing field, characterized by an improved understanding of intracranial pathophysiology and decreasing overall mortality largely because of improved neurocritical and surgical care. This article summarizes the classification system, management approaches, and recent controversies in the care of mild, moderate, and severe TBI.

Burns and environmental injuries are common as primary or secondary problems in survivors of natural disasters, terrorist incidents, and combat operations. In recent years, intensive military medical experience has resulted in substantial progress in treatment of these important problems. This article reviews practical applications of this new knowledge.

Historically, complex extremity injuries, otherwise known as mangled extremities, have been difficult management problems. This is especially true in multiply-injured patients where many priorities exist and where amputation is considered a failure of limb salvage. Over the past decade, advances in the total management of complex extremity injuries, from the placement of life-saving and limb-saving tourniquets in the prehospital setting to the advancement of prosthetics and rehabilitation months to years later, have resulted in superb functional results regardless of whether limb salvage or amputation is undertaken.

Efforts to develop trauma systems in the United States followed the publication of the landmark article, "Accidental Death and Disability: The Neglected Disease of Modern Society," by the National Academy of Sciences (1966) and have resulted in the implementation of a system of care for the seriously injured in most states and within the US military. In 2007, Hoyt and Coimbra published an article detailing the history, organization, and future directions of trauma systems within the United States. This article provides an update of the developments that have occurred in trauma systems in system verification and regionalization.

Israel is a small country with a unique trauma system that was developed from the experience gained in peace and in war. That trauma system was designed to fit the state's current health system, which is different from the European and American systems. This article describes the infrastructure of both prehospital and in-hospital trauma management, as well as the main cornerstones of their development. The experience that was gained from multiple mass casualty incidents is discussed. The protocols of mass casualty management in the prehospital and in-hospital setup are described.

Throughout history, wars have resulted in medical advancements, especially in trauma. Once clinical challenges are identified, they require documentation and analysis before changes to care are introduced. The wars in Afghanistan and Iraq led to the collection of clinically relevant data from the entire medical system into a formal trauma registry. Improvements in data collection and human research oversight have allowed more effective and efficient techniques to capture and analyze trauma data, which has enabled rapid development and dissemination of clinical practice guidelines in the midst of war. These data-driven experiences are influencing trauma practice patterns in the civilian community.

The increasing need for skilled emergency surgical providers, coupled with decreasing experience in emergency surgery among trainees, has led to significant shortages in the availability of such surgeons. In response to this crisis, surgical leaders have developed a comprehensive curriculum and a set of professional standards to guide the training of a new specialist: the acute care surgeon. This article reviews the development and goals for Fellowship training of this new specialty.

SURGICAL CLINICS
OF NORTH AMERICA

DOWNLOAD
Free App!

Review Articles
THE CLINICS

NOW AVAILABLE FOR YOUR iPhone and iPad

SURGICAL CLINICS
OF NORTH AMERICA

Foreword

Recent Advances and Future Directions in Trauma Care

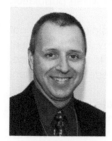

Ronald F. Martin, MD
Consulting Editor

Seven thousand eight hundred thirty-four is a large number. Of course, it is larger than some and smaller than others. Its relative magnitude might depend more on what it measures than the actual number itself. In this case, I could not begin to suggest that I could tell you how large of a number it is. You will have to decide. The number 7834 is the official number of coalition fatalities from Operation Enduring Freedom and Operation Iraqi Freedom that are recorded as of the day of the writing of this foreword. Of that number, 6484 of those killed in action were United States service members and 1350 were from other countries participating in the coalition forces. Nearly 2000 United States service members died in Afghanistan and 4486 died in Iraq. Somewhere in the ballpark of a log order greater than that were seriously wounded. Some of the wounded were able to return to duty, while many more were not. The numbers of other-than-Coalition personnel wounded or killed are not reliably calculable but estimated to be a substantially larger number even still.

Those numbers—those, in my opinion, very large numbers—are the price that we as a society have paid for the information that we share with you in this issue.

It is hardly a novel observation that many of the advances in surgery and surgical thought are derived from lessons learned on or from the battlefield. Whether we respond to the high-tech weapons of large, well-funded armies and the havoc they wreak or the reintroduction of the low-tech weapons of the insurgent, we still must learn and relearn lessons. As is always our hope, we wish to understand and store that which we have learned well and rapidly in order that others may benefit as quickly as possible.

Fewer than 5 of 1000 Americans have served in these recent armed conflicts. An even smaller fraction of American physicians or surgeons have served. The lessons shared in this issue have been collected from those who have been there and witnessed first hand

Surg Clin N Am 92 (2012) xiii–xiv
http://dx.doi.org/10.1016/j.suc.2012.06.005
0039-6109/12/$ – see front matter © 2012 Elsevier Inc. All rights reserved.

surgical.theclinics.com

the challenges of medicine at war. I have had the distinct honor and privilege of working with and for many of them, either here in the continental United States or in Iraq, Afghanistan, or both. The *Surgical Clinics of North America* is privileged to have these contributors share what they have learned with us.

It is my fervent hope that the majority of our readership will never have to use the information gathered in this issue under the circumstances under which it was collected. That said, much of what we have learned benefits our civilian population who suffer from traumatic injuries as well as other maladies.

The opinions I express in this foreword are absolutely my own opinions and do not necessarily reflect the opinions or positions of the United States Army, the Department of Defense, the United States Government, or the other contributors to this issue. Also, I have no financial disclosures other than that from time to time the federal government employed me during this process.

It has been 3917 days since these conflicts began and as stated 7800 coalition partners and countless others have died during this time. We have learned much and now we need to incorporate that knowledge into our everyday work in a meaningful and lasting way. It came at too great a price to do otherwise.

It is Memorial Day weekend 2012 as the final touches are put on this issue. I should like to commemorate this issue to all those who have fallen in service to their country. I would also like to thank and remember all those who served past and present.

Ronald F. Martin, MD
Department of Surgery
Marshfield Clinic
1000 North Oak Avenue
Marshfield, WI 54449, USA

Colonel, United States Army Reserves
Medical Corps Associate Dean
University of Wisconsin School of Medicine and Public Health

E-mail address:
martin.ronald@marshfield.org

Preface
Recent Advances and Future Directions in Trauma Care

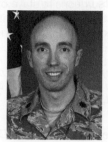

LtCOL Jeremy W. Cannon, MD, SM
Guest Editor

What a great time to be a trauma surgeon! In many ways, our specialty is now enjoying a sweeping revival. The insights and innovations of many years have culminated in a cascade of advances over the past decade with benefits demonstrated both on the battlefield and in our practices at home. Meanwhile, many bright surgeon-scientists are now unraveling the conundrums in trauma care that have puzzled us for years while also revealing a host of new and even more difficult questions.

Despite these positive developments, numerous challenges in trauma care remain. The uncertainty of how health care within this country will be delivered in the future weighs heavily on our surgical leadership. Many hospitals and surgical practices across the country continue to debate the optimal practice model for specialists in the fields of trauma surgery, acute care surgery, general surgery, and the surgical subspecialties. A comprehensive disaster management plan that permits both autonomy at the state level and nationwide organization has yet to be fully worked out. And, of course, severely injured patients continue to expire daily in community hospitals, trauma centers, and combat hospitals across the world despite the rigorous application of the best evidence in trauma systems and patient management.

After a decade of war with unprecedented military-civilian collaboration, this issue of *Surgical Clinics of North America* aims to chronicle the most important advances in trauma care and to address some of the challenges for the future. The articles that follow should thus serve as a benchmark for the state of the art in trauma care in 2012. To this end, this issue is subdivided into three areas of focus:

- Lessons learned in trauma care from prehospital to ICU management
- Advances in the signature injures of the last decade—traumatic brain injury, extremity trauma, and burns/environmental injuries
- Practical developments in trauma systems and trauma training.

Surg Clin N Am 92 (2012) xv–xvi
http://dx.doi.org/10.1016/j.suc.2012.06.004
0039-6109/12/$ – see front matter © 2012 Elsevier Inc. All rights reserved.

surgical.theclinics.com

The assembled authors include both military and civilian experts who have committed untold hours to this ambitious project. In some cases, the articles were drafted or revised on dusty computers with painfully slow network connections many thousands of miles from home. For this act of selfless service by those in uniform and for the tremendous wellspring of support by our civilian colleagues, the editors and readers of this issue owe a great debt of gratitude. Although this debt cannot be repaid, please know your efforts will enable many current and future trauma surgeons to stave off the grave indictment of Dr Edward Churchill: "...in every new war the same stupid mistakes are made again and soldiers lose their lives and limbs because the doctor was ignorant of past experience."

The opinions expressed in this document are solely those of the author and do not represent an endorsement by or the views of the United States Air Force, the Department of Defense, or the United States Government.

LtCOL Jeremy W. Cannon, MD, SM
Division of Trauma and Acute Care Surgery
San Antonio Military Medical Center
Fort Sam Houston, TX 78234, USA

Norman M. Rich Department of Surgery
Bethesda, MD 20814, USA

E-mail address:
jcannon@massmed.org

Invited Commentary

Recent Advances and Future Directions in Trauma Care

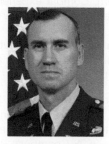

COL Lorne H. Blackbourne, MD
Invited Commentary

The authors in this issue of the *Surgical Clinics of North America* must be applauded not only collectively for providing an outstanding overview of recent advances and future directions for improvement in military medical care but also individually for their dedication to saving lives and limiting the suffering of those wounded in combat—many spending years in austere conditions away from their family, friends, and fellow countrymen.

This issue is of a historic stature at a historic time. As the overseas contingency operations in Iraq and Afghanistan come to an end, the time to document the advances and the areas for improvement in combat casualty care is indeed now.

Documenting the advances is extremely important to provide medical personnel in any future conflict the full benefit of "lessons learned" not only with unique techniques and methods but also with their application in treating vastly complex battlefield wounds.

Documenting the areas for improvement in combat casualty care, often referred to as "gaps," has taken on a new historical importance—especially in the United States. US military medical personnel now face the challenge of Executive Order No. 13139, signed September 30, 1999, which specifies that only products and medications approved by the US Food and Drug Administration (FDA) can be used on the battlefield. This order has changed the paradigm of major military medical advances from the time of active conflict to a time of relative peace that will allow the luxury of time during the prolonged process of research, development, and then FDA approval.

In the shadow of this new paradigm, this issue of *Surgical Clinics of North America* is an outstanding beacon of knowledge for those trying to elucidate and then bridge the unique "gaps" of military medical technology and capability.

Surg Clin N Am 92 (2012) xvii–xviii
http://dx.doi.org/10.1016/j.suc.2012.06.006
0039-6109/12/$ – see front matter Published by Elsevier Inc.

surgical.theclinics.com

Now is the time for all combat-experienced medical personnel to document all of the data we can analyze on our Wounded Warriors. Data are the most important element in substantiating areas of excellence and areas for improvement along the continuum of combat casualty care. Every medical facility needs to have efforts to document their local combat-wounded population as well as global efforts using the Department of Defense Trauma Registry (which was previously named the Joint Theater Trauma Registry) housed at the Joint Trauma System. Combat experience allows for unique insight into the areas for potential research and will allow for combat-relevant questions to be answered.

These authors have by their efforts, in essence, helped treat wounded in any future conflict. Sir Winston Churchill would likely have called this effort to help save lives and alleviate suffering in a time of war "glorious to both God and man."

COL Lorne H. Blackbourne, MD
Commander
US Army Institute of Surgical Research
3698 Chamber's Pass
Fort Sam Houston, TX 78234, USA

E-mail address:
lorne.h.blackbourne@us.army.mil

Prehospital Emergency Trauma Care and Management

Jeffrey D. Kerby, MD, PhD[a,b,*], Marianne V. Cusick, MD, MSPH[c]

KEYWORDS

- Trauma • Emergency care • Prehospital

KEY POINTS

- Use of endotracheal intubation in the prehospital care environment remains controversial. Well-designed randomized trials are necessary to assess the efficacy and risks associated with prehospital endotracheal intubation. Alternatives to endotracheal intubation for airway management are available and becoming more commonly used.
- Tourniquets should be considered, even in the civilian setting, when direct pressure fails to control bleeding from extremity wounds. Emergency medical service (EMS) systems should train medics in proper use and placement of tourniquets.
- Current trends are for limited crystalloid resuscitation and early use of blood and blood products before hemorrhage control. Randomized trials are currently under way to test limited crystalloid resuscitation in the prehospital environment for both blunt and penetrating injury. Several resuscitation adjuncts are currently being investigated for prehospital use.
- Traditional vital signs are limited in their ability to accurately identify patients in shock. Identification of patients in occult shock is an active area of investigation using point-of-care devices, assessment of heart-rate variability, and measurement of tissue oxygenation.
- Prehospital research infrastructure is being established and continuing to expand, which will allow for further growth of research activities to evaluate new products and resuscitative strategies.

This work was supported by Grant No. 5UO1H077881 from the National Heart, Lung, and Blood Institute.

Jeffrey D. Kerby, MD, PhD, is a principal investigator and director of the Alabama Regional Clinical Center for the National Heart, Lung, and Blood–sponsored Resuscitation Outcomes Consortium.

[a] Section of Trauma, Burns, and Surgical Critical Care, Department of Surgery, University of Alabama at Birmingham, 701 19th Street South, LHRB 112, Birmingham, AL 35294-0007, USA; [b] Alabama Resuscitation Center, University of Alabama at Birmingham, 619 19th Street South, Room 251, Birmingham, AL 35249, USA; [c] Department of Surgery, University of Alabama at Birmingham, 1922 7th Avenue South, KB 217, Birmingham, AL 35294-0007, USA
* Corresponding author. Section of Trauma, Burns, and Surgical Critical Care, Department of Surgery, University of Alabama at Birmingham, 701 19th Street South, LHRB 112, Birmingham, AL 35294-0007.
E-mail address: jeffrey.kerby@ccc.uab.edu

Surg Clin N Am 92 (2012) 823–841
doi:10.1016/j.suc.2012.04.009
0039-6109/12/$ – see front matter Published by Elsevier Inc.
surgical.theclinics.com

INTRODUCTION

Approximately 50% of injury-related deaths occur in the first 12 hours, and both mortality and late complications have been linked to the efficacy of early interventions. Consequently, improvements in prehospital treatment algorithms and resuscitation strategies have the potential to improve survival and reduce morbidity.[1–3] The indications and type of airway control maneuvers in the prehospital setting continue to evolve. Devices used to control exsanguinating hemorrhage and further innovation in the field of topical hemostatic agents are further refining prehospital and combat casualty care paradigms. Early detection of occult shock along with the use of resuscitation adjuncts and refinements of delayed resuscitation strategies are being investigated actively. With advancements in federal regulations governing informed consent procedures and development of the necessary infrastructure to perform randomized trials in the prehospital environment, research in the field of prehospital resuscitation of trauma patients has increased significantly. This article provides an overview of the current status of prehospital care and also highlights some of the recent advancements and future research in each of the following critical areas:

- Airway control
- Hemorrhage control
- Prehospital resuscitation and resuscitation adjuncts
- Identification of occult shock
- Prehospital research infrastructure.

AIRWAY CONTROL

Prehospital endotracheal intubation remains one of the more controversial interventions in the emergency medical service repertoire. Some investigators call into question the safety and efficacy of performing endotracheal intubation in the prehospital care setting whereas proponents of endotracheal intubation by EMS personnel report that first responders are capable of endotracheal intubation with low complication rates.[4–9] EMS systems with the highest reported endotracheal success rate are stringently trained with some systems requiring more than 20 live intubations before certification and a minimum of 12 field or prehospital intubations annually to remain certified and maintain adequate clinical experience.

More recent studies have reported successful prehospital intubation rates as high as 97% in regions where paralytics agents are routinely used.[4] Proponents of the use of paralytic agents suggest that allowing neuromuscular blockade allows for the expansion of the indications for intubation to a larger population from merely those that are comatose to those that are critically injured who may benefit from airway protection and controlled oxygenation and ventilation. The current use of neuromuscular blocking agents, however, is limited to all but a few ground EMS systems currently, whereas the practice is more common among aeromedical agencies under direct medical control.

The opponents of prehospital intubation have raised concerns regarding the safety and efficacy of prehospital intubation.[8,10–14] The leading arguments against the procedure are related to the level of complexity of the intervention, the lack of proved benefit, and the potential delay to definite care. Wang and colleagues[12] noted that more than 50 cognitive and psychomotor tasks are required for successful endotracheal intubation. Further opponents suggest that the national requirements for certification are inadequate and EMS responders are not prepared to perform endotracheal intubation in the chaotic environment of the prehospital resuscitation scene.[8] A main concern regarding prehospital intubation is the associated increased morbidity and mortality found in several retrospective and observational studies.

Only one randomized trial of prehospital intubation has been performed to date. The trial enrolled 830 pediatric patients and randomized patients to either endotracheal intubation or bag-valve mask ventilation.[15] Although the study did have significant limitations, it observed no difference in survival to hospital discharge and no difference in the rate of good neurologic outcome between groups. Other smaller and non-randomized studies have also concluded that in an urban EMS system endotracheal intubation offered no benefit versus bag-valve mask ventilation.[16,17]

The role of prehospital intubation in the brain injury population is a particular point of interest because brain-injured patients often have compromised mental status and concerns for maintaining an adequate airway. Only one study published to date has shown a survival advantage for head-injured patients undergoing intubation,[9] whereas several publications have shown the association between out-of-hospital intubation and higher morbidity and mortality.[7,13,14,17–20] All of these studies have limitations, including the retrospective or nonrandomized design, small populations with limited survivors to hospital discharge, and patients identified in the field by Glasgow Coma Scale score or retrospectively with head or head and neck Abbreviated Injury Severity Score. These factors are known to be poor identifiers of traumatic brain injury in the prehospital setting and, therefore, may have included a large number of patients without true head injury, therefore biasing the sample. In the only study to date that used CT data to identify head injury, the investigators concluded that nearly 90% of patients with prehospital Glasgow Coma Scale score less than or equal to 8 and CT-verified head injury required intubation either in the field or in the emergency department and that prehospital intubation resulted in no increased risk of mortality.[6]

At the current time, there is inconclusive evidence regarding the impact of prehospital intubation in trauma patients. Because endotracheal intubation is a skill that will remain in use by emergency medical providers, they should be adequately trained and maintain sufficient numbers of clinical intubations to remain certified. A large multicentered study is needed to accurately assess the efficacy and risks associated with prehospital endotracheal intubation.

Multiple alternatives to endotracheal intubation are available, including:

- Bag-valve mask
- Laryngeal mask
- Combitube
- King airway.

The alternatives listed previously are being used more commonly in the prehospital setting and not only require less training and skill for insertion but also have been shown to result in less delay to definitive care.[17,21] In addition, adjuncts to endotracheal intubation, such as video-assisted laryngoscopy, are being developed and tested for use in the prehospital setting.[22]

When a patient arrives at the authors' medical center with one of these alternative airways, if they are hemodynamically stable, the time is taken to secure a definitive airway with an endotracheal tube if possible or place a surgical airway if there is significant facial trauma. If a patient needs immediate surgery, the patient is transported to the operating room before manipulating these alternative airways.

An example of a prehospital airway management algorithm is provided in **Fig. 1**. Within this simple algorithm, prehospital personnel are encouraged to rapidly progress to the next step rather than repetitively attempting a given approach after initial failure. This algorithm also incorporates the alternative or rescue airways (discussed previously).

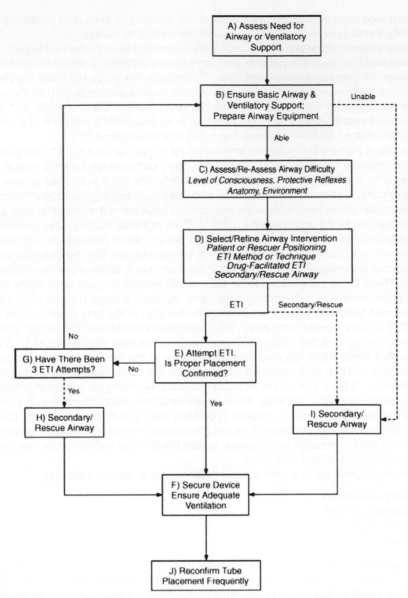

Fig. 1. Prehospital airway management algorithm. ETI, endotracheal intubation. (*From* Wang HE, Kupas DF, Greenwood MJ, et al. An algorithmic approach to prehospital airway management. Prehosp Emerg Care 2005;9(2):145–55; with permission.)

Some EMS groups may use a variation of this algorithm wherein alternative airway management strategies are the first-line approach.

HEMORRHAGE CONTROL

Uncontrolled hemorrhage is the leading cause of mortality among combat casualties and the second leading cause of death for civilian trauma.[1,23,24] Control of compressible hemorrhage is one of the first priorities for prehospital personnel when caring for an injured patient and takes precedence in Tactical Combat Casualty Care (TCCC). When hemorrhage cannot be stopped with direct pressure or simple maneuvers, then advanced maneuvers need to be used. Recently, there have been major advances in understanding of how to appropriately use tourniquets and also the development of deployable hemostatic agents that can be used as adjuncts for hemorrhage control.

Tourniquet Use

Hemorrhage from extremity wounds is common especially in wartime and with increasing numbers of penetrating trauma. There has been a long and ongoing debate over the use of tourniquets in the prehospital setting, specifically in the battlefield. Although tourniquets were commonly used in the US Civil War, Spanish Civil War, and World War I, they lost favor given the concerns of increased morbidity with their use.[25] With advancements in technology and more precise indications for its use, the tourniquet has once again come into favor and all military personnel in the active combat theater are provided tourniquets. Recent reports suggest that tourniquets used appropriately have a low morbidity risk and improved outcomes are seen when tourniquets are applied early, before the onset of shock.[25,26] Kragh and colleagues[27] performed a prospective review of tourniquet use during Operation Iraqi Freedom. Of 2838 patients admitted to a combat support hospital in Baghdad during 2006, 232 injured combatants had 429 tourniquets applied on 309 injured extremities. Tourniquet use in the prehospital care environment and before the development of shock was strongly associated with survival. No amputations resulted solely from tourniquet use. In the current TCCC guidelines, combat medics are encouraged to consider early application of the tourniquet for control of bleeding. The current recommendation is for placement of a Combat Application Tourniquet-1 (Composite Resources, Rock Hill, South Carolina) directly to the skin 2 inches to 3 inches above the wound. Preferably, placement occurs above the knee or the elbow of the injured extremity to insure adequate compression of inflow to the injured extremity.

Although commonly used in the military setting, tourniquet use in civilian prehospital trauma care currently is not common. This is primarily related to the differences in wounding mechanisms and patterns as well as short transport times, particularly in more urban locations. Current recommendations are to use a tourniquet if hemorrhage cannot be controlled with direct pressure, a pressure dressing, or selective clamping of bleeding vessels.[28] A recent review of experience with isolated exsanguinating extremity hemorrhage from penetrating injury in one community noted that although infrequent, more than half of the patients that succumbed to their injury had bleeding from a site that anatomically would have been amenable to tourniquet control.[29]

Based on the military experience and improvements in tourniquet technology, some emergency medical personnel are being trained in tourniquet application. The 6th edition of PHTLS: Prehospital Trauma Life Support endorses the use of tourniquets before extrication and transport if direct pressure or a pressure dressing fail to control hemorrhage.[30] Widespread familiarity with indications for tourniquet use and proper application technique could also have benefits in disaster or mass casualty situations in the future where extremity injuries amenable to tourniquet application.

Approaches to Noncompressible Hemorrhage

The issue of noncompressible torso hemorrhage is discussed in detail by Morrison and Rasmussen elsewhere in this issue. A brief review, however, of the prehospital management of this problem is also warranted.

A new variety of tourniquet has recently been developed to compress the abdominal aorta in instances of exsanguinating lower-extremity junctional hemorrhage, massive blood loss from areas proximal to the inguinal ligaments, buttocks, perineum, gluteal, and pelvic areas. The tourniquet is designed to wrap around the abdomen and has a wedge shaped anterior portion inflated by a hand pump to compress the aorta near the umbilicus.[31] The device has recently been given premarket clearance by the US Food and Drug Administration (FDA) and has started production for orders received by the US military and other law enforcement agencies.[32] The concept for this device is supported in part by research by Blaivas and colleagues,[33] who evaluated cessation of blood flow in the common femoral arteries during external compression and showed that a weight of 140 pounds to the distal abdominal aorta or 120 pounds to the proximal iliac artery was adequate to stop blood through the common femoral artery.

Aortic occlusion to increase or preserve central perfusion can also be attained via an endovascular technique.[34–36] Although not yet adopted in resuscitative practices, the technique for endovascular occlusion of the aorta has been well described.[34] When comparing the two techniques to no aortic occlusion in a large animal hemorrhagic shock model, endovascular occlusion animals had more normal pH, had lower serum lactate, and required less fluid and vasopressor resuscitation than the aortic clamping group while maintaining similar aortic pressure, carotid blood flow, and brain oximetry.[36] Although neither technique is currently used in the prehospital setting, as the technology and expertise with femoral access techniques improve along with the capabilities of providers in the prehospital environment, it is interesting to speculate whether or not this maneuver could find its way into the prehospital environment as a means of providing control for noncompressible hemorrhage.

The role of topical hemostatic agents in controlling hemorrhage had been limited to primarily combat resuscitation; however, more recently, their use has become more commonplace in civilian prehospital practice. In general, the compounds are useful in curtailing massive hemorrhage from deep, penetrating wounds, particularly in junctional zones, such as the groin, axilla, and base of the neck. The ideal topical hemostatic agent has been described as having the ability to stop both arterial and venous hemorrhage, working quickly, packaged ready-to-use, simple to apply, lightweight, durable, risk-free, and inexpensive.[37,38] Although an agent that meets these exact specifications has not yet been developed, the three most common classes of topical hemostatic compounds are:

- Mucoadhesive agents (eg, WoundStat, HemCon, and Celox)
- Procoagulant supplementors (eg, QuikClot Combat Gauze)
- Clotting factor concentrators (eg, QuikClot Zeolite granular and QuikClot ACS+).

Mucoadhesive agents work by creating a seal over bleeding wounds, specifically the positively charged complex binds to the negatively charged red blood cells and forms a clot that hardens. Procoagulant supplementors deliver additional clotting factors or active existing clotting factors directly at the point of hemorrhage. Lastly, the clotting factor concentrators work through the rapid hemoconcentration at the bleeding site, resulting in concentration of platelets and clotting factor proteins.

All agents have shown benefit over traditional field dressing gauze application in animal models of hemorrhage.[37,39–41] In a recent comparison of hemostatic agents, Clay and colleagues[39] investigated the effectiveness of several topical hemostatic agents compared with traditional gauze in a swine extremity hemorrhage model and found all topical hemostatic agents resulted in less blood loss and improved survival versus standard gauze field dressing. Specifically, WoundStat achieved 100% survival whereas Celox, HemCon, and QuikClot ACS+ attained 85% survival. Traditional field gauze application resulted in 100% mortality. Furthermore, in a recent comprehensive review of hemostatic dressings, Granville-Chapman and colleagues reviewed 60 articles comparing hemostatic agents in venous, arterial, mixed venous-arterial hemorrhage. They report that although the early topical hemostatics (HemCon and QuikClot) improved hemostasis in animal hemorrhage models versus traditional gauze application; the newer agents (WoundStat, QuikClot Combat Gauze, and Celox) delivered more superior hemorrhage control, with WoundStat 100% effective in controlling hemorrhage.[37]

Although they show efficacy, there are safety concerns that have been outlined related to these agents. The initial formulation of QuikClot, made from Zeolite granules, created a significant exothermic reaction related to the rapid dehydration effect of the product that could lead to thermal injury and necrosis of tissues.[42] This reaction was confirmed in case reports documenting significant burns to the skin and surrounding tissues. In earlier experiments with WoundStat, granular particles were identified in the tissues by histology, raising the possibility of thrombogenic potential. On further investigation by Kheirabadi and colleagues,[43] they noted WoundStat caused occlusive thrombus in injured vessels and significant irreparable damage to the endothelium precluding surgical repair. WoundStat granules were also seen in systemic circulation as emboli in the lungs. An additional concern is ease of removal of the product as the powder-based and granule-based products require multiple surgical washouts to remove compared with the gauze type products. Due to these concerns, the first-generation formulation of QuikClot has been replaced with second-generation and third-generation products and WoundStat has been removed from the market. Currently, QuikClot Combat Gauze is the hemostatic agent of choice for military use and is incorporated in TCCC guidelines. Similar to tourniquet application, the use of hemostatic agents in the civilian prehospital care setting is currently limited in scope and application compared with military use.

PREHOSPITAL RESUSCITATION

In conjunction with airway control and controlling external hemorrhage, a primary goal of emergency medical service providers is to restore perfusion. Prompt and appropriate access to the intravascular space is crucial for resuscitation with administration of fluids and medications. The placement of large-bore peripheral intravenous catheters is still the standard of care. Vascular access, however, is not always feasible and an alternative approach must be used. The use of intraosseous (IO) devices has steadily increased over time and become more commonplace. The concept of accessing the bone marrow, which can act as a noncollapsible conduit to the central circulation, was first described in 1922.[44] Although IO devices were often used in the 1930s and 1940s, their use dissipated with the advent of plastic catheters and better techniques for intravascular access. In recent years, however, there has been a resurgence of interest in the IO route for resuscitation and the FDA has approved several IO catheters and insertion systems, including automatic and spring-loaded systems for insertion into the tibia, sternum, and humerus.[45–47] Use of the IO devices, with focus on sternal placement, has been incorporated in TCCC guidelines and training and are commonly deployed in EMS systems for use in the both pediatric and adult civilian trauma.

The traditional treatment regimen for trauma patients is aggressive fluid resuscitation to restore circulating volume and systolic blood pressure (SBP) to a minimum of 90 mm Hg. The current guideline endorsed by the American College of Surgeons Committee on Trauma and the Advanced Trauma Life Support (ATLS) course is to resuscitate all trauma patients with 2 L or more of crystalloid after injury.[28,48] Since the 1960s, both crystalloid and colloid solutions have been used to correct hypotension during the resuscitation of injured patients. The principle of aggressive fluid resuscitation is based on the belief that the administration of fluids results in greater likelihood of survival after severe hemorrhage compared with no treatment. These original experiments were fraught with limitations because the studies were animal trials designed to control hemorrhage before the initiation of fluid resuscitation. In these trials there was improved survival with early administration of intravenous fluids. Although external control of compressible hemorrhage is a tenet of prehospital resuscitation, patients with life-threatening surgical bleeding not amenable to compression do not achieve hemostasis before fluid administration in the field. Aggressive resuscitation in this scenario could in theory lead to more blood loss than a strategy of limited volume resuscitation.

Although there is a growing body of evidence regarding the issue of prehospital fluid administration, there is no consensus and little has changed with the approach in the prehospital arena. For example, conventional civilian prehospital practice uses either normal saline (NS) or lactated Ringer (LR) solution for resuscitation, but there is ongoing debate regarding which solution is better, which patients require fluid administration, and how much fluid to give. Currently there are several options under consideration and investigation.

- No fluids
- Crystalloid (isotonic or hypertonic)
- Colloids
- Oxygen-carrying solutions
- Blood products.

The concept of withholding resuscitation and allowing for permissive hypotension in patients with ongoing hemorrhage dates back to World War I.[49] This concept has been adopted into the management of several medical conditions, including major gastrointestinal hemorrhage and aortic aneurysm rupture, and has been shown to increase survival in select groups of injured patients.[50,51] The theory of worsening hemorrhage associated with intravenous fluid administration is based on the concept that excess fluid dilutes clotting factors and increased hydraulic pressure leads to "popping the clot."[49,52] Permissive hypotensive resuscitation or delayed resuscitation may result in early reintroduction of clotting factors and minimize tissue edema with improved oxygen exchange.[53,54] In a systematic review of the literature, it was observed that in all animal trials investigating hypotensive resuscitation, restriction of fluid was associated with reduced risk of death.[54] In the most well-known and described clinical study to date evaluating delayed resuscitation in a human clinical trial, standard resuscitation in the field was compared with delayed resuscitation initiated only after the patient reached the operating room in 598 hypotensive patients with penetrating injury to the torso. Mean SBP on hospital arrival was 79 ± 46 mm Hg in the immediate group and 72 ± 43 mm Hg in the delayed group ($P = .02$). Blood pressure on arrival to the operating room was similar. Mortality was 62% in the delayed resuscitation group versus 70% in the standard resuscitation group, a statistically significant difference.[50] Although these results are compelling, this study was a single institution study in an urban setting that enrolled only those with penetrating torso injury. Despite the evidence showing benefit, these limitations have kept this approach from becoming more widely adopted. A multicenter trial evaluating limited crystalloid resuscitation in both blunt and penetrating trauma patients in mixed urban and rural settings organized by the Resuscitation Outcomes Consortium (ROC)[55] is currently under way. This study will limit the use of crystalloid infusion for hypotensive patients in both the prehospital setting and for up to 2 hours in hospital or until surgical control of hemorrhage has been achieved. In contrast to the civilian setting, permissive hypotension with administration of limited amounts of fluids (maximum of two 500-mL boluses of Hextend a minimum of 30 minutes apart) is the current standard of care in the field for treatment of combat casualties and has been adopted in TCCC guidelines. Although the basis for this decision is in part related to judicious use of a limited resource in the far forward military environment, the cumulative literature regarding limited resuscitation provides additional rationale for this approach.

Regarding the NS versus LR debate, several studies, both human and animal, have evaluated the difference between the two, with NS resuscitation resulting in significantly higher sodium and chloride values with lower bicarbonate and pH levels.[56–58] Additionally, in a porcine animal study where resuscitation was initiated after animals sustained a grade V liver injury, the animals resuscitated with NS after 30 minutes of uncontrolled hemorrhage lost twice as much blood as those resuscitated with LR, required more fluid to maintain adequate blood pressure, and were more coagulopathic.[58] Currently, ATLS guidelines recommend LR as the initial resuscitative fluid and NS as an alternative.[28] Despite this recommendation, however, a majority of EMS agencies continue to use NS exclusively in the prehospital arena, mostly because of the compatibility of NS with medication administration in medical emergencies and the logistic and cost issues associated with deploying two different types of crystalloids. Further research and clinical trials need to be performed to evaluate the relative safety and efficacy of both fluids as well as other newer generation isotonic alternatives in prehospital trauma care.

Several studies, including a large multicenter, randomized controlled trial have investigated the potential benefits of hypertonic saline (HS) resuscitation after injury.[5,59–62] HS has been shown to decrease inflammation, improve organ perfusion, and limit organ injury in many animal studies; however, the clinical trials of HS resuscitation compared with isotonic fluids have not shown improvements in survival. In the largest and most recent randomized placebo-controlled trial investigating the effectiveness of HS solutions to date, 7.5% HS with and without 6% dextran-70 was compared with NS in patients with hemorrhagic shock or traumatic brain injury. A total of 853 patients were enrolled in the hemorrhagic shock arm and 1282 patients in the traumatic brain injury arm. Both studies were stopped early, however, on the basis of futility, because there was no observed benefit in survival or neurologic outcome.[60,63]

There are some promising data suggesting select colloid solutions may provide survival benefit. Hextend, 6% hetastarch in lactated electrolyte buffer, is a colloid solution approved for use in hypovolemic patients undergoing elective surgery. In the first report discussing the safety and efficacy of hetastarch during the initial resuscitation of trauma patients, Ogilvie and colleagues[64,65] determined hetastarch was safe and resulted in reduced deaths and overall mortality compared with standard crystalloid resuscitation. Despite its potential benefit, there are concerns related to the use of colloid solutions, including the potential for anaphylaxis and coagulopathy.[66] As discussed previously, Hextend is currently the initial fluid used in limited quantities for combat casualty resuscitation in the field under TCCC guidelines. It is currently not commonly used in civilian prehospital practice.

All the fluids discussed previously can provide some volume expansion capabilities and improve blood pressure; however, none of these agents possesses any oxygen carrying capability. Third-generation hemoglobin-based oxygen carriers, acellular hemoglobin solutions derived from either outdated human blood stores (PolyHeme) or from bovine blood (Hemopure), held great promise as candidate resuscitative agents for prehospital use.[67–70] In addition to their oxygen-carrying capacity, they had the additional benefit of being heat stable with long shelf lives and the ability to adequately resuscitate after hemorrhage in low volumes.[71] All of these characteristics made them ideal for use in the prehospital civilian and combat casualty care situations. A randomized clinical trial using PolyHeme, however, failed to show a mortality benefit[72] and the FDA did not approve the planned Navy-sponsored RESUS prehospital trauma study using Hemopure.[73] The primary concern with these products is the nitric oxide scavenging effect associated with the cell-free hemoglobin with the end result of increased blood pressure and concerns for increased bleeding, stroke, and myocardial infarction in at risk populations. The potential for use of oxygen-carrying solutions in prehospital resuscitation is at the current time limited and will rely on the development of newer products capable of oxygen-carrying capacity with limited nitric oxide scavenging potential.

The deployment of blood components in the prehospital setting is becoming more frequent, particularly in rotary wing transport. Currently, there are multiple air services that carry packed red blood cells with a few also carrying plasma. Although contemporary data on experience with the use of prehospital blood products are currently limited, more information about the utility of this approach should become available as these sites gain clinical expertise and ultimately publish their experience. Additionally, the Department of Defense has recently funded research grants to evaluate the prehospital use of plasma for traumatic hemorrhage.[74] The development of lyophilized formulations of fresh frozen plasma will also make prehospital plasma use logistically more appealing.[75,76]

In addition to the primary resuscitation agents discussed previously, there are several potential resuscitative adjuncts that could be used prehospital to improve outcomes for trauma patients, with some undergoing active investigation. The prehospital administration of arginine vasopressin in injured patients who do not respond to standard resuscitation fluids may be beneficial through enhancing and prolonging the compensatory mechanisms that respond to shock and by shunting blood centrally to maintain blood flow to the heart, brain, and kidneys.[77–80] Arginine vasopressin is an endogenous hormone that is known to be beneficial in septic shock and cardiopulmonary arrest.[81] In a small, randomized, double-blinded study, hypotensive trauma patients who were given a low-dose arginine vasopressin infusion compared with saline alone required less fluid for resuscitation and trended toward early survival advantage, although no statistical difference was observed.[80] A large international multicenter, randomized controlled trial (Vasopressin in Refractory Traumatic Hemorrhagic Shock [VITRIS]) has been designed to investigate the effects of prehospital arginine vasopressin in injured hemorrhagic shock patients and is currently enrolling patients.[82]

Tranexamic acid (TXA), an antifibrinolytic agent that has been used since the 1960s to control bleeding from blood dyscrasias, gastrointestinal sources, and surgical sites, is also being evaluated as an adjunct to trauma resuscitation of trauma patients.[83] TXA inhibits both plasminogen activation and plasmin activity, thus preventing the breakdown of formed clot. In a recent large, multicenter, randomized, double-blind, placebo-controlled trial (Clinical Randomisation of an Antifibrinolytic in Significant Haemorrhage 2 [CRASH 2]), more than 20,000 adult trauma patients were enrolled and randomized. The population who received TXA had a significant reduction in all-cause mortality and an overall reduction in death secondary to hemorrhage. There was no observed difference in amount of blood transfusions administered between groups. Further analysis suggested greater benefit was observed if TXA was administered within 3 hours of injury.[83,84] A recent retrospective military-based study comparing outcomes in patients who had received TXA with those who did not receive TXA showed improved mortality in the group that received the drug, particularly for those who received a massive transfusion.[85] Although studies to date have focused primarily on in hospital administration of the drug, prehospital trials have been discussed to evaluate if early administration of TXA would extend the reported benefits of in hospital treatment.

Basic scientific studies have long espoused the beneficial effect of administration of estrogen after trauma regardless of gender or age.[86,87] Of particular interest to prehospital care is the ability of a single dose of 17β-estradiol to improve survival in male animals after trauma hemorrhage even in the absence of fluid administration.[88] There are currently 2 pilot studies being performed in ROC, 1 in patients with hemorrhagic shock and another in patients with traumatic brain injury (Resuscitative Endocrinology: Single-dose Clinical Uses for Estrogen [RESCUE]). The purpose of these initial studies is to assess the feasibility and safety of a single dose of intravenous Premarin prior to moving forward with larger, multicenter prehospital trials.

IDENTIFICATION OF OCCULT SHOCK

Since the mid-twentieth century, hypotension and shock were defined as an SBP less than or equal to 90 mm Hg. Little scientific evidence is available, however, to support the belief that actual tissue hypoperfusion or ischemia is first observed or limited to patients with SBP less than or equal to 90 mm Hg. More recent reports suggest that SBP less than or equal to 110 mm Hg more accurately reflects the first clinical evidence of hypoperfusion.[89–92] Furthermore, some investigators suggest the use of SBP alone is unreliable and cannot accurately assess tissue hypoperfusion or shock.[93,94]

Adjuncts to traditional vital signs are commercially available for prehospital use and are being tested in the prehospital setting. Simple point-of-care devices (similar to glucometers) along with specific monitors to analyze heart rate variability and tissue oxygenation saturations are promising and will undoubtedly provide additional benefit in recognizing hypoperfusion and shock, even in the chaotic prehospital setting. Adjuncts, specifically point-of-care blood lactate, have been studied by several investigators and found a reliable predictor of postinjury hemorrhage. Lactate elevations are associated with the need for hospital admission, ICU admission, emergent intervention, and death.[95,96] In a study of more than 2000 patients with borderline hypotension, defined as SBP between 90 mm Hg and 110 mm Hg, serum lactate obtained immediately on arrival to the emergency department was more predictive than blood pressure, obtained either prehospital or on arrival to the emergency department, in predicting the need for greater than 6 units of red blood cell transfusion within 24 hours of arrival and mortality.[95] Furthermore, Guyette and colleagues[96] measured prehospital point-of-care blood lactate in more than 1000 patients and found that higher values are predictive and that addition of blood lactate levels to initial vital signs and Glasgow Coma Scale score significantly increased the predictability of need for urgent operation, multiple organ dysfunction syndrome, and mortality. This study has now been extended to a multicenter prehospital trial (Biomarker Lactate Assessment of Shock in Trauma [BLAST]). The primary aim of the study is to evaluate prehospital lactate in comparison to SBP for the ability to predict the need for resuscitative care (the administration of packed red blood cells or emergent intervention for hemorrhage control using thoracotomy, laparotomy, pelvic fixation, or interventional radiologic control) or death within 6 hours of emergency department arrival.

The noninvasive prehospital adjuncts have been useful in identifying patients with increased mortality or need for massive transfusion. The shock index (SI), a calculation of heart rate divided SBP, is a simple method that has been shown to be more predictive of mortality within 48 hours than heart rate or SBP alone. In a study of more than 8000 normotensive patients with SBP greater than 90 mm Hg, prehospital vital signs were used to calculate SI, and SI greater than 0.9 was associated with significant increase likelihood of needed massive transfusion, longer length of stay, and not surviving the injuries sustained. From this analysis, the investigators concluded the SI was able to identify patients at high risk for needing massive transfusion although they were reported to be hemodynamically stable en route.[97] Zarzaur and colleagues[98] further investigated the utility of the SI in the older populations greater than 54 years old and found that age × SI was the best predictor of mortality and need for at least 4 units of blood transfusion. Although these studies suggest a that SI may be a useful adjunct in predicting sicker patients, further prospective studies will need to be performed to determine the practical utility of this measure with regard to field trauma triage.

In a study by Sagraves and colleagues,[99] use of the InSpectra StO_2 (Hutchinson Technology) tissue oxygen monitor was evaluated in the prehospital environment for feasibility and predictive ability. They concluded that the monitors were easy to use without interference from other monitoring systems or avionics. The device was able to distinguish between survivors and nonsurvivors with a 3-fold increase in mortality for every 10% drop in StO_2 reading.

The ability of an injured patient to compensate and maintain blood pressure during hemorrhagic blood loss is secondary to the inherent autonomic responses of the patient. Heart rate variability, as determined by ECG analysis, may be able to characterize the autonomic compensation of a patient to loss of blood volume and, therefore, be used in field triage of trauma victims. Cooke and colleagues[100] have investigated heart rate variability in the prehospital environment. In their study, ECG tracings from on-board monitors obtained during transport from the scene of injury to the emergency department were analyzed using commercially available software. Heart rate variability of patients who died was compared with the tracings of those who survived and differences in R-R intervals were reported in the patients who died from hemorrhagic shock. This study was limited by its retrospective nature and the need for clean ECG data that excluded a large number of patients from the analysis. Although these results are intriguing, it is unknown at this time whether these measures will add any additional real-time information and triage accuracy to the field provider.

PREHOSPITAL RESEARCH INFRASTRUCTURE

In the care of severely injured trauma patients, timely intervention and transport to an appropriate level of care are paramount to improve the chance of survival. Although prehospital care has greatly improved with the development of trauma systems of care, the infrastructure to evaluate new interventions in the field and to translate promising scientific and clinical advances into improved outcomes has only been recently developed. The ROC is a clinical trial network focusing on research in the area of prehospital cardiopulmonary arrest and severe traumatic injury. The National Heart, Lung, and Blood Institute primarily funds the network with additional support from the American Heart Association, the United States Army Medical Research and Materiel Command, the Canadian Institutes of Health Research, the Heart and Stroke Foundation of Canada, and Defence Research and Development Canada. The network consists of 10 primary regional clinical centers along with many satellite centers and is tasked with performing both prehospital trauma and cardiac arrest trials. The network has allowed the clinical sites involved in the research to actively engage their prehospital care providers in the design and implementation of studies aimed at prehospital care. Along with interventional clinical trials, the network has an ongoing observational data collection and evaluation component. The end result of these collaborations is establishment of a sustainable research infrastructure able to rapidly design and implement needed studies as well as the fostering of a prehospital research culture that will stimulate further ideas and organized approaches to systematically evaluate prehospital care. The cumulative effect has great potential to rapidly transform prehospital care in the coming years.

Much of the difficulty in performance of prehospital research lies in the ability to obtain informed consent. Although informed consent is a fundamental of human research subjects, there are instances when it is not possible. Inherently, research in the prehospital or emergency setting is difficult because the critical nature of the patient population and limited amount of time to enroll patients. Research on emergency patients was traditionally performed using deferred consent; however, the ability to perform emergency research using this mechanism was halted in 1993. With the passage of the Final Rule in 1996 by the FDA, which has oversight authority for medical research, emergency and prehospital research was allowed under what has become known as exception from informed consent.

The FDA Final Rule (21 CFR 50.24) has several conditions that all must be met and justified to perform emergency research under this mechanism:

1. The human subjects are in a life-threatening condition and valid scientific evidence is available that indicates the safety and effectiveness of the intervention.
2. Obtaining informed consent from patients or their legally authorized representative is not feasible because of a patient's condition; the intervention must be administered before obtaining consent is possible; or there is no way to prospectively identify the individuals likely to become eligible for the research.
3. Participation in the research holds the prospect of direct benefit based on the life-threatening condition of the patient, appropriate preclinical and clinical evidence of benefit, and an appropriate risk-to-benefit ratio.
4. The research could not practically be performed without the waiver.
5. The research protocol defines the therapeutic window and the investigator is committed to the obtaining the legally authorized representative consent during the window.
6. The local institutional review board has approved informed consent documents that could be used during the therapeutic window.
7. Additional protections of a patient's rights and welfare will be provided to include community consultation, public disclosure, and a commitment from the research team to contact family members if the patient cannot consent or the legally authorized representative is not available.

In the years after passage of the Final Rule, an increasing number of research trials have been conducted in all areas of emergency care, but there are limitations. In addition to the expanded cost, time, and administration to supply community consultation, there is a concern of introducing bias in study results if patients or their legally authorized representative does not consent to allow review of records after initial enrollment under the waiver of consent. Nichol and colleagues[101] state the importance of further review of the medical records as endpoints, such as survival to discharge. Furthermore, they suggest the exception of consent should extend to allow review of the medical record, because the benefit would include a more thorough assessment of outcomes and adverse effects; this would allow a reduction in bias at the expense of minimal risk related to confidentiality.[101] The regulations allowing waiver of informed consent included specific clauses to protect enrollment of racial and ethnic minorities in emergency research. In a recent study, Sugarman and colleagues[102] retrospectively compared registry enrollment with trial enrollment from sites participating in the ROC HS trial. After comparison of the patients enrolled in the observational trial registry, there were no racial or ethnical differences observed among those enrolled in the interventional trials.

Performance of research in the prehospital setting is an evolving process. As more studies are performed, more will be learned about the effectiveness of the community consultation and public disclosure practices and the acceptance of the public regarding these studies and consent procedures.[103,104]

REFERENCES

1. Stewart RM, Myers JG, Dent DL, et al. Seven hundred fifty-three consecutive deaths in a level I trauma center: the argument for injury prevention. J Trauma 2003;54(1):66–70 [discussion: 70–1].
2. MacLeod JB, Cohn SM, Johnson EW, et al. Trauma deaths in the first hour: are they all unsalvageable injuries? Am J Surg 2007;193(2):195–9.
3. Trunkey DD. Trauma. Accidental and intentional injuries account for more years of life lost in the U.S. than cancer and heart disease. Among the prescribed remedies are improved preventive efforts, speedier surgery and further research. Sci Am 1983;249(2):28–35.
4. Bulger EM, Copass MK, Maier RV, et al. An analysis of advanced prehospital airway management. J Emerg Med 2002;23(2):183–9.
5. Bulger EM, Nathens AB, Rivara FP, et al. National variability in out-of-hospital treatment after traumatic injury. Ann Emerg Med 2007;49(3):293–301.
6. Vandromme MJ, Melton SM, Griffin R, et al. Intubation patterns and outcomes in patients with computed tomography-verified traumatic brain injury. J Trauma 2011;71(6):1615–9.
7. Davis DP, Koprowicz KM, Newgard CD, et al. The relationship between out-of-hospital airway management and outcome among trauma patients with Glasgow Coma Scale Scores of 8 or less. Prehosp Emerg Care 2011;15(2): 184–92.
8. Strote J, Roth R, Cone DC, et al. Prehospital endotracheal intubation: the controversy continues (conference proceedings). Am J Emerg Med 2009;27(9):1142–7.
9. Winchell RJ, Hoyt DB. Endotracheal intubation in the field improves survival in patients with severe head injury. Trauma Research and Education Foundation of San Diego. Arch Surg 1997;132(6):592–7.
10. Davis DP, Fakhry SM, Wang HE, et al. Paramedic rapid sequence intubation for severe traumatic brain injury: perspectives from an expert panel. Prehosp Emerg Care 2007;11(1):1–8.
11. Wang HE, Kupas DF, Paris PM, et al. Multivariate predictors of failed prehospital endotracheal intubation. Acad Emerg Med 2003;10(7):717–24.
12. Wang HE, Kupas DF, Greenwood MJ, et al. An algorithmic approach to prehospital airway management. Prehosp Emerg Care 2005;9(2):145–55.
13. Bochicchio GV, Ilahi O, Joshi M, et al. Endotracheal intubation in the field does not improve outcome in trauma patients who present without an acutely lethal traumatic brain injury. J Trauma 2003;54(2):307–11.
14. Wang HE, Peitzman AB, Cassidy LD, et al. Out-of-hospital endotracheal intubation and outcome after traumatic brain injury. Ann Emerg Med 2004;44(5): 439–50.

15. Gausche M, Lewis RJ, Stratton SJ, et al. Effect of out-of-hospital pediatric endotracheal intubation on survival and neurological outcome: a controlled clinical trial. JAMA 2000;283(6):783–90.
16. Cobas MA, De la Peña MA, Manning R, et al. Prehospital intubations and mortality: a level 1 trauma center perspective. Anesth Analg 2009;109(2):489–93.
17. Stockinger ZT, McSwain NE. Prehospital endotracheal intubation for trauma does not improve survival over bag-valve-mask ventilation. J Trauma 2004; 56(3):531–6.
18. Davis DP, Hoyt DB, Ochs M, et al. The effect of paramedic rapid sequence intubation on outcome in patients with severe traumatic brain injury. J Trauma 2003; 54(3):444–53.
19. Davis DP, Peay J, Sise MJ, et al. The impact of prehospital endotracheal intubation on outcome in moderate to severe traumatic brain injury. J Trauma 2005; 58(5):933–9.
20. Sloane C, Vilke GM, Chan TC, et al. Rapid sequence intubation in the field versus hospital in trauma patients. J Emerg Med 2000;19(3):259–64.
21. Langeron O, Birenbaum A, Amour J. Airway management in trauma. Minerva Anestesiol 2009;75(5):307–11.
22. Bjoernsen LP, Lindsay B. Video laryngoscopy in the prehospital setting. Prehosp Disaster Med 2009;24(3):265–70.
23. Bellamy RF. The causes of death in conventional land warfare: implications for combat casualty care research. Mil Med 1984;149(2):55–62.
24. Acosta JA, Yang JC, Winchell RJ, et al. Lethal injuries and time to death in a level I trauma center. J Am Coll Surg 1998;186(5):528–33.
25. Welling DR, McKay PL, Rasmussen TE, et al. A brief history of the tourniquet. J Vasc Surg 2012;55(1):286–90.
26. Kragh JF, Walters TJ, Baer DG, et al. Practical use of emergency tourniquets to stop bleeding in major limb trauma. J Trauma 2008;64(Suppl 2):S38–49 [discussion: S49–50].
27. Kragh JF Jr, Walters TJ, Baer DG, et al. Survival with emergency tourniquet use to stop bleeding in major limb trauma. Ann Surg 2009;249(1):1–7.
28. Surgeons ACo. Advanced trauma life support for doctors—student course manual. 8th edition. Chicago: American College of Surgeons; 2010.
29. Dorlac WC, DeBakey ME, Holcomb JB, et al. Mortality from isolated civilian penetrating extremity injury. J Trauma 2005;59(1):217–22.
30. NAEMT's PHTLS: Prehospital Trauma Life Support. 6th edition. Mosby; 2007.
31. Greenfield EM, Schwartz RB, Croushorn JM, et al. Efficacy and safety of a novel abdominal tourniquet device for the control of pelvic and lower extremity hemorrhage. Paper presented at: 16th World Congress for Disaster and Emergency Medicine. Victoria, BC, Canada, May 12–15, 2009.
32. Baker T. Emergency medicine physicians develop device to stop lethal bleeding in soldiers. 2012. Available at: http://news.georgiahealth.edu/archives/5001. Accessed January 25, 2012.
33. Blaivas M, Shiver S, Lyon M, et al. Control of hemorrhage in critical femoral or inguinal penetrating wounds–an ultrasound evaluation. Prehosp Disaster Med 2006;21(6):379–82.
34. Stannard A, Eliason JL, Rasmussen TE. Resuscitative Endovascular Balloon Occlusion of the Aorta (REBOA) as an Adjunct for Hemorrhagic Shock. J Trauma 2011;71(6):1869–72.
35. White JM, Cannon JW, Stannard A, et al. A porcine model for evaluating the management of noncompressible torso hemorrhage. J Trauma 2011;71(Suppl 1):S131–8.

36. White JM, Cannon JW, Stannard A, et al. Endovascular balloon occlusion of the aorta is superior to resuscitative thoracotomy with aortic clamping in a porcine model of hemorrhagic shock. Surgery 2011;150(3):400–9.

37. Granville-Chapman J, Jacobs N, Midwinter MJ. Pre-hospital haemostatic dressings: a systematic review. Injury 2011;42(5):447–59.

38. Pusateri AE, McCarthy SJ, Gregory KW, et al. Effect of a chitosan-based hemostatic dressing on blood loss and survival in a model of severe venous hemorrhage and hepatic injury in swine. J Trauma 2003;54(1):177–82.

39. Clay JG, Grayson JK, Zierold D. Comparative testing of new hemostatic agents in a swine model of extremity arterial and venous hemorrhage. Mil Med 2010; 175(4):280–4.

40. Ward KR, Tiba MH, Holbert WH, et al. Comparison of a new hemostatic agent to current combat hemostatic agents in a Swine model of lethal extremity arterial hemorrhage. J Trauma 2007;63(2):276–83 [discussion: 283–4].

41. Alam HB, Uy GB, Miller D, et al. Comparative analysis of hemostatic agents in a swine model of lethal groin injury. J Trauma 2003;54(6):1077–82.

42. Wright JK, Kalns J, Wolf EA, et al. Thermal injury resulting from application of a granular mineral hemostatic agent. J Trauma 2004;57(2):224–30.

43. Kheirabadi BS, Mace JE, Terrazas IB, et al. Safety evaluation of new hemostatic agents, smectite granules, and kaolin-coated gauze in a vascular injury wound model in swine. J Trauma 2010;68(2):269–78.

44. Drinker CK, Drinker KR, Lund CC. The circulation in the mammalian bone marrow. Am J Physiol 1922;62:92.

45. Byars DV, Tsuchitani SN, Erwin E, et al. Evaluation of success rate and access time for an adult sternal intraosseous device deployed in the prehospital setting. Prehosp Disaster Med 2011;26(2):127–9.

46. Paxton JH, Knuth TE, Klausner HA. Proximal humerus intraosseous infusion: a preferred emergency venous access. J Trauma 2009;67(3):606–11.

47. Hulse EJ, Thomas GO. Vascular access on the 21st century military battlefield. J R Army Med Corps 2010;156(4 Suppl 1):385–90.

48. Kortbeek JB, Al Turki SA, Ali J, et al. Advanced trauma life support, 8th edition, the evidence for change. J Trauma 2008;64(6):1638–50.

49. Cannon WB, Fraser J, Cowell EM. The preventive treatment of wound shock. J Am Med Assoc 1918;70:618–21.

50. Bickell WH, Wall MJ, Pepe PE, et al. Immediate versus delayed fluid resuscitation for hypotensive patients with penetrating torso injuries. N Engl J Med 1994; 331(17):1105–9.

51. Dutton RP, Mackenzie CF, Scalea TM. Hypotensive resuscitation during active hemorrhage: impact on in-hospital mortality. J Trauma 2002;52(6): 1141–6.

52. Sondeen JL, Coppes VG, Holcomb JB. Blood pressure at which rebleeding occurs after resuscitation in swine with aortic injury. J Trauma 2003;54(Suppl 5): S110–7.

53. Stern SA, Wang X, Mertz M, et al. Under-resuscitation of near-lethal uncontrolled hemorrhage: effects on mortality and end-organ function at 72 hours. Shock 2001;15(1):16–23.

54. Mapstone J, Roberts I, Evans P. Fluid resuscitation strategies: a systematic review of animal trials. J Trauma 2003;55(3):571–89.

55. Resuscitation outcomes consortium. Available at: https://roc.uwctc.org. Accessed January 16, 2012.

56. Reid F, Lobo DN, Williams RN, et al. (Ab)normal saline and physiological Hart-mann's solution: a randomized double-blind crossover study. Clin Sci (Lond) 2003;104(1):17–24.

57. Scheingraber S, Rehm M, Sehmisch C, et al. Rapid saline infusion produces hy-perchloremic acidosis in patients undergoing gynecologic surgery. Anesthesi-ology 1999;90(5):1265–70.

58. Kiraly LN, Differding JA, Enomoto TM, et al. Resuscitation with normal saline (NS) vs. lactated ringers (LR) modulates hypercoagulability and leads to increased blood loss in an uncontrolled hemorrhagic shock swine model. J Trauma 2006;61(1):57–64 [discussion: 64–5].

59. Brasel KJ, Bulger E, Cook AJ, et al. Hypertonic resuscitation: design and im-plementation of a prehospital intervention trial. J Am Coll Surg 2008;206(2):220–32.

60. Bulger EM, May S, Brasel KJ, et al. Out-of-hospital hypertonic resuscitation following severe traumatic brain injury: a randomized controlled trial. JAMA 2010;304(13):1455–64.

61. Vassar MJ, Perry CA, Holcroft JW. Analysis of potential risks associated with 7.5% sodium chloride resuscitation of traumatic shock. Arch Surg 1990;125(10):1309–15.

62. Vassar MJ, Perry CA, Holcroft JW. Prehospital resuscitation of hypotensive trauma patients with 7.5% NaCl versus 7.5% NaCl with added dextran: a controlled trial. J Trauma 1993;34(5):622–32 [discussion: 632–3].

63. Bulger EM, May S, Kerby JD, et al. Out-of-hospital hypertonic resuscitation after traumatic hypovolemic shock: a randomized, placebo controlled trial. Ann Surg 2011;253(3):431–41.

64. Ogilvie MP, Pereira BM, McKenney MG, et al. First report on safety and efficacy of hetastarch solution for initial fluid resuscitation at a level 1 trauma center. J Am Coll Surg 2010;210(5):870–80, 880–72.

65. Ogilvie MP, Ryan ML, Proctor KG. Hetastarch during initial resuscitation from trauma. J Trauma 2011;70(Suppl 5):S19–21.

66. Bunn F, Trivedi D, Ashraf S. Colloid solutions for fluid resuscitation. Cochrane Database Syst Rev 2011;3:CD001319.

67. Manning JE, Katz LM, Brownstein MR, et al. Bovine hemoglobin-based oxygen carrier (HBOC-201) for resuscitation of uncontrolled, exsanguinating liver injury in swine. Carolina Resuscitation Research Group. Shock 2000;13(2):152–9.

68. York GB, Eggers JS, Smith DL, et al. Low-volume resuscitation with a polymer-ized bovine hemoglobin-based oxygen-carrying solution (HBOC-201) provides adequate tissue oxygenation for survival in a porcine model of controlled hemor-rhage. J Trauma 2003;55(5):873–85.

69. Gould SA, Moore EE, Hoyt DB, et al. The first randomized trial of human poly-merized hemoglobin as a blood substitute in acute trauma and emergent surgery. J Am Coll Surg 1998;187(2):113–20 [discussion: 120–2].

70. Rice J, Philbin N, Handrigan M, et al. Vasoactivity of bovine polymerized hemo-globin (HBOC-201) in swine with traumatic hemorrhagic shock with and without brain injury. J Trauma 2006;61(5):1085–99.

71. Fitzpatrick CM, Biggs KL, Atkins BZ, et al. Prolonged low-volume resuscitation with HBOC-201 in a large-animal survival model of controlled hemorrhage. J Trauma 2005;59(2):273–81 [discussion: 281–3].

72. Moore EE, Moore FA, Fabian TC, et al. Human polymerized hemoglobin for the treatment of hemorrhagic shock when blood is unavailable: the USA multicenter trial. J Am Coll Surg 2009;208(1):1–13.

73. Quick summary—blood products advisory committee 88th Meeting. 2006. Available at: http://www.fda.gov/ohrms/dockets/ac/06/minutes/2006-4270M.htm. Accessed January 22, 2012.

74. Prehospital use of plasma for traumatic hemorrhage (PUPTH); 2011. Funding Opportunity Number: W81XWH-11-PUPTH-IAA.

75. Spoerke N, Zink K, Cho SD, et al. Lyophilized plasma for resuscitation in a swine model of severe injury. Arch Surg 2009;144(9):829–34.

76. Shuja F, Shults C, Duggan M, et al. Development and testing of freeze-dried plasma for the treatment of trauma-associated coagulopathy. J Trauma 2008; 65(5):975–85.

77. Krismer AC, Wenzel V, Voelckel WG, et al. Employing vasopressin as an adjunct vasopressor in uncontrolled traumatic hemorrhagic shock. Three cases and a brief analysis of the literature. Anaesthesist 2005;54(3):220–4.

78. Voelckel WG, Convertino VA, Lurie KG, et al. Vasopressin for hemorrhagic shock management: revisiting the potential value in civilian and combat casualty care. J Trauma 2010;69(Suppl 1):S69–74.

79. Raab H, Lindner KH, Wenzel V. Preventing cardiac arrest during hemorrhagic shock with vasopressin. Crit Care Med 2008;36(Suppl 11):S474–80.

80. Cohn SM, McCarthy J, Stewart RM, et al. Impact of low-dose vasopressin on trauma outcome: prospective randomized study. World J Surg 2011;35(2): 430–9.

81. Dünser MW, Hasibeder WR, Wenzel V. Vasopressin in septic shock. N Engl J Med 2008;358(25):2736 [author reply: 2737–8].

82. Lienhart HG, Lindner KH, Wenzel V. Developing alternative strategies for the treatment of traumatic haemorrhagic shock. Curr Opin Crit Care 2008;14(3): 247–53.

83. Cap AP, Baer DG, Orman JA, et al. Tranexamic acid for trauma patients: a critical review of the literature. J Trauma 2011;71(Suppl 1):S9–14.

84. Shakur H, Roberts I, Bautista R, et al. Effects of tranexamic acid on death, vascular occlusive events, and blood transfusion in trauma patients with significant haemorrhage (CRASH-2): a randomised, placebo-controlled trial. Lancet 2010;376(9734):23–32.

85. Morrison JJ, Dubose JJ, Rasmussen TE, et al. Military Application of Tranexamic Acid in Trauma Emergency Resuscitation (MATTERs) Study. Arch Surg 2012; 147(2):113–9 [Epub 2011 Oct 17].

86. Angele MK, Schwacha MG, Ayala A, et al. Effect of gender and sex hormones on immune responses following shock. Shock 2000;14(2):81–90.

87. Knoferl MW, Angele MK, Diodato MD, et al. Female sex hormones regulate macrophage function after trauma-hemorrhage and prevent increased death rate from subsequent sepsis. Ann Surg 2002;235(1):105–12.

88. Chen JG, Not L, Ng T, et al. 17 b-estradiol (E2) administration after major blood loss improves liver ATP, 3-hour survival and also long-term survival following prolonged hypotension (3 hour) and fluid resuscitation. Shock 2006;25(Suppl 1):11.

89. Eastridge BJ, Salinas J, McManus JG, et al. Hypotension begins at 110 mm Hg: redefining "hypotension" with data. J Trauma 2007;63(2):291–7 [discussion: 297–9].

90. Eastridge BJ, Salinas J, Wade CE, et al. Hypotension is 100 mm Hg on the battlefield. Am J Surg 2011;202(4):404–8.

91. Edelman DA, White MT, Tyburski JG, et al. Post-traumatic hypotension: should systolic blood pressure of 90-109 mmHg be included? Shock 2007;27(2):134–8.

92. Bruns B, Gentilello L, Elliott A, et al. Prehospital hypotension redefined. J Trauma 2008;65(6):1217–21.
93. Hick JL, Rodgerson JD, Heegaard WG, et al. Vital signs fail to correlate with hemoperitoneum from ruptured ectopic pregnancy. Am J Emerg Med 2001; 19(6):488–91.
94. McGee S, Abernethy WB, Simel DL. The rational clinical examination. Is this patient hypovolemic? JAMA 1999;281(11):1022–9.
95. Vandromme MJ, Griffin RL, Weinberg JA, et al. Lactate is a better predictor than systolic blood pressure for determining blood requirement and mortality: could prehospital measures improve trauma triage? J Am Coll Surg 2010;210(5): 861–7, 867–9.
96. Guyette F, Suffoletto B, Castillo JL, et al. Prehospital serum lactate as a predictor of outcomes in trauma patients: a retrospective observational study. J Trauma 2011;70(4):782–6.
97. Vandromme MJ, Griffin RL, Kerby JD, et al. Identifying risk for massive transfusion in the relatively normotensive patient: utility of the prehospital shock index. J Trauma 2011;70(2):384–8 [discussion: 388–90].
98. Zarzaur BL, Croce MA, Fischer PE, et al. New vitals after injury: shock index for the young and age x shock index for the old. J Surg Res 2008;147(2):229–36.
99. Sagraves SG, Newell MA, Bard MR, et al. Tissue oxygenation monitoring in the field: a new EMS vital sign. J Trauma 2009;67(3):441–3 [discussion: 443–4].
100. Cooke WH, Salinas J, Convertino VA, et al. Heart rate variability and its association with mortality in prehospital trauma patients. J Trauma 2006;60(2):363–70 [discussion: 370].
101. Nichol G, Powell J, van Ottingham L, et al. Consent in resuscitation trials: benefit or harm for patients and society? Resuscitation 2006;70(3):360–8.
102. Sugarman J, Sitlani C, Andrusiek D, et al. Is the enrollment of racial and ethnic minorities in research in the emergency setting equitable? Resuscitation 2009; 80(6):644–9.
103. Holcomb JB, Weiskopf R, Champion H, et al. Challenges to effective research in acute trauma resuscitation: consent and endpoints. Shock 2011;35(2):107–13.
104. Bulger EM, Schmidt TA, Cook AJ, et al. The random dialing survey as a tool for community consultation for research involving the emergency medicine exception from informed consent. Ann Emerg Med 2009;53(3):341–50, e341–2.

Noncompressible Torso Hemorrhage

A Review with Contemporary Definitions and Management Strategies

Jonathan J. Morrison, MB, ChB, MRCS[a,b],
Todd E. Rasmussen, MD[b,c,d],*

KEYWORDS

- Noncompressible torso hemorrhage • Trauma surgery • Military surgery
- Damage-control surgery • Damage-control resuscitation

KEY POINTS

- Vascular disruption with concomitant hemorrhage is the leading cause of potentially preventable death in both civilian and military trauma. If this occurs in the torso or in a junctional area, it is termed noncompressible torso hemorrhage (NCTH).
- Although the concept of NCTH is intuitive, there remains no formal definition by which to characterize the scope of the problem and compare interventions.
- A novel and inclusive definition using anatomic, physiologic, and procedural criteria enables the identification of patients with NCTH.
- Management requires rapid intervention including damage-control resuscitation and surgery with an emphasis on early hemostasis.
- Despite the emergence of new strategies such as damage-control resuscitation and adjuncts such as endovascular surgery, the principles of proximal and distal vascular control are essential.

The authors have nothing to disclose. The views and opinions expressed in this article are those of the authors and do not reflect the official policy or position of the US Air Force, US Department of Defense, or the US Government.
[a] The Academic Department of Military Surgery & Trauma, Royal Centre for Defence Medicine, Birmingham Research Park, Vincent Drive, Edgbaston, Birmingham B15 2SQ, United Kingdom; [b] U.S. Army Institute of Surgical Research, 3400 Rawley East Chambers Avenue, Suite B, Fort Sam Houston, TX 78234, USA; [c] U.S. Air Force Medical Service, 59th Medical Deployment Wing, Science and Technology Section, 2200 Bergquist Drive, Suite 1, Lackland Air Force Base, TX 78236, USA; [d] The Norman M. Rich Department of Surgery, the Uniformed Services University of the Health Sciences, 4301 Jones Bridge Road, Bethesda, MD 20814, USA
* Corresponding author. US Army Institute of Surgical Research, 3400 Rawley East Chambers Avenue, Suite B, Fort Sam Houston, TX 78234-6315.
E-mail address: todd.rasmussen@amedd.army.mil

Surg Clin N Am 92 (2012) 843–858
doi:10.1016/j.suc.2012.05.002
0039-6109/12/$ – see front matter Published by Elsevier Inc.

surgical.theclinics.com

INTRODUCTION

Vascular disruption with hemorrhage remains a leading cause of death in both civilian[1,2] and wartime trauma.[3,4] Broadly classified, hemorrhage occurs from either compressible sites, meaning those locations amenable to immediate control with manual pressure or tourniquet application, or from noncompressible sites, meaning locations not amenable to control with direct pressure or tourniquet application (**Fig. 1**).[5] In the civilian setting, hemorrhage is present in 15% to 25% of admissions, and studies from the wars in Afghanistan and Iraq show that the rate of vascular injury in combat is approximately 10%.[4–6] Although extremity injury is overall most common, the focus of this review is on the management of vascular disruption and hemorrhage from sources within the torso, including the thorax, abdomen and pelvis, once these patients reach definitive care. An excellent review of the prehospital management strategies for these injuries is provided by Kerby and Cusick elsewhere in this issue.[7]

HEMORRHAGE AS A PROBLEM IN TRAUMA

Control of bleeding from vascular disruption within the torso is not readily amenable to control with direct pressure and is therefore referred to as noncompressible torso

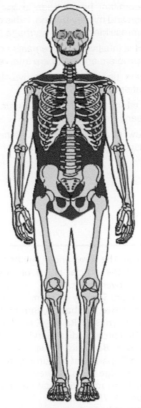

Fig. 1. The shaded area denotes the region where noncompressible torso hemorrhage is anatomically located. (*From* Blackbourne LH, Czarnik J, Mabry R, et al. Decreasing killed in action and died of wounds rates in combat wounded. J Trauma Inj Infect Crit Care 2010;69(1):S1; with permission.)

hemorrhage (NCTH). Civilian studies demonstrating that NCTH accounts for 60% to 70% of mortality following otherwise survivable injuries (ie, no lethal head or cardiac wounds) clearly emphasizes the lethality of this injury pattern.[1,2] Hemorrhage is also a significant problem in the wartime setting, accounting for up to 60% of deaths in potentially survivable injury scenario.[7,8] Studies on those killed in action in Afghanistan and Iraq have shown that of deaths occurring in the setting of otherwise survivable injuries,[3] 80% were a result of bleeding from within the torso.[4,5] The distinction between compressible extremity hemorrhage and NCTH is notable. There has been a demonstrable reduction in mortality from extremity injury with a better understanding of its epidemiology and the need to rapidly control hemorrhage with tourniquets and/or topical hemostatic agents.[8] To date, there has been no such reduction in mortality in the setting of NCTH.

DEFINITION

These observations have resulted in a thrust within the combat casualty care research community to better define and classify locations and patterns of NCTH. Despite its obvious significance, until the wars in Afghanistan and Iraq a consensus definition of NCTH was lacking. Recently reports have emerged from the military's Joint Trauma System and select civilian institutions proposing a unifying classification of this injury pattern. It has been the aim of these studies to establish a cohesive definition allowing for study of the epidemiology of this problem and comparison of management strategies, in hopes of reducing mortality. Until these recent reports, studies of injuries within the torso focused on specific organ injuries such as a series of liver injuries or fell along specialty boundaries such as a vascular surgeon's approach to iliac artery repair.

The wartime perspective on NCTH works from the premise that vascular disruption with bleeding can arise from an array of anatomic sites:

- Large axial vessels
- Solid organ injuries
- Pulmonary parenchymal injuries
- Complex pelvic fractures.

As such, the contemporary definition of NCTH begins with the presence of vascular disruption from 1 or more of 4 anatomic categories listed in **Table 1**. Cardiac wounds are not included within this definition, given their high mortality.

To identify only patients with active hemorrhage from these anatomic categories, the definition of NCTH includes the presence of physiologic measures or operative procedures that reflect hemodynamic instability and/or the need for urgent hemorrhage control. These include hypotension or shock and the need for emergent laparotomy, thoracotomy, or a procedure to manage bleeding from a complex pelvic fracture.

Table 1 Noncompressible torso hemorrhage (NCTH)	
Anatomic Criteria	**Hemodynamic/Procedural Criteria**
1. Thoracic cavity (including lung)	
2. Solid organ injury ≥grade 4 (liver, kidney, spleen)	Hemorrhagic shock[a]; or need for immediate operation
3. Named axial torso vessel	
4. Pelvic fracture with ring disruption	

[a] Defined as a systolic blood pressure <90 mm Hg.

Absent the physiologic or procedural inclusion criteria, the definition of NCTH would be prone to include injuries with the at-risk anatomic category that were not actively bleeding. This article reviews the military and civilian experience with noncompressible torso hemorrhage, and provides an overview of surgical and resuscitative strategies.

MILITARY AND CIVILIAN PERSPECTIVES

One of the first studies to recognize the importance of uncontrolled truncal was by Holcomb and colleagues,[5] who reviewed autopsy findings of special operations forces personnel killed early in the wars in Afghanistan and Iraq, between 2001 and 2004. A panel of experts reviewed the records of 82 fatalities and judged them as nonsurvivable (eg, lethal head or cardiac wounds) or potentially salvageable. This study was one of the first to specifically use the term "noncompressible truncal hemorrhage," although it was not specifically defined. NCTH was found to be the cause of death in 50% of patients judged to have sustained potentially survivable injuries.

Kelly and colleagues[4] used a similar methodology to analyze 997 United States military deaths that occurred within 2 time periods: 2003 to 2004 and 2006. Hemorrhage was the leading cause of death in those with otherwise survivable injuries, and accounted for 87% and 83% of deaths during these respective periods. Airway problems, head injury, and sepsis constituted the remaining causes of death.

Within the hemorrhage group, 50% were due to NCTH and 33% to extremity hemorrhage (amenable to tourniquet application). This study also introduced hemorrhage from another distinct anatomic and clinically important location: junctional areas between the torso and the extremities. Junctional vascular injury or hemorrhage from the proximal femoral or axillobrachial vessels is often not amenable to direct pressure or application of a tourniquet, and therefore poses an especially difficult problem. In the study by Kelly and colleagues,[4] 20% of deaths from hemorrhage occurred from injuries to these junctional zones. Again, in these early studies from the war, NCTH was not explicitly defined but encompassed disruption of any torso-associated vascular structure or viscera.

It is interesting that these figures remained unchanged when Eastridge and colleagues[6] expanded this analysis to all US military personnel who died of wounds between 2001 and 2009. While lethal head injury was the dominant pattern of trauma in the nonsurvivable cases, hemorrhage again accounted for 80% of potentially survivable deaths. Truncal hemorrhage accounted for 48% of deaths in this cohort of casualties. The publication of these studies provided an important characterization of battlefield injury, and illustrated the high and early lethality of NCTH in those who could have otherwise survived their injuries. In parallel with postmortem studies, several clinical studies have examined the incidence of hemorrhage in particular organ systems.

In a study using the US Joint Theater Trauma Registry (JTTR), White and colleagues[9] reported the incidence of vascular injury in US troops between 2002 and 2009. The investigators observed a specific vascular injury rate of 12% (1570 of 13,075), which was 5 times higher than that described in previous wartime reports. Named large vessel injury accounted for 12% of the torso vascular injuries in this study, with iliac, aortic, and subclavian vessels being the most commonly injured.

In a separate study also using the JTTR, Propper and colleagues[10] examined wartime thoracic injury from 2002 to 2009. The investigators found that thoracic injury of any type occurred in 5% of wartime casualties. In this cohort, mean Injury Severity Score (ISS) was 15 and crude mortality was 12%. The most common thoracic injury pattern in this study was pulmonary contusion (32%), followed by hemopneumothorax (19%).

A report by Morrison and colleagues[11] from a single combat support hospital in Afghanistan analyzed 12 months of consecutive episodes of abdominal trauma. More than half (65 patients, 52.0%) required immediate laparotomy, with hemorrhage from solid organs identified in 46 patients (70.8%). There were 15 deaths (23%) in patients undergoing immediate laparotomy, with a median New ISS of 29 and range of 1 to 67.

Despite the value of these studies, they do not specifically emphasize the potential lethality from vascular disruption resulting in NCTH. In this context and given the undeniable association of NCTH with early mortality in those with otherwise survivable injuries, military researchers and civilian collaborators have aggressively sought to establish a unifying definition of this injury pattern. Table 1 shows the initial definition of NCTH developed at the US Army's Institute of Surgical Research, which is based on the previously mentioned anatomic categories of vascular disruption linked to either a physiologic or procedural criterion. A procedure in this definition is defined as an emergent laparotomy, thoracotomy, or procedure undertaken to control bleeding from a complex pelvic injury.

EPIDEMIOLOGY OF NONCOMPRESSIBLE TORSO HEMORRHAGE

A recent study of the US JTTR presented at the American Association for the Surgery of Trauma in 2011 used the definition presented in Table 1 to characterize the epidemiology of NCTH in patients injured in Iraq and Afghanistan between 2002 and 2010. Using the injury pattern criteria alone, 1936 patients were identified as having an injury putting them at risk for NCTH, which was nearly 13% of battle-related casualties. When the physiologic and procedural inclusion criteria were applied to this cohort, 331 patients with a mean ISS ± SD of 30 ± 13 were identified as having NCTH. The most common pattern of hemorrhage was pulmonary parenchyma (32%), followed by bleeding from a named, large vessel within the torso (20%). High-grade solid organ injury (grade IV or V liver, kidney, or spleen) also constituted 20% of cases, and pelvic fracture with vascular disruption accounted for 15%. The most lethal injury pattern (odds ratio; 95% confidence interval) in this study was that to a named large vessel within the torso (3.42; 1.91–6.10), followed by injury to the pulmonary parenchyma (1.89; 1.08–3.33), and complex pelvic fracture with vessel disruption (0.80; 0.36–1.80).

The same investigators applied this definition to British troops injured in Iraq and Afghanistan from 2001 to 2010 using the United Kingdom's Trauma Registry. This analysis included patients who died before receiving treatment at a military surgical hospital (ie, killed in action) and thus did not apply the physiologic or procedural inclusion criteria. This report identified 234 patients with the anatomic injury profile at risk for NCTH, which was 13% of UK battle-related injuries, a number nearly identical to the incidence of this injury pattern in the US JTTR. The overall case fatality rate of UK patients with NCTH was 83%, compared with 25% for any battle-related injury, underscoring the significant mortality burden posed by vascular disruption of any type within the torso.

The civilian experience with NCTH carries a similar message, albeit with a different injury pattern. Specifically, vascular injury or disruption within the torso in the civilian population consists predominantly of blunt rather than penetrating or explosive mechanisms.[2] Hemorrhage remains the leading cause of potentially preventable death in civilian settings, accounting for 30% to 40% of mortality, with 33% to 56% of such deaths occurring in the prehospital phase of injury.[1] Tien and colleagues[12] examined 558 consecutive trauma deaths at a Canadian level-I trauma center. While the most numerous cause of death was related to central nervous system injury, 15% were due to hemorrhage, with 16% of such deaths judged to be preventable. Delay in identifying the bleeding source was cited as the most common preventable reason, with pelvic hemorrhage the most common source. These findings were confirmed and extended by investigators at Los Angeles County + University of Southern California Medical Center, which identified delayed pelvic hemorrhage control as the most frequent cause of preventable deaths from hemorrhage.[13]

CLINICAL MANAGEMENT STRATEGIES IN TORSO HEMORRHAGE CONTROL

The aim of this section is to provide a summary of tools and adjuncts available for the control of torso hemorrhage within the context of current literature. Despite advances in surgical understanding, technique, and technology, one fundamental tenet remains: proximal and distal control are essential when managing suspected vascular injury.

Damage-Control Surgery and Damage-Control Resuscitation

Damage-control surgery (DCS) is a surgical strategy originally described in the context of exsanguinating abdominal trauma, whereby the completeness of operative repair is sacrificed to limit physiologic deterioration.[14,15] This technique has been extended to include other body regions.[16] Definitive operative repair is then completed in a staged fashion following resuscitation and warming in the intensive care unit. DCS is an extreme surgical strategy that carries a risk of infection; intra-abdominal abscess, wound dehiscence, incisional hernia, and enterocutaneous fistulas are common.[17-19] Consequently, this approach should only be used in select patients, as discussed in the review by Chovanes and colleagues elsewhere in this issue.

Military experience in Iraq identified a survival benefit in patients receiving a higher ratio of packed red blood cells (PRBC) to fresh frozen plasma (FFP), who had a significantly lower mortality than patients receiving the lower ratio (19% vs 65%; $P<.001$).[20] This finding has brought about the concept of a balanced or hemostatic resuscitation whereby major trauma patients are resuscitated with a unit ratio of around 1:1 PRBC to FFP. This concept has evolved into a coherent strategy incorporating additional hemorrhage-control adjuncts and is termed damage-control resuscitation (DCR).[21] Most DCR protocols incorporate techniques such as permissive hypotension, minimal use of crystalloid, aggressive warming, and novel infusible hemostatic drugs such as tranexamic acid, paired with DCS for early hemorrhage control.[22]

It is important that DCS should be considered a tool within DCR, which may be used in circumstances of extreme physiology or significant anatomic injury burden.[23] The evidence thus far suggests that the adoption of DCR confers a survival advantage, and is associated with a reduction in the use of DCS techniques.[18,24,25] The specific elements of DCR are well reviewed by Cohen elsewhere in this issue.

However, although DCR demonstrates significant promise, it does liberally use precious resources exposing patients to the risks associated with blood products. Work is being undertaken on product ratios[26,27] and the use of novel compounds to reduce this reliance, such as lyophilized fibrinogen and platelets.[28]

Resuscitative Surgical Maneuvers

A proportion of patients with NCTH present with circulatory collapse, either profoundly hypotensive or in cardiac arrest. Management of patients presenting in such a fashion has been extensively studied.[29-32] The current civilian standard of care is to perform a resuscitative thoracotomy (RT), which permits the following maneuvers[33]:

- Release of cardiac tamponade
- Management of thoracic bleeding

- Control of massive air-leaks
- Internal cardiac massage
- Thoracic aortic occlusion.

The latter maneuver is undoubtedly the most practiced, as aortic control theoretically enhances cerebral and myocardial perfusion.

Although RT is typically performed for thoracic wounding, it has been explored for use in patients with a tense hemoperitoneum in physiologic distress.[34,35] The aim is to obtain control of the vascular inflow of the abdomen while enhancing central pressure, before laparotomy and abdominal hemostasis. This approach is now being challenged because of its poor survival rate, although the physiologic principle of aortic occlusion supporting central pressure remains.

Resuscitative techniques whereby proximal control is remote to the site of injury should not be used liberally, as direct vascular control, when possible, results in a lesser ischemic burden. A recent animal study examined thoracic clamping versus aortic clamping versus direct control of an iliac arterial injury identified a significantly reduced burden of global ischemia with direct control.[36]

Aortic occlusion can also be achieved by endovascular balloon occlusion, as demonstrated by the use of percutaneous devices used to control the neck of abdominal aortic aneurysms during endovascular repair.[37,38] This technique enables the physiologic benefit to be realized without the additional burden of entering a body cavity. Such a technique has been used in trauma as early as the Korean War[39] and since.[40] To date, it has not been used widely or systematically evaluated. However, with recent improvements in endovascular devices and resuscitation in general, there is a renewed interest in this approach, which has been termed resuscitative endovascular balloon occlusion of the aorta (REBOA).[41]

Recent animal work has characterized the reduced physiologic burden of REBOA compared with RT.[42] Animals in class IV shock were allocated to aortic occlusion by a balloon or clamp via thoracotomy. The balloon group demonstrated the same improvement in mean aortic pressure as the clamp group, but with a lower lactate, base excess, and pH measurements after intervention. A different group has identified 40 minutes as the optimum time for aortic balloon occlusion in hypovolemic animals using similar end points.[43]

Operative Exposures in Noncompressible Torso Hemorrhage

The majority of patients with these types of injuries qualify for management in a damage-control fashion, and the appropriate surgical maneuvers depends primarily on the location of hemorrhage within the torso. Certain techniques are described well by Chovanes and colleagues in this issue.

Thorax

For hemorrhage control within the thoracic cavity, access to the ipsilateral side is best via an anterolateral thoracotomy, through the fourth interspace, with the patient in the supine position, tilted up on a roll (**Fig. 2**). This approach also allows extension of this incision across the sternum into the right hemithorax or the clam-shell incision, permitting access to either of the other 2 compartments in the chest (mediastinum and contralateral thoracic cavity) if required (**Fig. 3**). It is important that a surgeon performing this maneuver must also have the ability to concomitantly explore the abdomen, so this must be included when preparing the surgical field.

Once within the chest, hemorrhage control is the priority. Pulmonary bleeding can be controlled using several techniques, depending on location. Injury to the periphery

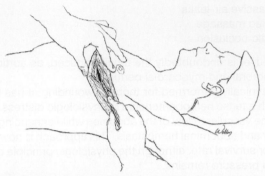

Fig. 2. Anterolateral thoracotomy through the fourth intercostal space permitting access to the left hemithorax, aorta, and cardiac structures. (*From* Hirshberg A, Mattox KL. The no-nonsense trauma thoracotomy. In: Top knife. Shrewsbury: TFM Publishing Ltd; 2005. p. 160. © January 2005, Asher Hirshberg MD & Kenneth L. Mattox MD; with permission from TFM Publishing Ltd. [www.tfmpublishing.com]).

of the lung can be stapled off in a nonanatomic fashion using a linear stapler. Bleeding from within a wound tract is effectively managed following tractotomy, whereby a linear stapler or clamp is introduced down the length of the wound tract and then deployed. This action opens the tract, permitting direct oversewing of disrupted vessels using 3-0 or 4-0 polypropylene sutures on a larger tapered needle (eg, SH) or control with a stapling device.

If hemorrhage from the lung is from the deeper hilar structures, the lung itself (after mobilization) can be compressed or even twisted on itself to occlude the hilar vessel.

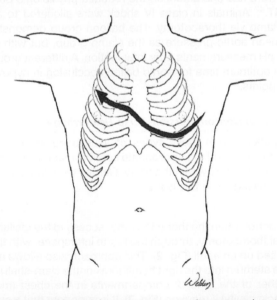

Fig. 3. Extension of the anterolateral thoracotomy across the sternum into the right intercostal space, facilitating access to the mediastinum and right hemithorax. (*From* Hirshberg A, Mattox KL. The no-nonsense trauma thoracotomy. In: Top knife. Shrewsbury: TFM Publishing Ltd; 2005. p. 161. © January 2005, Asher Hirshberg MD & Kenneth L. Mattox MD; with permission from TFM Publishing Ltd. [www.tfmpublishing.com]).

Because such a hilar twist results in a physiologic burden similar to a pneumonectomy (ie, significant elevation in right heart afterload), it should be performed only as a last resort. In cases where the injury significantly compromises a patient's pulmonary reserve, extracorporeal life support (ECLS) may also be a useful adjunct.[44]

Abdomen

The abdomen should be opened through a midline incision from the xiphoid process to the pubic symphysis to permit access to all 4 quadrants. Initial packing remains the best method of initial hemostasis, allowing for the resuscitation to restore the circulating volume. An additional useful adjunct for patients in extremis is resuscitative aortic occlusion of the aorta at the diaphragmatic hiatus. The next key step is sequential evaluation of the abdomen and a decision regarding local control of hemorrhage and contamination.

Hemorrhage from the solid organs of the abdomen is managed differently, depending on the organ in question. Exposure and removal of the spleen is fairly straightforward and well tolerated by the patient, and thus splenectomy is the favored maneuver for the hemorrhaging spleen.

By contrast, hemorrhage from the liver necessitates packing to control venous bleeding in most instances. Control of the porta hepatus at the gastrohepatic ligament and application of the Pringle maneuver is often used as an adjunct to liver packing to control inflow to the organ. Depending on the nature of the wound and the location of the hepatic bleeding, the liver can be mobilized by dividing the coronary and triangular ligaments and allowing the left and right lobes to be drawn or compressed together. If this maneuver is successful, a Vicryl mesh can be used to wrap the liver and maintain apposition of the lobes for hemostasis. If the bleeding liver wound is a defined tract, a tractotomy can be performed to allow exposure and ligation of specific vessels deeper within the wound, or a Penrose drain can be tied over a nasogastric tube to allow inflation of the Penrose within the tract and application of a balloon tamponade.

Mesenteric vessels can be controlled by Forgarty thrombectomy balloons, inserted proximally through small to mid-sized vessels and inflated for proximal control in some cases. Collateral flow to the bowel is generally robust, and ligation of branches of the superior mesenteric artery distal to the middle colic artery is often tolerated. Similarly, proximal branches of the celiac artery or the artery itself can be ligated as a damage-control maneuver with serial observation of the bowel. If the superior and inferior mesenteric and internal iliac arteries are patent and uninjured, ligation of proximal celiac artery branches or the celiac artery itself is often tolerated. Although temporary vascular shunts are mainly used in extremity vessels, there are case reports of their application to mesenteric vessel injuries.[45]

Retroperitoneum

Posterior to the peritoneal sac lies the retroperitoneum, which can be divided into 4 zones. Zone I is centrally located and contains the aorta and inferior vena cava (IVC). Hemorrhage often manifests as a hematoma and should always be explored in this zone. Management of such injuries should adhere to standard principles of proximal and distal control of the vessel. The aorta can be widely exposed through a left medial visceral rotation (the Mattox maneuver, **Fig. 4**) by mobilizing the left colon and kidney. The IVC can be explored through a right visceral rotation (the Cattel-Braasch maneuver, **Fig. 5**), mobilizing the large and small bowel fully to the root of the mesentery.

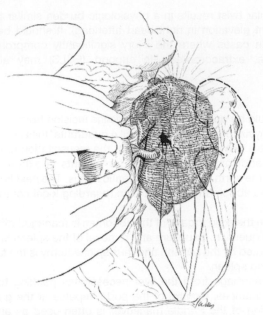

Fig. 4. The left medical visceral rotation (the Mattox maneuver) where the left colon and kidney are mobilized to permit access to the aorta and left-sided retroperitoneal structures. (*From* Hirshberg A, Mattox KL. The no-nonsense trauma thoracotomy. In: Top knife. Shrewsbury: TFM Publishing Ltd; 2005. p. 63. © January 2005, Asher Hirshberg MD & Kenneth L. Mattox MD; with permission from TFM Publishing Ltd. [www.tfmpublishing.com]).

Approaching large-vein injuries in the abdomen is often more challenging than controlling and repairing arterial hemorrhage. Like bleeding from large arteries, one must be prepared with multiple suction devices and a good retraction device, and be sure that the anesthesia team is prepared with warmed rapid transfusion devices. Because large veins often do not tolerate clamps in the setting of trauma and hematoma, direct pressure should be applied with sponge-sticks or the smaller Kittner dissector sponges. These devices substitute for manual pressure and allow one to create more visibility in the operative field.

In situations of large-vein injuries, one should prepare to use a larger tapered needle (eg, SH) on 4-0 polypropylene suture. Larger needles are necessary to see and manipulate within the copious amounts of dark blood that pool between placement of the sutures. Using needles that are too small or suture that is too fine is often frustrating, and results in tearing of the vein and worsening of the injury. When approaching the vena cava or iliac veins one must also be cognizant of the posterior lumbar or lumbosacral branches, which are often quite large and not visible from the anterior approach. If the defect in the vena cava or iliac veins is large enough to cause a greater than 50% narrowing on primary repair, the option of shunting or ligation should be considered.

Zone II is perirenal in location and generally should be managed conservatively in blunt trauma, provided there is no expansion and the patient is hemodynamically stable. Penetrating trauma requires a different approach, with an emphasis on exploration and repair of the kidney if possible, or nephrectomy. If there is concern of injury to or violation of the collecting system, drains should be left in the perinephric or retroperitoneal space.

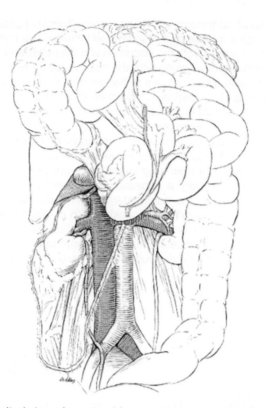

Fig. 5. The right medical visceral rotation (the Cattel-Braasch maneuver) whereby the right colon and duodenum is mobilized to the base of the small bowel mesentery to permit access to the inferior vena cava and right-sided retroperitoneal structures. (*From* Hirshberg A, Mattox KL. The no-nonsense trauma thoracotomy. In: Top knife. Shrewsbury: TFM Publishing Ltd; 2005. p. 67. © January 2005, Asher Hirshberg MD & Kenneth L. Mattox MD; with permission from TFM Publishing Ltd. [www.tfmpublishing.com]).

Zone III originates from within the pelvis, although these injuries can be extensive, tracking all the way up to the supracolic compartment. Pelvic hematomas are best managed conservatively in blunt trauma, and opening them should be avoided. Further management options are outlined below. In penetrating, vascular control is vital, especially if a direct vessel injury is suspected, and may require mobilization of the terminal aorta.

Operative management of bleeding from the portal-retrohepatic zone (sometimes referred to as Zone IV) is fraught with difficulty. Control of bleeding from the retrohepatic vena cava is especially challenging and is associated with high mortality. Contained hematomas should be left undisturbed, and expanding lesions should be packed in the first instance.

Pelvis

The pelvis is a complex compartment containing several unique anatomic structures typically managed in the elective setting by specialists from a range of disciplines (eg, urology, orthopedic surgery, vascular surgery, and general/colorectal surgery). Operative exposure of the pelvic space can be achieved through either a transperitoneal approach at the time of laparotomy or with an extraperitoneal approach, which can be accomplished through a midline or a Pfannenstiel incision. The former is the quicker approach, enabling access to both the abdomen and the pelvis and permitting access to the aorta and distal vascular along with the hollow viscera within that region. The extraperitoneal approach allows access to the external iliac vasculature for suprainguinal arterial control and for packing of the preperitoneal space (**Fig. 6**). The latter is a useful adjunct to managing venous bleeding in complex pelvic fractures once boney stabilization has been achieved.

Arterial bleeding from the pelvis is most commonly managed with endovascular techniques such as coil embolization in cases of complex pelvic fracture. In rare instances of pelvic fracture or open fragmentation or gunshot wounds to the pelvis, ligation of the internal iliac artery is necessary as a hemorrhage-control maneuver. Because of cross-filling from the contralateral internal iliac artery, ligation of one side must typically be accompanied by packing with or without topical hemostatic agents to achieve hemostasis. Ligation of both internal iliac arteries is rarely necessary and is associated with very poor outcomes, related both to the complex nature of the wound and to the subsequent pelvic, buttock, and peroneal ischemia.

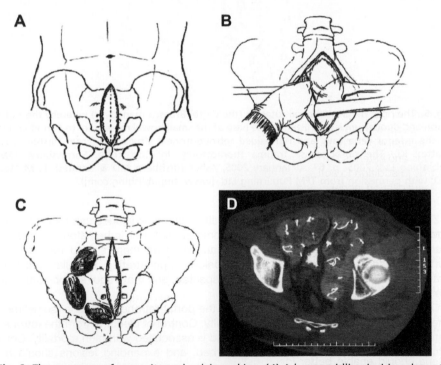

Fig. 6. The sequence of preperitoneal pelvic packing. (*A*) A lower midline incision down to the peritoneum. (*B*) Blunt dissection of preperitoneal space. (*C*) Packing of the preperitoneal space. (*D*) A representative computed tomography scan demonstrating the packs in situ. ([*A–C*] *From* Cothren CC, Osborn PM, Moore EE, et al. Preperitoneal pelvic packing for hemodynamically unstable pelvic fractures: a paradigm shift. J Trauma 2007;62(4):836; with permission; [*D*] *From* Totterman A, Madsen JE, Skaga NO, et al. Extraperitoneal pelvic packing:a salvage procedure to control massive traumatic pelvic hemorrhage. J Trauma 2007;62(4):845; with permission).

PUTTING IT ALL TOGETHER: CURRENT APPLICATIONS AND FUTURE DIRECTIONS

NCTH will continue to challenge clinicians, and future research strategies require a novel approach to reduce the mortality of this injury complex. The first step requires recognition and characterization of the problem, best served by a unifying definition enabling investigators to compare true like with like. Efforts to develop such a definition are under way in both military and civilian settings. In addition, it is important to characterize not only mortal injury patterns in relation to NCTH but also the temporal distribution of deaths. With this approach, both prehospital and hospital interventions can be developed appropriately.

The identification and quantification of specific injuries will allow a tailoring of resuscitation strategies. Meanwhile, several promising new technologies designed to facilitate the management of NCTH are emerging. As an example, REBOA has been discussed already in the context of early animal work, and this technique is now starting to appear in clinical practice. It is also very important that this transition from preliminary evidence to clinical application be done in such a way that reliable data can be captured to ensure robust analysis of its clinical impact.

REBOA is one example of how endovascular approaches may offer novel solutions to difficult problems in trauma care. Expansion of other endovascular or minimally invasive approaches will only continue with traditional elective techniques being used and modified for trauma. This aspect is epitomized by the advent of the Hybrid Operating Room, where physicians can seamlessly change approach from operative to endovascular and vice versa without having to change location.[46,47] This approach may prove to be exceptionally useful in junctional trauma, such as in the pelvis, where approaches are often performed in parallel.

Yet further in the future is the potential application of ECLS[44,48] in combination with hypothermia for patients who suffer a traumatic arrest from NCTH. Following promising animal data and human evidence from nontraumatic cardiac arrest, a multicenter trial of ECLS with deep hypothermia for the management of polytrauma patients has been conceived.[49] The application of this technology theoretically reduces metabolic demand and extends the time frame within which a surgeon must achieve hemorrhage control. In addition to active thermoregulation, the extracorporeal circuit can be used for resuscitation access and the introduction of agents to ameliorate reperfusion injury, among other functions.

SUMMARY

Vascular disruption with concomitant hemorrhage is the leading cause of potentially preventable death in both civilian and military trauma. NCTH is a particularly challenging entity which, despite being an intuitive concept, lacks a formal definition. Management requires rapid decision making, aggressive resuscitation, and surgery with an emphasis on early hemostasis. Despite the emergence of DCR and adjuncts such as endovascular surgery, the principles of proximal and distal control remain.

The use a novel and inclusive definition of NCTH based on anatomic and physiologic criteria should enable better identification of this important patient population and enable comparisons of treatment modalities in the future.

REFERENCES

1. Kauvar D, Lefering R. Impact of hemorrhage on trauma outcome: an overview of epidemiology, clinical presentations, and therapeutic considerations. J Trauma 2006;60(6):3–11.

2. Kauvar DS, Wade CE. The epidemiology and modern management of traumatic hemorrhage: US and international perspectives. Crit Care 2005;9(5):S1–9.

3. Martin M, Oh J, Currier H, et al. An analysis of in-hospital deaths at a modern combat support hospital. J Trauma 2009;66(4):S51.

4. Kelly JF, Ritenour AE, Mclaughlin DF, et al. Injury severity and causes of death from Operation Iraqi Freedom and Operation Enduring Freedom: 2003-2004 versus 2006. J Trauma 2008;64(2):11–5.

5. Holcomb JB, McMullin NR, Pearse L, et al. Causes of death in U.S. Special Operations Forces in the global war on terrorism: 2001-2004. Ann Surg 2007;245(6):986–91.

6. Eastridge BJ, Hardin M, Cantrell J, et al. Died of wounds on the battlefield: causation and implications for improving combat casualty care. J Trauma 2011;71(1):4–8.

7. Kotwal R, Montgomery H, Kotwal B, et al. Eliminating preventable death on the battlefield. Arch Surg 2011;146(12):1350–8.

8. Kragh JF, Walters TJ, Baer DG, et al. Survival with emergency tourniquet use to stop bleeding in major limb trauma. Ann Surg 2009;249(1):1–7.

9. White JM, Stannard A, Burkhardt GE, et al. The epidemiology of vascular injury in the wars in Iraq and Afghanistan. Ann Surg 2011;253(6):1184–9.

10. Propper BW, Gifford SM, Calhoon JH, et al. Wartime thoracic injury: perspectives in modern warfare. Annals Thorac Surg 2010;89(4):1032–5.

11. Morrison JJ, Clasper JC, Gibb I, et al. Management of penetrating abdominal trauma in the conflict environment: the role of computed tomography scanning. World J Surg 2011;35(1):27–33.

12. Tien H, Spencer F, Tremblay L. Preventable deaths from hemorrhage at a level I Canadian trauma center. J Trauma 2007;62:142–6.

13. Teixeira PG, Inaba K, Hadjizacharia P, et al. Preventable or potentially preventable mortality at a mature trauma center. J Trauma 2007;63:1338–47.

14. Rotondo MF, Zonies DH. The damage control sequence and underlying logic. Surg Clin N Am 1997;77(4):761.

15. Shapiro MB, Jenkins DH, Schwab CW, et al. Damage control: collective review. J Trauma 2000;49(5):969–78.

16. Loveland JA, Boffard KD. Damage control in the abdomen and beyond. Brit J Surg 2004;91(9):1095–101.

17. Hatch QM, Osterhout LM, Podbielski J, et al. Impact of closure at the first take back: complication burden and potential overutilization of damage control laparotomy. J Trauma 2011;71(6):1503–11.

18. Higa G, Friese R, O'Keeffe T, et al. Damage control laparotomy: a vital tool once overused. J Trauma 2010;69(1):53–9.

19. Miller RS, Morris JA, Diaz JJ, et al. Complications after 344 damage-control open celiotomies. J Trauma 2005;59(6):1365–74.

20. Borgman MA, Spinella PC, Perkins JG, et al. The ratio of blood products transfused affects mortality in patients receiving massive transfusions at a combat support hospital. J Trauma 2007;63(4):805–13.

21. Duchesne JC, McSwain NE, Cotton BA, et al. Damage control resuscitation: the new face of damage control. J Trauma 2010;69(4):976–90.

22. Hodgetts TJ. Damage control resuscitation. J Roy Army Med Corps 2008;153(4):299–300.

23. Midwinter MJ. Damage control surgery in the era of damage control resuscitation. J Roy Army Med Corps 2009;155(4):323–6.

24. Duchesne JC, Kimonis K, Marr AB, et al. Damage control resuscitation in combination with damage control laparotomy: a survival advantage. J Trauma 2010;69(1):46–52.

25. Cotton BA, Reddy N, Hatch QM, et al. Damage control resuscitation is associated with a reduction in resuscitation volumes and improvement in survival in 390 damage control laparotomy patients. Ann Surg 2011;254(4):598–605.
26. Davenport R, Curry N, Manson J. Hemostatic effects of fresh frozen plasma may be maximal at red cell ratios of 1:2. J Trauma 2011;70:90–6.
27. Holcomb JB, Zarzabal LA, Michalek JE, et al. Increased platelet: RBC ratios are associated with improved survival after massive transfusion. J Trauma 2011; 71(2):S318–28.
28. Duchesne JC. Lyophilized fibrinogen for hemorrhage after trauma. J Trauma 2011;70(5):S50–2.
29. Edens JW, Beekley AC, Chung KK, et al. Long term outcomes after combat casualty emergency department thoracotomy. J Am Coll Surg 2009;209(2):188–97.
30. Frezza E, Mezghebe H. Is 30 minutes the golden period to perform emergency room thoracotomy (ERT) in penetrating chest injuries? J Cardiovasc Surg (Torino) 1999;40(1):147–51.
31. Moore EE, Knudson MM, Burlew CC, et al. Defining the limits of resuscitative emergency department. J Trauma 2011;70(2):334–9.
32. Passos EM, Engels PT, Doyle JD, et al. Societal costs of inappropriate emergency department thoracotomy. J Am Coll Surg 2012;214(1):18–25.
33. Asensio J, Wall M, Minei J. Practice management guidelines for emergency department thoracotomy. J Am Coll Surg 2001;193(3):303–9.
34. Ledgerwood A, Kazmers M, Lucas C. The role of thoracic aortic occlusion for massive hemoperitoneum. J Trauma 1976;16(8):610–5.
35. Seamon MJ, Pathak AS, Bradley KM, et al. Emergency department thoracotomy: still useful after abdominal exsanguination? J Trauma 2008;64(1):1–7.
36. White JM, Cannon JW, Stannard A, et al. Direct vascular control results in less physiologic derangement than proximal aortic clamping in a porcine model of noncompressible extrathoracic torso hemorrhage. J Trauma 2011;71(5):1278–87.
37. Arthurs Z, Starnes B, See C, et al. Clamp before you cut: proximal control of ruptured abdominal aortic aneurysms using endovascular balloon occlusion: case reports. Vasc Endovasc Surg 2006;40(2):149–55.
38. Assar A, Zarins C. Endovascular proximal control of ruptured abdominal aortic aneurysms: the internal aortic clamp. J Cardiovasc Surg 2009;50(3):381.
39. Hughes C. Use of an intra-aortic balloon catheter tamponade for controlling intra-abdominal hemorrhage in man. Surgery 1954;36(1):65.
40. Gupta BK, Khaneja SC, Flores L, et al. The role of intra-aortic balloon occlusion in penetrating abdominal trauma. J Trauma 1989;29(6):861.
41. Stannard A, Eliason JL, Rasmussen TE. Resuscitative endovascular balloon occlusion of the aorta (REBOA) as an adjunct for hemorrhagic shock. J Trauma 2011;71(6):1869–72.
42. White J, Cannon J, Stannard A, et al. Endovascular balloon occlusion of the aorta is superior to resuscitative thoracotomy with aortic clamping in a porcine model of hemorrhagic shock. Surgery 2011;150:400–9.
43. Avaro JP, Mardelle V, Roch A, et al. Forty-minute endovascular aortic occlusion increases survival in an experimental model of uncontrolled hemorrhagic shock caused by abdominal trauma. J Trauma 2011;71(3):720–5.
44. Arlt M, Philipp A, Voelkel S, et al. Extracorporeal membrane oxygenation in severe trauma patients with bleeding shock. Resuscitation 2010;81(7):804–9.
45. Reilly P, Rotondo M, Carpenter J. Temporary vascular continuity during damage control: intraluminal shunting for proximal superior mesenteric artery injury. J Trauma 1995;39(4):757–60.

46. Urbanowicz BJ, Taylor G. Hybrid OR: is it in your future? Nurs Manage 2010;5:
    22–6.
47. Zhao DX, Leacche M, Balaguer JM, et al. Routine intraoperative completion angi-
    ography after coronary artery bypass grafting and 1-stop hybrid revasculariza-
    tion results from a fully integrated hybrid catheterization laboratory/operating
    room. J Am Coll Cardiol 2009;53(3):232–41.
48. Perchinsky M, Long W, Hill J. Extracorporeal cardiopulmonary life support with
    heparin-bonded circuitry in the resuscitation of massively injured trauma patients.
    J Am Coll Surg 1995;169:488–91.
49. Tisherman SA. Emergency preservation and resuscitation (EPR) for cardiac
    arrest from trauma (EPR-CAT). Clinical trials identifier: 1042015.

The Evolution of Damage Control Surgery

John Chovanes, DO[a], Jeremy W. Cannon, MD, SM[b,c],
Timothy C. Nunez, MD[b],*

KEYWORDS

- Damage control surgery • Abbreviated laparotomy • Temporary abdominal closure
- Temporary chest closure • Shunt • Combat surgery

KEY POINTS

- "Patient alive at all costs" is the philosophy of damage control.
- Damage control should begin at the point of injury. Prehospital personnel must be educated on damage control and their performance evaluated.
- Damage control implementation should be limited to clear indications. There are many objective parameters to guide clinicians in the appropriate use of damage control.
- Damage control can be implemented on the battlefield and across a transcontinental health care system. The patient in this system gets care at several locations by numerous providers.
- Damage control has clearly expanded outside the abdomen with a clear presence in other surgical specialties and resuscitation.

INTRODUCTION

Over the last decade, there has been one constant in the implementation of damage control: change. In this decade, damage control surgery has become a tool clinicians probably use too often.[1,2] At the same time, the United States military has shown that damage control surgery can be safely and effectively used across a transcontinental health care system.[3,4] Furthermore, damage control has expanded outside the

The opinions expressed in this document are solely those of the authors and do not represent an endorsement by or the views of the United States Army, the United States Air Force, the Department of Defense, or the United States Government.
The authors have nothing to disclose.
[a] Department of Surgery, Cooper University Hospital, One Cooper Plaza, Camden, NJ 08103, USA; [b] Division of Trauma and Acute Care Surgery, San Antonio Military Medical Center, 3551 Roger Brooke Drive, Fort Sam Houston, TX 78234, USA; [c] Norman M. Rich Department of Surgery, Uniformed Services University of the Health Sciences, Bethesda, MD, USA
* Corresponding author.
E-mail address: timothy.nunez@us.army.mil

doi:10.1016/j.suc.2012.04.002
0039-6109/12/$ – see front matter Published by Elsevier Inc.
surgical.theclinics.com

abdomen to include management of thoracic injuries, vascular injuries, and overall patient resuscitation. In this article, our aim is to give a historical perspective on the origins of damage control surgery and how it has significantly changed in the past decade.

HISTORIC PERSPECTIVE

A decisive operation completed at one setting has long been the hallmark of modern surgery.[5] In this paradigm, the injured patient arrives at the hospital, is taken to the operating room, the areas of injury are located, resections and anastomoses are completed, and the patient is definitively "closed." However, over time, many clinicians came to recognize that some very seriously injured patients, when subjected to this approach, ultimately succumbed either during the operation or shortly thereafter in the intensive care unit.

In the 1980s, several investigators began to challenge the traditional algorithm of definitive surgery completed at the first operation. Initially, the focus was on severe hepatic trauma, and the idea of hepatic packing began to take hold.[6–9] It was at this time that Stone and colleagues[10] presented a small series of patients with onset of major coagulopathy during laparotomy. These investigators proposed temporarily closing the patient with intra-abdominal packing in place to tamponade any ongoing coagulopathic bleeding. After a period of resuscitation, the patient was taken to the operating room for definitive management. In 1992, Burch and colleagues[11] presented a series of 200 critically injured patients in which they identified the triad of hypothermia, acidosis, and coagulopathy as rapidly fatal if left uninterrupted. These investigators further describe techniques to abbreviate the traditional laparotomy, including the use of intravascular shunts, attenuation of enteric injury spillage by the use of Presley vascular clamps, and skin-only closure of the abdominal wall. Furthermore, they described transporting the patient to the surgical intensive care unit for attempted treatment of metabolic derangements and coagulopathy. Of the original 200 patients, 68 died within 2 hours of the initial operation and only 66 survived to hospital discharge. Despite the overall high mortality, these data did support the use of an abbreviated laparotomy in extreme situations.

In 1993, Rotondo and colleagues[12] applied the term damage control to this concept of an abbreviated laparotomy followed by intensive resuscitation. This phrase was adopted from the US navy, which teaches its sailors to use all available means to keep a battle-damaged ship afloat.[13] The investigators applied this same philosophy to their management of critically injured patients from West and Southwest Philadelphia during the emergence of the 9-mm semiautomatic weapon in the civilian population.[14] In this retrospective study of multiply injured patients, all of whom required a massive transfusion, 22 patients underwent standard laparotomy and closure, whereas 24 underwent damage control. Although survival was similar in the damage control versus standard management groups (55% vs 58%), a subset of 22 patients with multiple visceral injuries and a vascular injury showed improved survival when the damage control approach was used (77% vs 11%). These investigators went on to codify 3 distinct areas of care, which are now commonly termed damage control stages 1 (DC1), 2 (DC2), and 3 (DC3) (**Box 1**).

The term damage control has since been applied broadly to a surgical management philosophy and numerous surgical techniques across multiple disciplines, including orthopedic surgery, neurosurgery, emergency general surgery, vascular surgery, and burn surgery. It has also extended to both the prehospital and early resuscitation

> **Box 1**
> **Initial damage control stages as described**
>
> *Stage 1: DC1*
>
> • Control hemorrhage
>
> • Limit peritoneal contamination
>
> • Temporary abdominal closure
>
> *Stage 2: DC2*
>
> • Hypothermia prevention/treatment
>
> • Correction of coagulopathy
>
> • Correction of acidosis
>
> *Stage 3: DC3*
>
> • Definitive surgery
>
> • May require multiple surgeries
>
> • Creation of ostomies, feeding access, fascial closure
>
> • No longer than 72 hours from Stage 1
>
> *Data from* Rotondo MF, Schwab CW, McGonigal MD, et al. 'Damage control': an approach for improved survival in exsanguinating penetrating abdominal injury. J Trauma 1993;35(3):375.

phase (damage control zero [DC0]) and to reconstructive surgery (damage control 4 [DC4]).[15–17]

MILITARY APPLICATIONS OF DAMAGE CONTROL

Between 1985 and 1999, large urban centers experienced an increase in the number of gunshot wounded and the number of ballistic injuries per patient theoretically attributable to the ready availability of semiautomatic handguns.[18] In this environment, many of the damage control principles described earlier were pioneered; however, few realized the great benefit the combat wounded would gain from the application of these concepts.[19,20]

In contrast to Vietnam, the primary wounding mechanism in Operation Iraqi Freedom and Operation Enduring Freedom has been blast injury with multiple fragmentation wounds.[21] This catastrophic injury pattern and the need to rapidly evacuate these patients out of the combat zone make abbreviated staged surgical interventions[22] and damage control resuscitation[23,24] the ideal approach.

In contrast to civilian applications of damage control surgery, military damage control unfolds over at least 10 stages during modern combat casualty care (**Fig. 1**).[3] When a soldier is injured by an improvised explosive device (IED), DC0 is initiated by a combat medic or corpsman, and the soldier is rapidly evacuated to the nearest combat surgical facility where DC1 is performed. The patient then enters DC2 and is evacuated to a higher echelon of care. DC3 is then initiated at either a Level III facility (eg, Craig Joint Theater Hospital, Bagram, Afghanistan) before evacuation from the combat theater or on arrival at a Level IV facility (eg, Landstuhl Regional Medical Center, Germany) with DC2 performed during transport. The echelon IV facility reevaluates the needs for continuation of DC2 or the initiation of DC3, after which the patient is then transported to the continental United States for ongoing DC3, DC4,[25] and rehabilitation.[26]

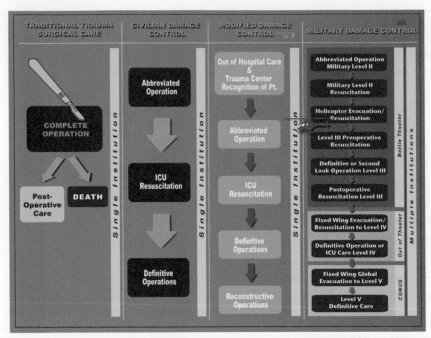

Fig 1. Damage control management contrasts with the traditional model of definitive surgery at the index operation. Military application of this approach is staged in both time and space with the casualty moving sequentially through the chain of evacuation as both damage control resuscitation and surgery are being conducted.

These combat experiences have solidified the concept of staged interventions and resuscitation in high-acuity combat casualty care. Despite the lethality of injuries, if a wounded solider survives the rapid transport to a military medical facility with surgical capability, the likelihood of survival is now higher than any previous recorded conflict.[4]

PATHOPHYSIOLOGY

Multiply traumatized patients with severe wounds typically mount a vigorous immunologic response.[27,28] Over the past 2 decades, the role of cytokines in this response has been elucidated. Pape and colleagues[29] demonstrated that elevations in inflammatory markers correlate with the severity of organ failure in patients with multiple injuries. Perl and colleagues[30] supported this idea and showed that significant higher interleukin (IL) 6 plasma levels were observed in nonsurvivors than in survivors. Furthermore, these increased levels are present early after injury and correlate with the injury severity score, increased morbidity, and increased mortality.[31] Elevated IL-6 levels also correlate with the development of acute respiratory distress syndrome after fracture stabilization with intramedullary nailing.[32–34]

Other cytokines, such as IL-10, granulocyte-monocyte colony-stimulating factor, tissue necrosis factor α and its receptors, and IL-1, also contribute to the inflammatory state. However, the ability to accurately measure the inflammatory state in the acute clinical setting is limited. The complex interplay between the inciting event, the host immune response, and mediators and any genetic predispositions are theorized to be lessened by delaying definitive surgery.[35] Staged interventions may result in a more even balance between injury response and native repair mechanisms.

The acute coagulopathy of trauma is firmly tied to this cytokine burden. It is known that the higher a patient's injury severity score, in civilian and combat injuries, the more likely that patient will have coagulopathy.[36–38] This coagulopathy presents early, similar to the early rise in IL-6 levels. Multiple investigators have elucidated mechanisms for the development of this early coagulopathy, which include hypoperfusion, tissue trauma, and systemic shock among others.[39] Furthermore, this tissue injury and hypoperfusion results in hyperfibrinolysis and activation of the protein C pathway leading to fibrinogen depletion and systemic anticoagulation. Thus, damage control resuscitation needs to be directed specifically at these mechanisms,[40,41] whereas damage control surgery is performed to limit any ongoing hemorrhage or soilage contributing to these derangements.

DAMAGE CONTROL RESUSCITATION

Damage control resuscitation, the idea of whole blood or attempted whole blood reconstitution coupled with early identification of the need for hypotensive resuscitation, limited crystalloid, and hypothermia prevention, demonstrates further expansion of the damage control philosophy and is now recognized as critical to the success of damage control surgery.[15,41–44] Although Lucas and colleagues[45] had shown the benefit of plasma supplementation during hemorrhagic shock in an animal model, this concept did not expand dramatically until recent conflicts. The merits of this approach was well demonstrated in the landmark study by Borgman and colleagues,[46] which showed a significant mortality benefit to wounded soldiers who received a high ratio of plasma to packed cells. Similarly, the concept of permissive hypotension during resuscitation is also not new. It had been described as early as World War I by US Army Captain Cannon along with his coworkers.[47] Bickell and colleagues[48] expanded on this concept nearly 80 years later in a landmark study demonstrating benefit to this approach in patients with penetrating torso injuries.

Adjuncts to damage control resuscitation include topical hemostatic agents such as combat gauze.[49] The CRASH-2 (Clinical Randomisation of an Antifibrinolytic in Significant Haemorrhage 2) trial has now added tranexamic acid as another damage control adjunct to the armamentarium of the trauma surgeon.[50] Some investigators believe that other pharmacologic agents may emerge as future therapies in the care of massively injured patients in extremis.[51] These principles of damage control resuscitation are discussed at length in an article by Cohen in this issue.

INDICATIONS

"An alive patient at all costs" is the philosophy of damage control.[51] However, patient selection and application of damage control surgery continue to evolve.[52] Most trauma patients who present to the modern day trauma center will not require a damage control approach. Only a select few who are seriously injured should require damage control resuscitation and surgical management. Current indications for damage control resuscitation and surgery are outlined in **Box 2**.[12,43,44,52–56]

Ultimately, the decision to enter a damage control mode with a particular patient represents the height of surgical judgment and should take into consideration several factors. First, the patient's physiology and trauma burden should be considered as described earlier. Second, the experience of the surgeon with the particular injury pattern and the capabilities of the surgical team must be considered. Last, logistical factors such as the hospital capacity and availability of a tertiary or quaternary referral center must be considered.

Box 2
Indications for damage control resuscitation and surgery

Damage control resuscitation (civilian)

- ABC score (2 or more positive elements)
  - HR>120
  - SBP<90
  - Positive FAST
  - Penetrating mechanism
- Prehospital shock index>0.9
  - HR/SBP

Damage control resuscitation (military)

- McLaughlin score (2 positive elements)
  - HR>105
  - SBP<110
  - pH<7.25
  - Hematocrit<32%
- High energy–dismounted IED blast injury
- 2 proximal amputations
- 1 proximal amputation and a penetrating torso injury

Damage control surgery

- Multiple life-threatening injuries
- pH<7.2
- Temperature<34°C
- Coagulopathy (clinical or demonstrated on laboratory evaluation)
- Hypotension/shock
- Combined hollow viscous injury and vascular or vascularized organ injury
- Transfusion volume of >4 L of PRBC or >5 L of PRBC combined with whole blood
- Combined crystalloid and blood product resuscitation of >12 L
- Lack of clinical experience/resources to complete procedure
- Need to reassess viability
- Mass casualty situations

Abbreviations: ABC, assessment of blood consumption; FAST, focused assessment with sonography for trauma; HR, heart rate; SBP, systolic blood pressure.
   Data from Refs.[12,43,44,52–56]

Recent publications emphasize that surgeons have probably become too comfortable with damage control techniques, leading to the over use of this approach. Higa and colleagues[1] decreased the use of damage control laparotomy from 36.0% to 8.8%, with a significant decrease in mortality. Hatch and colleagues[2] reviewed their damage control experience over a 4-year period and found that 20% of the patients with open abdomens after initial laparotomy did not have a clear indication for damage control. In time, as surgeons gain experience with damage control and as more groups identify appropriate triggers, patient selection should become more refined, resulting in the optimal application of this approach.

DAMAGE CONTROL LAPAROTOMY

The quintessential damage control techniques are applied in severe abdominal trauma where this approach was first described. It is essential that the entire operating room team be prepared for the critically ill patient who requires damage control. The damage control principles in this initial operation include[57]:

- Obtaining control of hemorrhage
- Limiting peritoneal contamination
- Applying temporary abdominal closure.

A variety of techniques may be required to control hemorrhage. Initially, the patient should undergo packing of all 4 quadrants. This may need to be paired with vascular control for the abdominal hemorrhage. Ledgerwood and colleagues[58] originally described performing a left anterior lateral thoracotomy for proximal aortic control for hemorrhagic control before laparotomy. Recent preclinical evidence suggests that the physiologic cost of this thoracotomy is greater than direct control or endovascular occlusion techniques.[59,60] The use of deep hypothermia (with extracorporeal support) to afford cerebral protection and a relatively bloodless field is also on the horizon.[61–64] Both these concepts are early in development and should not be broadly applied until the risks and benefits are clearly delineated in the context of a clinical trial. If these innovative approaches show validity, resuscitative anterolateral thoracotomies will have a diminished role in the management of extrathoracic torso trauma.

Damage control management of solid organ bleeding involves either removal or compression of the source. If bleeding is primarily from the spleen, splenectomy is preferred during damage control as opposed to a time-consuming splenorrhaphy. Massive bleeding from the liver is best controlled by packs from above and below. Expanding lateral retroperitoneal hematomas are best approached laterally to medially. If one kidney is the source, quick palpation of the contralateral renal fossa to confirm the presence of a normal kidney is preferred to an on-table intravenous pyelography before nephrectomy.

Repair of vessels, if time permits, is the preferred method for controlling major truncal arterial and venous injuries. However, ligation of truncal vessels may need to be considered. Shunting is also an option for control of a major vascular injury. This approach is more typically applied for peripheral vascular injuries, but it is a valid option in truncal hemorrhage.[65] Shunting can be done rapidly to control hemorrhage and maintain distal perfusion.

Control of contamination is essential, although many argue as to how early in the first operative procedure this has to be done. With respect to stool and other enteric contents, the surgeon has many tools that can rapidly control the contamination. Linear stapling devices, skin staplers, Allis clamps, and umbilical tapes can all be used to control leakage. Alternatively, if faced with noncircumferential holes in the bowel, the defect may be quickly repaired with 2-0 or 3-0 silk sutures.

Injuries to the pancreas and duodenum can present the surgeon with an exceptionally challenging clinical scenario. Patients with pancreaticoduodenal injuries typically have major associated solid organ or vascular injuries. Rickard and colleagues[66] in a 30-month review of pancreatic and duodenal injuries stressed the complex nature of these injuries and the need to prevent metabolic failure by "keeping it simple"(and quick). When faced with duodenal injuries, primary repair with 1- or 2-layers may be attempted if the patient is not on the brink of physiologic collapse. In the damage control situation, rapid debridement and closure of the injured duodenum should be accomplished. Nasogastric decompression is sufficient, and consideration of pyloric exclusion should be tabled until definitive reconstruction. Proximal pancreatic injuries with or without a ductal injury and distal injuries without ductal involvement should be treated with closed suction drainage.[66] Distal pancreatic injuries with clear ductal involvement are best addressed with distal pancreatectomy with splenectomy. We prefer leaving a drain in this situation. Our opinion is that preservation of the spleen is too time consuming in a patient with marginal physiologic reserve. High-grade pancreatic injuries (Grade IV and V) should be addressed in a staged manner. Pancreaticoduodenectomy at the index procedure is usually an exercise in futility. In a recent report, Seamon and colleagues[67] studied only pancreatic injuries in 42 patients treated using the damage control procedure. These investigators recommended either resection and drainage or drainage alone in this situation rather than simply packing the abdomen without closed suction drains near the pancreatic injury. Sharpe and colleagues[68] studied all pancreatic injuries over a 13-year period after they had established a simple management algorithm. Only distal injuries with clear ductal involvement were resected. The proximal and low probability distal injuries were treated with closed suction drainage alone. Compared with a previous report from the same institution, these investigators showed a significant reduction in pancreatic-associated morbidity and mortality.[68,69]

If the decision has been made to perform a damage control procedure, then primary fascial reapproximation should not be attempted. Many temporary abdominal closure methods such as towel clip or Bogotá bag closure (suturing plastic bag to the skin to avoid compromising the fascia) have been described,[70] but these are mainly of historical interest. One of the most common methods used at present is the "vac-pack" technique[71] reviewed in an article by Cannon and colleagues elsewhere in this issue. Commercially available negative pressure devices are also frequently used to address the open abdomen at the completion of DC1.

DAMAGE CONTROL THORACOTOMY

Thoracic damage control, although not a new concept, has not been as well described in the literature as abdominal damage control. The principles, however, are the same: an abbreviated operation with rapid transport to the intensive care unit in an effort to restore the patient's physiologic condition to normal (or near-normal) before definitive repair.[72]

An abbreviated thoracic operation is triggered by the same factors as described earlier. For positioning, even when the primary surgical concern is in the chest cavity, the supine position is the most practical and flexible approach. Extending the arms out at 90° or placing the patient into a "taxi-hailing" position with a slight "bump" under the left chest may assist in exposure.[73] However, given the potential for an emergent celiotomy (even in those in whom it is not anticipated preoperatively), the supine position is the most universal position.[72,74]

Patients who require resuscitative thoracotomy in the emergency department are almost always candidates for thoracic damage control because this procedure is typically performed in patients who have had penetrating injuries and are in extremis.[75–78] This temporizing measure allows the surgeon to expeditiously move the patient to the operating room for more secure control of hemorrhage if vital signs are restored.

An anterolateral thoracotomy is the optimal incision for patients who present in extremis. This procedure allows rapid identification of injuries in the left chest or mediastinum. It can also identify injuries in the right chest when the anterolateral thoracotomy is extended across midline. Once the chest is opened, several maneuvers can be used to quickly address life-threatening issues[72]:

- Releasing cardiac tamponade
- Compressing the proximal aorta
- Packing the chest cavity for general hemorrhage control.

If pericardial tamponade is encountered and released, control of cardiac/great vessel bleeding is then immediately required. This control can be accomplished by applying a finger over the area with gentle pressure or by rapid suture or staple closure. With large defects, some investigators have described balloon occlusion with a bladder catheter placed into the defect,[73] although this can also worsen the situation by extending the laceration. In cases in which intravenous access is limited or nonexistent, a large-bore catheter (or simply a length of IV tubing) can be placed directly into the right atrium to facilitate resuscitation.[79]

Injuries to vascular structures in the chest are approached in the same manner as we have described for other vascular injuries. A lengthy operation to primarily repair a vascular injury in a tenuous patient is generally ill advised. Simple lateral repair, shunt placement, and ligation are the best options. In some instances, placement of a covered endovascular stent can be both expeditious and definitive.[80,81]

Lung injuries are typically the easiest to deal with from a technical standpoint. Twisting the lung around its hilum has been described in cases of significant hemorrhage from the lung and pulmonary vessels. The inferior pulmonary ligament must first be released after which the damaged lung is twisted 180° to provide compression of the main pulmonary artery and vein.[82] This can also be achieved with a pulmonary hilar clamp. Both of these maneuvers can be used as a temporary intraoperative adjunct or can be used for an extended period while other injuries are being addressed and the patient is undergoing resuscitation. Massive hemorrhage from through-and-through pulmonary parenchymal injuries are best approached by unroofing the overlying lung tissue between clamps or with a linear stapler, a so-called tractotomy.[83] Following this maneuver, the bleeding source can be more readily identified and directly sutured.

Esophageal injuries encountered in a patient with severe physiologic disturbances can be challenging. Primary repair is ideal if the patient's physiologic condition permits. Most investigators recommend primary closure with wide drainage for such injuries with reinforcement of the repair with pericardium or intercostal muscle.[84–87] If the patient is too unstable or the defect too large to perform a primary repair, wide drainage with at least 2 large-bore chest tubes and a nasogastric tube placed at the site of injury connected to continuous low wall suction is a viable damage control option in this situation.

Most upper airway injuries are amendable to passing the endotracheal tube past the site of injury. Occasionally, a penetrating injury with an anteroposterior trajectory can make an anterior defect in the trachea that can be managed by passing an endotracheal or tracheostomy tube through this defect.

Temporary chest wall closure may take some creative techniques depending on the incision made and the degree of chest wall damage from the original injury. The goals in chest wall closure are to maintain adequate perfusion and oxygenation while also controlling any diffuse coagulopathic hemorrhage. A closure is also needed that will allow the clinician to know if the hemorrhage is not controlled. Packing the thoracic cavity with towel clip closure is acceptable. A recent review did not show any deleterious effects from thoracic packing in comparison with a definitive closure.[88] However, because the chest does not have the ability to "swell," a thoracic compartment syndrome may develop during DC2, resulting in a significant setback for the patient.

Consequently, we prefer a modified "vac-pack" or black sponge vacuum-assisted closure (discussed in the aforementioned article by Cannon and colleagues elsewhere in the same issue). This closure is fashioned by first placing chest tubes into the thoracic cavity to monitor any ongoing blood loss. A bowel bag or another sterile plastic cover (without perforations) is then placed over the lung to serve as the pleura. A negative pressure dressing is then applied over the open wound to seal the chest cavity.

DAMAGE CONTROL VASCULAR SURGERY

Vascular injuries in the torso and extremities can result in a significant physiologic burden for the patient, which sometimes necessitates a damage control approach. In 1988, Feliciano and colleagues[89] demonstrated that in 300 consecutive laparotomies for gunshot wounds, the survival rate dropped by nearly 30% when a vascular injury was present. Historically, the primary techniques to control hemorrhage included direct pressure, packing, vascular repair, or ligation.

More recently, placement of a vascular shunt into the injured vessel has been promoted as an ideal damage control approach for extremity vascular trauma.[90–92] In their study describing the US military experience in managing vascular injury, Rasmussen and colleagues[93] reported that 30 shunts (26 arterial and 4 venous injuries; 22 in proximal extremity vessels and 8 in distal vessels) were placed for vascular damage control over 12 months of combat operations. In these patients, thrombectomy was performed before shunt placement and regional anticoagulation with heparinized saline was used, and a fasciotomy was performed in all cases. Definitive vascular repair with autologous conduit was performed after resuscitation. In these patients, 86% of proximal shunts remained patent (as compared with only 12% of distal shunts), with an overall limb salvage rate of 93%. These results have been replicated in both military[94] and civilian[65] settings, firmly establishing vascular shunting as the damage control vascular injury management technique of choice for proximal extremity vascular injuries.

A range of different conduits can be used as a shunt. In Rasmussen's series, of 30 shunts, 16 were Javid shunts, 12 were Argyle shunts, and 2 were Sundt shunts. Pruitt-Inahara shunts have also been described for this purpose.[65] Alternatively, intravenous catheters (with the hub removed), intravenous tubing, and chest tubes can be used for this purpose. The shunt should be sized to avoid kinking of the proximal or distal vessels while also limiting the intraluminal length of tubing because this section of the vessel must be excised at the time of definitive repair (**Fig. 2**). The shunt is secured on either end typically with silk ties or a vessel loop and should be tagged for easy identification at the subsequent operation.

Intraluminal stents can be used as a damage control intervention in selected cases of vascular trauma as discussed earlier. The primary indication for stent placement is for injuries to the thoracic aorta, although survivors with these injuries are generally managed with blood pressure control initially to prevent early rupture followed by interval repair.[95,96] In junctional areas, such as the distal subclavian artery or the iliac artery, placement of a covered stent may be a lifesaving damage control maneuver.[80] However, this approach has yet to be systematically evaluated.

COMPLICATIONS

Damage control surgery does carry significant risks as demonstrated by both the historic and recent literature on this topic. For damage control abdominal surgery, the rate of wound complications is as high as 25%.[97] Others have reported high rates of intra-abdominal abscesses following abdominal closure in these cases.[98]

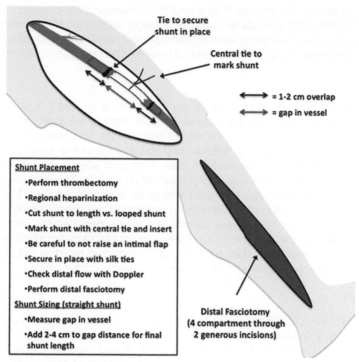

Tie to secure shunt in place

Central tie to mark shunt

⟷ = 1-2 cm overlap

←⟶ = gap in vessel

Shunt Placement
- •Perform thrombectomy
- •Regional heparinization
- •Cut shunt to length vs. looped shunt
- •Mark shunt with central tie and insert
- •Be careful to not raise an intimal flap
- •Secure in place with silk ties
- •Check distal flow with Doppler
- •Perform distal fasciotomy

Shunt Sizing (straight shunt)
- •Measure gap in vessel
- •Add 2-4 cm to gap distance for final shunt length

Distal Fasciotomy
(4 compartment through 2 generous incisions)

Fig. 2. Technique for vascular shunt placement.

Enteroatmospheric fistulae can also complicate these procedures when abdominal domain is lost. Sriussadaporn and colleagues[99] performed a retrospective study in such patients and found that the following factors predict fistulae formation:

- Prolonged exposure of viscera
- Frequent dressing changes
- Type of prosthetic placed
- Fascial dehiscence.

Loss of abdominal domain in these patients results in a giant ventral hernia. Novel approaches to both preventing this complication and managing those that have already developed have been described. The VAC abdominal dressing (Kinetic Concepts, Inc, San Antonio, TX, USA), ABRA elastic tensioning system (ABRA, Canica, Almonte, Ontario, Canada), and the use of a variety of biological grafts all have been used to facilitate abdominal closure.[100] In patients who develop giant hernias, separation of components has been applied to re-establish coverage with native tissue.[25,101]

Complications of thoracic damage control similarly include infections and wound complications. In addition, retained hemothorax, prolonged air leaks, bronchopleural fistulae, and spit fistulae can all result depending on the original injury and the surgery performed.

After vascular damage control, the primary complications include distal ischemia from either ligation or subsequent thrombosis of the injured vessel, venous hypertension, infection, and limb loss. As noted earlier, shunt insertion has become a mainstay in vascular damage control with very few complications attributable specifically to shunt placement. Shunt occlusion occurs in about 5% of cases and is more common if placed in a distal extremity vessel (eg, the anterior tibial artery).[65,93] However, limb loss following shunt placement is difficult to attribute to shunt use or failure rather than to the original injury. Other complications of extremity vascular damage control relate to limb salvage. These include chronic pain, neuropathy, malunion of bony injuries, and limb dysfunction.

SUMMARY

Damage control surgery, regardless of the body cavity to which it is applied, is a concept that promotes unconventional surgical techniques that restore normal anatomy and physiology over several staged procedures. The goal is to stay out of trouble rather than to get out of trouble, and this approach has been successfully applied in military and civilian practices alike. Profound physiologic derangements can be avoided by abbreviating the index surgical procedure. This permits adequate resuscitation after hemorrhage and gross soilage have been controlled. More recent concepts in this approach include identifying patients at risk for physiologic exhaustion, novel methods of hemorrhage control and injury management, expansion of temporary closure to the chest, and use of vascular shunts. Ongoing study is required to better identify candidate patients for damage control and to refine the techniques that result in functional survivors with the fewest possible complications.

REFERENCES

1. Higa G, Friese R, O'Keeffe T, et al. Damage control laparotomy: a vital tool once overused. J Trauma 2010;69(1):53.
2. Hatch QM, Osterhout LM, Podbielski J, et al. Impact of closure at the first take back: complication burden and potential overutilization of damage control laparotomy. J Trauma 2011;71(6):1503.
3. Blackbourne LH. Combat damage control surgery. Crit Care Med 2008; 36(Suppl 7):S304.
4. Eastridge BJ, Jenkins D, Flaherty S, et al. Trauma system development in a theater of war: experiences from Operation Iraqi Freedom and Operation Enduring Freedom. J Trauma 2006;61(6):1366.
5. Moore W. The knife man: the extraordinary life and times of John Hunter, father of modern surgery. New York: Broadway Books; 2005.
6. Stone HH, Lamb JM. Use of pedicled omentum as an autogenous pack for control of hemorrhage in major injuries of the liver. Surg Gynecol Obstet 1975; 141(1):92.
7. Carmona RH, Peck DZ, Lim RC Jr. The role of packing and planned reoperation in severe hepatic trauma. J Trauma 1984;24(9):779.
8. Feliciano DV, Mattox KL, Jordan GL Jr, et al. Management of 1000 consecutive cases of hepatic trauma (1979-1984). Ann Surg 1986;204(4):438.
9. Feliciano DV, Mattox KL, Burch JM, et al. Packing for control of hepatic hemorrhage. J Trauma 1986;26(8):738.
10. Stone HH, Strom PR, Mullins RJ. Management of the major coagulopathy with onset during laparotomy. Ann Surg 1983;197(5):532.
11. Burch JM, Ortiz VB, Richardson RJ, et al. Abbreviated laparotomy and planned reoperation for critically injured patients. Ann Surg 1992;215(5):476.
12. Rotondo MF, Schwab CW, McGonigal MD, et al. 'Damage control': an approach for improved survival in exsanguinating penetrating abdominal injury. J Trauma 1993;35(3):375.
13. Department of defense surface ship survivabilty. Washington, DC: Naval Warfare Publication; 1989. p. 3–20, 31.

14. Schwab CW. Violence: America's uncivil war—presidential address, Sixth Scientific Assembly of the Eastern Association for the Surgery of Trauma. J Trauma 1993;35(5):657.
15. Beekley AC. Damage control resuscitation: a sensible approach to the exsanguinating surgical patient. Crit Care Med 2008;36(7):S267.
16. Johnson JW, Gracias VH, Schwab CW, et al. Evolution in damage control for exsanguinating penetrating abdominal injury. J Trauma 2001;51(2):261.
17. Le Noel A, Merat S, Ausset S, et al. The damage control resuscitation concept. Ann Fr Anesth Reanim 2011;30(9):665 [in French].
18. McGonigal MD, Cole J, Schwab CW, et al. Urban firearm deaths: a five-year perspective. J Trauma 1993;35(4):532.
19. Pruitt BA Jr. Combat casualty care and surgical progress. Ann Surg 2006; 243(6):715.
20. Simmons JW, White CE, Eastridge BJ, et al. Impact of improved combat casualty care on combat wounded undergoing exploratory laparotomy and massive transfusion. J Trauma 2011;71(Suppl 1):S82.
21. Kelly JF, Ritenour AE, McLaughlin DF, et al. Injury severity and causes of death from Operation Iraqi Freedom and Operation Enduring Freedom: 2003-2004 versus 2006. J Trauma 2008;64(Suppl 2):S21.
22. Schwab CW. Crises and war: stepping stones to the future. J Trauma 2007; 62(1):1.
23. Fox CJ, Gillespie DL, Cox ED, et al. The effectiveness of a damage control resuscitation strategy for vascular injury in a combat support hospital: results of a case control study. J Trauma 2008;64(Suppl 2):S99.
24. Spinella PC. Warm fresh whole blood transfusion for severe hemorrhage: U.S. military and potential civilian applications. Crit Care Med 2008;36(Suppl 7): S340.
25. Vertrees A, Greer L, Pickett C, et al. Modern management of complex open abdominal wounds of war: a 5-year experience. J Am Coll Surg 2008; 207(6):801.
26. Stinner DJ, Burns TC, Kirk KL, et al. Return to duty rate of amputee soldiers in the current conflicts in Afghanistan and Iraq. J Trauma 2010;68(6):1476.
27. Cuthbertson DP. Post-shock metabolic response. Lancet 1942;239(6189):433.
28. Cuthbertson DP. The physiology of convalescence after injury. Br Med Bull 1945; 3:96.
29. Pape HC, van Griensven M, Rice J, et al. Major secondary surgery in blunt trauma patients and perioperative cytokine liberation: determination of the clinical relevance of biochemical markers. J Trauma 2001;50(6):989.
30. Perl M, Gebhard F, Bruckner UB, et al. Pulmonary contusion causes impairment of macrophage and lymphocyte immune functions and increases mortality associated with a subsequent septic challenge. Crit Care Med 2005;33(6): 1351.
31. Pape HC, Remmers D, Grotz M, et al. Levels of antibodies to endotoxin and cytokine release in patients with severe trauma: does posttraumatic dysergy contribute to organ failure? J Trauma 1999;46(5):907.
32. Harwood PJ, Giannoudis PV, van Griensven M, et al. Alterations in the systemic inflammatory response after early total care and damage control procedures for femoral shaft fracture in severely injured patients. J Trauma 2005;58(3):446.
33. Michaels AJ. Management of post traumatic respiratory failure. Crit Care Clin 2004;20(1):83.

34. Gebhard F, Pfetsch H, Steinbach G, et al. Is interleukin 6 an early marker of injury severity following major trauma in humans? Arch Surg 2000; 135(3):291.
35. van Griensven M. Pathogenetic changes: isolated extremity trauma and polytrauma. In: Pape HC, Peitzman AB, Schwab CW, editors. Damage control management in the polytrauma patient. 1st edition. New York: Springer; 2010.
36. Brohi K, Singh J, Heron M, et al. Acute traumatic coagulopathy. J Trauma 2003; 54(6):1127.
37. Niles SE, McLaughlin DF, Perkins JG, et al. Increased mortality associated with the early coagulopathy of trauma in combat casualties. J Trauma 2008;64(6):1459.
38. MacLeod JB, Lynn M, McKenney MG, et al. Early coagulopathy predicts mortality in trauma. J Trauma 2003;55(1):39.
39. Hess JR, Brohi K, Dutton RP, et al. The coagulopathy of trauma: a review of mechanisms. J Trauma 2008;65(4):748.
40. Brohi K, Cohen MJ, Ganter MT, et al. Acute coagulopathy of trauma: hypoperfusion induces systemic anticoagulation and hyperfibrinolysis. J Trauma 2008; 64(5):1211.
41. Duchesne JC, McSwain NE Jr, Cotton BA, et al. Damage control resuscitation: the new face of damage control. J Trauma 2010;69(4):976.
42. Holcomb JB, Jenkins D, Rhee P, et al. Damage control resuscitation: directly addressing the early coagulopathy of trauma. J Trauma 2007;62(2):307.
43. Nunez TC, Voskresensky IV, Dossett LA, et al. Early prediction of massive transfusion: simple as ABC? J Trauma 2009;66(2):346–52.
44. Vandromme MJ, Griffin RL, Kerby JD, et al. Identifying risk for massive transfusion in the relatively normotensive patient: utility of the prehospital shock index. J Trauma 2011;70(2):384.
45. Lucas CE, Ledgerwood AM, Saxe JM, et al. Plasma Supplementation is beneficial for coagulation during severe hemorrhagic shock. Am J Surg 1996;171(4): 399–404.
46. Borgman MA, Spinella PC, Perkins JG, et al. The ratio of blood products transfused affects mortality in patients receiving massive transfusions at a combat support hospital. J Trauma 2007;63(4):805.
47. Cannon W, Fraser J, Cowell E. The preventive treatment of wound shock. JAMA 1918;70(9):618.
48. Bickell WH, Wall MJ Jr, Pepe PE, et al. Immediate versus delayed fluid resuscitation for hypotensive patients with penetrating torso injuries. N Engl J Med 1994;331(17):1105.
49. Butler FK. Tactical Combat Casualty Care: update 2009. J Trauma 2010; 69(Suppl 1):S10.
50. Shakur H, Roberts I, Bautista R, et al. Effects of tranexamic acid on death, vascular occlusive events, and blood transfusion in trauma patients with significant haemorrhage (CRASH-2): a randomised, placebo-controlled trial. Lancet 2010;376(9734):23.
51. Schwab C. Master surgeon lecture. How I do it. Damage control surgery. 69th Annual Meeting of the American Association for the Surgery of Trauma. Boston, September 22–25, 2010.
52. Cirocchi R, Abraha I, Montedori A, et al. Damage control surgery for abdominal trauma. Cochrane Database Syst Rev 2010;1:CD007438.
53. Asensio JA, McDuffie L, Petrone P, et al. Reliable variables in the exsanguinated patient which indicate damage control and predict outcome. Am J Surg 2001; 182(6):743.

54. Asensio JA, Petrone P, Roldan G, et al. Has evolution in awareness of guidelines for institution of damage control improved outcome in the management of the posttraumatic open abdomen? Arch Surg 2004;139(2):209.
55. Ivatury RR, Diebel L, Porter JM, et al. Intra-abdominal hypertension and the abdominal compartment syndrome. Surg Clin North Am 1997; 77(4):783.
56. McLaughlin DF, Niles SE, Salinas J, et al. A predictive model for massive transfusion in combat casualty patients. J Trauma 2008;64(Suppl 2):S57.
57. Rotondo MF, Zonies DH. The damage control sequence and underlying logic. Surg Clin North Am 1997;77(4):761.
58. Ledgerwood AM, Kazmers M, Lucas CE. The role of thoracic aortic occlusion for massive hemoperitoneum. J Trauma 1976;16(08):610.
59. White JM, Cannon JW, Stannard A, et al. Endovascular balloon occlusion of the aorta is superior to resuscitative thoracotomy with aortic clamping in a porcine model of hemorrhagic shock. Surgery 2011;150(3):400.
60. White JM, Cannon JW, Stannard A, et al. Direct vascular control results in less physiologic derangement than proximal aortic clamping in a porcine model of noncompressible extrathoracic torso hemorrhage. J Trauma 2011; 71(5):1278.
61. Bellamy R, Safar P, Tisherman SA, et al. Suspended animation for delayed resuscitation. Crit Care Med 1996;24(Suppl 2):S24.
62. Tisherman SA, Safar P, Radovsky A, et al. Therapeutic deep hypothermic circulatory arrest in dogs: a resuscitation modality for hemorrhagic shock with 'irreparable' injury. J Trauma 1990;30(7):836.
63. Tisherman SA. Hypothermia and injury. Curr Opin Crit Care 2004;10(6):512.
64. Alam HB, Bowyer MW, Koustova E, et al. Learning and memory is preserved after induced asanguineous hyperkalemic hypothermic arrest in a swine model of traumatic exsanguination. Surgery 2002;132(2):278.
65. Subramanian A, Vercruysse G, Dente C, et al. A decade's experience with temporary intravascular shunts at a civilian level I trauma center. J Trauma 2008;65(2):316.
66. Rickard MJ, Brohi K, Bautz PC. Pancreatic and duodenal injuries: keep it simple. ANZ J Surg 2005;75(7):581.
67. Seamon MJ, Kim PK, Stawicki SP, et al. Pancreatic injury in damage control laparotomies: is pancreatic resection safe during the initial laparotomy? Injury 2009;40(1):61.
68. Sharpe JP, Magnotti LJ, Weinberg JA, et al. Impact of a defined management algorithm on outcome after traumatic pancreatic injury. J Trauma Acute Care Surg 2012;72(1):100.
69. Patton JH Jr, Lyden SP, Croce MA, et al. Pancreatic trauma: a simplified management guideline. J Trauma 1997;43(2):234.
70. Boele van Hensbroek P, Wind J, Dijkgraaf MG, et al. Temporary closure of the open abdomen: a systematic review on delayed primary fascial closure in patients with an open abdomen. World J Surg 2009;33(2):199.
71. Barker DE, Kaufman HJ, Smith LA, et al. Vacuum pack technique of temporary abdominal closure: a 7-year experience with 112 patients. J Trauma 2000;48(2): 201.
72. Wall MJ Jr, Soltero E. Damage control for thoracic injuries. Surg Clin North Am 1997;77(4):863.
73. Rotondo MF, Bard MR. Damage control surgery for thoracic injuries. Injury 2004; 35(7):649.

74. Hirshberg A, Wall MJ Jr, Allen MK, et al. Double jeopardy: thoracoabdominal injuries requiring surgical intervention in both chest and abdomen. J Trauma 1995;39(2):225.

75. Cogbill TH, Moore EE, Millikan JS, et al. Rationale for selective application of Emergency Department thoracotomy in trauma. J Trauma 1983;23(6):453.

76. Moore EE, Moore JB, Galloway AC, et al. Postinjury thoracotomy in the emergency department: a critical evaluation. Surgery 1979;86(4):590.

77. Baker CC, Thomas AN, Trunkey DD. The role of emergency room thoracotomy in trauma. J Trauma 1980;20(10):848.

78. Beall AC Jr, Diethrich EB, Cooley DA, et al. Surgical management of penetrating cardiovascular trauma. South Med J 1967;60(7):698.

79. Renz BM, Stout MJ. Rapid right atrial cannulation for fluid infusion during resuscitative emergency department thoracotomy. Am Surg 1994;60(12):946.

80. Avery LE, Stahlfeld KR, Corcos AC, et al. Evolving role of endovascular techniques for traumatic vascular injury: a changing landscape? J Trauma Acute Care Surg 2012;72(1):41.

81. Reuben BC, Whitten MG, Sarfati M, et al. Increasing use of endovascular therapy in acute arterial injuries: analysis of the National Trauma Data Bank. J Vasc Surg 2007;46(6):1222.

82. Wilson A, Wall MJ Jr, Maxson R, et al. The pulmonary hilum twist as a thoracic damage control procedure. Am J Surg 2003;186(1):49.

83. Wall MJ Jr, Villavicencio RT, Miller CC 3rd, et al. Pulmonary tractotomy as an abbreviated thoracotomy technique. J Trauma 1998;45(6):1015.

84. Gupta NM, Kaman L. Personal management of 57 consecutive patients with esophageal perforation. Am J Surg 2004;187(1):58.

85. Bhatia P, Fortin D, Inculet RI, et al. Current concepts in the management of esophageal perforations: a twenty-seven year Canadian experience. Ann Thorac Surg 2011;92(1):209.

86. Skinner DB, Little AG, DeMeester TR. Management of esophageal perforation. Am J Surg 1980;139(6):760.

87. Brinster CJ, Singhal S, Lee L, et al. Evolving options in the management of esophageal perforation. Ann Thorac Surg 2004;77(4):1475.

88. Lang JL, Gonzalez RP, Aldy KN, et al. Does temporary chest wall closure with or without chest packing improve survival for trauma patients in shock after emergent thoracotomy? J Trauma 2011;70(3):705.

89. Feliciano DV, Mattox KL, Jordan GL Jr. Intra-abdominal packing for control of hepatic hemorrhage: a reappraisal. J Trauma 1981;21(4):285.

90. Clouse WD, Rasmussen TE, Peck MA, et al. In-theater management of vascular injury: 2 years of the balad vascular registry. J Am Coll Surg 2007; 204(4):625.

91. Eger M, Golcman L, Goldstein A, et al. The use of a temporary shunt in the management of arterial vascular injuries. Surg Gynecol Obstet 1971;132(1):67.

92. Johansen K, Bandyk D, Thiele B, et al. Temporary intraluminal shunts: resolution of a management dilemma in complex vascular injuries. J Trauma 1982; 22(5):395.

93. Rasmussen TE, Clouse WD, Jenkins DH, et al. The use of temporary vascular shunts as a damage control adjunct in the management of wartime vascular injury. J Trauma 2006;61(1):8.

94. Taller J, Kamdar JP, Greene JA, et al. Temporary vascular shunts as initial treatment of proximal extremity vascular injuries during combat operations: the new standard of care at Echelon II facilities? J Trauma 2008;65(3):595.

95. Tadlock MD, Sise MJ, Riccoboni ST, et al. Damage control in the management of ruptured abdominal aortic aneurysm: preliminary results. Vasc Endovascular Surg 2010;44(8):638.

96. Demetriades D. Blunt thoracic aortic injuries: crossing the Rubicon. J Am Coll Surg 2012;214(3):247.

97. Miller RS, Morris JA Jr, Diaz JJ Jr, et al. Complications after 344 damage-control open celiotomies. J Trauma 2005;59(6):1365.

98. Montalvo JA, Acosta JA, Rodriguez P, et al. Surgical complications and causes of death in trauma patients that require temporary abdominal closure. Am Surg 2005;71(3):219.

99. Sriussadaporn S, Kritayakirana K, Pak-art R. Operative management of small bowel fistulae associated with open abdomen. Asian J Surg 2006;29(1):1.

100. Verdam FJ, Dolmans DE, Loos MJ, et al. Delayed primary closure of the septic open abdomen with a dynamic closure system. World J Surg 2011;35(10):2348.

101. Shapiro MB, Jenkins DH, Schwab CW, et al. Damage control: collective review. J Trauma 2000;49(5):969.

Towards Hemostatic Resuscitation
The Changing Understanding of Acute Traumatic Biology, Massive Bleeding, and Damage-Control Resuscitation

Mitchell Jay Cohen, MD

KEYWORDS

- Trauma • Acute traumatic coagulopathy • Coagulation • Bleeding
- Massive transfusion

KEY POINTS

- By the close of the 1990s, severely injured trauma patients were routinely resuscitated with large volumes of salt water and red blood cells with little attention paid to coagulation abnormalities or correcting coagulopathy.
- Acute traumatic coagulopathy (ATC) results from both severe tissue injury and blood loss resulting in shock. ATC has a very high associated mortality.
- ATC is partially mediated by activation of the protein C system. Activated protein C affects coagulopathy by both inhibiting clot formation and de-repressing fibrinolysis.
- Taken together, the recognition of ATC and the benefits of plasma-based resuscitation represent a paradigm shift in the resuscitative conduct after severe trauma.

INTRODUCTION

Transfusion and resuscitation practices in military and civilian trauma have undergone revolutionary shift over the past decade. New understandings of posttrauma physiology and biology have occurred in parallel with the acquisition of new clinical data on resuscitation practices. Together these understandings have radically changed the resuscitation and treatment patterns of severely injured solders and civilians resulting in decreased morbidity and reduced mortality and a fundamental reassessment of both the underlying biology and clinical manifestations of injury and resuscitation.

The author has nothing to disclose.
Department of Surgery, San Francisco General Hospital and the University of California, San Francisco, 1001 Potrero Avenue, Ward 3A, San Francisco, CA 94110, USA
E-mail address: mcohen@sfghsurg.ucsf.edu

Surg Clin N Am 92 (2012) 877–891
http://dx.doi.org/10.1016/j.suc.2012.06.001
0039-6109/12/$ – see front matter © 2012 Published by Elsevier Inc.

surgical.theclinics.com

Those lucky enough to both clinically practice and conduct research during this period have experienced a true paradigm shift in the understanding of posttrauma biology and physiology and a revolutionary change in the manner in which patients are resuscitated. Together, these have fundamentally changed the way patients, both military and civilian, behave in the operating room (OR), ICU, hospital and after discharge. This article aims to outline the history of resuscitation and transfusion practices in trauma and the changes in the understanding of the biology of coagulation and inflammation as well as clinical data that have driven changes in resuscitative conduct. Finally, the current state of the science (clinical and biological) is examined, suggesting future basic science and clinical investigation that will drive further changes in transfusion and resuscitation in severely injured military personnel and civilian patients.

THE HISTORY OF RESUSCITATION

The history of resuscitation parallels the history of armed conflict and its examination is essential to understanding how trauma resuscitation evolved to the current era. A complete history of trauma resuscitation is far beyond the scope of this article and has been covered well elsewhere.[1,2] Briefly, the modern understanding of resuscitation begins during the early to middle 1900s.[3] Before and continuing through World War I, there was essentially little or no resuscitation after injury. The prevailing belief regarding why injured solders did poorly centered on deleterious mediators (evil humors) and wound toxins. In this era, significant injury most often led to death.

Beginning in World War II, there was an understanding of resuscitation with blood and colloid (albumin) with a resultant increase in early survival.[4] Shock was better understood as an entity; however, there was little understanding of its underlying biology or mechanistic physiology. In keeping with this knowledge deficit, there was no understanding of differential resuscitation of the intravascular and intracellular compartments and, as a result, the reduced early mortality from blood transfusion was often followed by significant organ failure (generally renal and pulmonary failure), infection (if patients lived long enough), and late death. This was in the context of limited forward surgical care; difficult, slow, and often impossible evacuation; and increasing injury severity. Although there were significant advances in forward care, rapid surgical care, and evacuation to formal treatment, the World War II resuscitation paradigm continued through the Korean War.

Further improvements in field triage, forward surgical care, and casualty evacuation continued through the Vietnam Conflict. Additionally, advances in understanding of posttrauma physiology and biology, as well as blood banking, emerged during this time.[3,5] There was now an understanding of intravascular and intercellular physiology. Concurrently, there was, for the first time, the availability of banked blood and plentiful crystalloid. The combined early large-volume blood and crystalloid resuscitation resulted in better early survival and a significant reduction of the organ failure seen during World War II and Korea. Unfortunately, the early survival and reduction in renal failure unmasked a new entity of rapid and devastating pulmonary failure. This new entity, then termed Da Nang lung, now known as acute lung injury (ALI) or acute respiratory distress syndrome (ARDS), manifested as early survival followed by rapid pulmonary collapse.[6]

Through the 1970s and 1980s, two events and paradigms led to a resuscitation regime that was maintained for years. First, the advent of blood banking and component separation eliminated whole blood from the resuscitation supply. Indeed, by the early 1980s, because of resource allocation and cost concerns, the blood supply was converted from whole blood to components.[5,7] Hence, a unit of whole blood was processed into a unit of packed red blood cells (PRBC), a unit of fresh frozen plasma (FFP), a unit of cryoprecipitate, and some part of a unit (see later discussion) of platelets. The white blood cell component was essentially (variably) washed away. Although initially done for resource allocation and financial reasons, the HIV-AIDS and hepatitis crisis of the late 1980s and 1990s essentially eliminated any possibility of a rapidly screened, clean, whole blood supply. Left with components in the blood bank and crystalloid on the shelf, the second part of the paradigm shift toward modern resuscitation occurred as a result of a new understanding in the physiology of shock. A large body of literature led by ground-breaking work from Shires, Carrico, Shoemaker, and other investigators began to codify shock and quantify measures of survivable physiology, which pushed trauma resuscitation toward large-volume crystalloid and multiple PRBC transfusion resuscitation.[8–16] Trauma resuscitation was aimed at restoring flow and maximizing perfusion, with goals of normal or even supernormal perfusion.[16–18]

In keeping with this practice, the American College of Surgeons Advanced Trauma Life Support guidelines[19] suggested perturbing all injured patients with an initial 2 L of isotonic crystalloid. Patients who were transient responders (corresponding to class II and III shock) and nonresponders (corresponding to class III and IV shock) were given additional crystalloid and PRBCs. Little or secondary attention was given to plasma or other blood components. Indeed, until the most recent version of the Advanced Trauma Life Support guidelines, it was suggested that coagulopathy was uncommon after trauma; hence, plasma, platelet, and cryoprecipitate resuscitation was deemed unnecessary.

There was, additionally, a large retrospective literature suggesting that every unit of blood product was associated with poorer outcomes.[20–23] Although it made sense that additional blood cells were associated with worse outcomes because the need for blood was a marker for a sicker and more injured patient population, the mantra among the trauma community was that plasma and platelets were inherently deleterious—directly causing lung injury, organ dysfunction, and a propensity toward infection. Of course, little unconfounded, direct clinical data supported this conjecture and there was a dearth of actual mechanistic basic science data to explain inflammatory or immunologic perturbations. Undeterred, trauma practitioners believed that plasma was harmful.

Whether blood product resuscitation is directly harmful or the harm is linked to historical resuscitation practices remains an important question being addressed in the current era of balanced ratio resuscitation. Most of the data from the era suggest morbidity from plasma or platelet transfusions was confounded because these products were always administered as part of large-volume resuscitation. Hence, although regression analyses from these investigations found associations between blood product transfusions and morbidity, it remains unclear whether these were from the blood products themselves or from product resuscitation in the setting of large-volume, low ratio resuscitation (see later discussion). Either way, taken together, these factors were solidified by the 1990s and patients were routinely resuscitated with large volumes of salt water and red blood cells.[24,25]

PROBLEMS WITH LARGE-VOLUME RESUSCITATION: THE ADVENT OF DAMAGE CONTROL

Crystalloid and PRBC-based resuscitation were aimed at saving lives through restoration of circulatory homeostasis. That said, increasing injury severity, shorter transport times, and superior prehospital care all resulted in sicker patients arriving at the hospital. At the same time, more aggressive resuscitation was resulting in more patients surviving their initial injuries only to enter and then perish from the lethal triad of hypothermia, acidosis, coagulopathy, and subsequent physiologic collapse. Those who survived the acute postinjury phase were plagued by significant organ failure, lung injury, and infection. Damage control surgery developed to combat this physiologic collapse. Originally coined by Stone and colleagues in 1983,[26] and expanded and repopularized by Rotondo and colleagues[27] in 1993, the principle of damage control suggests that patients are just as likely to perish from physiologic exhaustion from definitive surgery as from their actual injuries.

The goals and steps of damage control were threefold and were aimed at restoration of physiologic homeostasis (see the articles by Chovanes and colleagues elsewhere in this issue for further exploration of this topic). First, quick, abbreviated surgery was performed to control lethal bleeding, gross spillage, and contamination while reestablishing peripheral perfusion. After this initial quick phase, patients were transferred to the ICU where they were resuscitated and warmed to established (although changing and often controversial) endpoints of resuscitation.[28] During this phase, coagulopathy was corrected, patients were warmed, and protective ventilator strategies were used toward the goal of balancing and attenuating the physiologic and inflammatory perturbations from the injury and initial surgical conduct. Finally, when patients were deemed stable, they were brought back to the operating room for formal repair of injuries. This iterative process was varied depending on the severity of the injuries and the resuscitative status of the patient.[28]

Several techniques, such as packing of solid organ injuries, shunts, and temporary abdominal closures, were used and indeed popularized. Over time, several groups reported on their successes using these techniques and damage control became the standard of care for the most severely injured. Ultimately, damage control was no longer a revolutionary idea because it soon developed into the standard of care after large-volume resuscitation.[29]

Although damage control surgery became the de facto norm, the survival of these patients was not without morbidity and controversy. The large-volume resuscitation and new surgical techniques led to a large number of surviving patients with significant increases in multiple organ failure, ALI or ARDS, infections, and open abdomens.[30,31] In particular, the number of patients with open abdomens and resulting complications, such as anastomotic breakdown, hernias, and (the most dreaded) enteroatmospheric fistulae, increased dramatically.[32,33] From this came an extensive literature characterizing this change while also suggesting ways to combat the sequelae of the resuscitative and damage control surgical conduct that had become standard of care within the civilian and military trauma community.[34–36] This was the state of the knowledge and the standard of care un til the early 2000s. Data on two fronts began to change this and led to the current concept of hemostatic damage control resuscitation. The first was the discovery and initial characterization of acute traumatic coagulopathy (ATC). The second, which transpired concurrently, was the discovery of the benefits of directly addressing hemostatic resuscitation. The following sections review advances in these specific areas. Additional aspects of damage control resuscitation, including permissive hypotension and recent advances in the science of crystalloid solutions, has been expertly reviewed by others.[37]

ATC: NEW UNDERSTANDINGS

There is a vast literature detailing iatrogenic coagulopathy after trauma.[38–46] The triad of hypothermia (which impairs thrombin production and platelet function), acidosis (impaired thrombin production), and dilution (clotting factor depletion) is well documented and clearly important. These factors (dilution, hypothermia, and acidosis) result in what is termed the lethal triad; however, these phenomena are better termed resuscitation-associated coagulopathy.[47]

From this data, however, came a strong and longstanding mantra that trauma patients bleed and become coagulopathic only because of the things that physicians do during resuscitation. Indeed, if trauma surgeons were polled, until just a few years ago they would have said that trauma patients coagulopathically bleed because of iatrogenic coagulopathy. It was anecdotally clear to the trauma community as a whole that patients are exposed and body cavities operatively opened (hypothermia), are given large volumes of relatively cool crystalloid (dilution and hypothermia) and PRBCs (additional dilution and resuscitation and factor depletion), and that these sick patients are acidotic (metabolic acidosis with impaired clotting function).

In the traumatic brain injury world, the mantra regarding traumatic coagulopathy is even stronger. Ask most neurosurgeons or neurologists why traumatic brain injury patients bleed and they will tell you that this is because of a disseminated intravascular coagulation-like consumptive coagulopathy resulting from a large release of tissue thromboplastin.[48,49] There is a similarly vast literature describing the incidence of brain injury-associated coagulopathy[48]; however, interestingly, there is little to no actual data to support this conjecture. Indeed, massive tissue factor (TF) release—the putative trigger for this coagulopathy—has never been conclusively assayed after traumatic brain injury. Instead this mantra is based on the fact that most of the early TF extracts were derived from porcine brain tissue, which resulted in the extrapolation that there must be massive TF release from direct brain injury.[49] As a result of the belief that coagulation abnormalities in polytrauma and traumatic brain injury were iatrogenic and resuscitation-associated, little attention was paid to early recognition of an endogenous coagulopathy. Instead, attenuating coagulopathy became secondary in importance to a resuscitative practice that was primarily aimed at producing flow, reversing shock states, and enhancing oxygen-carrying capacity through large-volume crystalloid resuscitation and PRBC transfusion.

That said, in the midst of this period of large-volume resuscitation, physicians caring for trauma patients were seeing and discussing a cohort of patients who were coagulopathic nearly immediately after injury, despite the absence of any iatrogenic reasons for coagulation perturbations. These anecdotally described patients were coagulopathic essentially immediately after injury and had significantly worse outcomes. In 2003, two nearly concurrent papers codified and began to define these phenomena. Brohi and colleagues[50] studied over 1000 severely injured patients who were brought by helicopter service to the Royal London Hospital. Of these, 24.4% were coagulopathic on arrival before or independent of the presence of resuscitation-associated coagulopathy. Patients with this ATC had nearly four times the mortality rate (46.0% vs 10.9%) At the same time, MacLeod and colleagues[51] retrospectively examined a database of over 20,000 patients and found that 28% of patients were coagulopathic on arrival. Like Brohi and colleagues[50] data, patients with coagulopathy had a much higher mortality (19.3% vs 6.3%). Subsequent data from multiple other groups have corroborated these data showing ATC after severe injury and shock.

In an attempt to characterize this ATC, the group at the University of California San Francisco–San Francisco General Hospital performed a study of 209 severely injured patients.[52] In this study, laboratory samples were collected immediately on arrival. Due to short transport times in San Francisco, patients arrived less than 30 minutes after injury and received essentially no prehospital resuscitation fluid. Patients who were severely injured with an injury severity score greater than 15 and tissue hypoperfusion (base deficit >6) were coagulopathic.

Interestingly, the results indicated that both tissue injury and hypoperfusion were necessary to affect this coagulopathy. Neither the blunt trauma patient with severe tissue injury but no shock nor the penetrating trauma patient with massive blood loss but no tissue injury were coagulopathic. However, in cases where both were combined, ATC occurred. As expected, patients who had ATC had more transfusion requirements, higher morbidity, and fourfold the mortality.

Further work by several groups showed that ATC was associated with and partially mediated by activation of the protein C system.[39,47,53] Protein C is a serine protease that is activated from its inactive zymogen in a mechanism involving thrombomodulin, endothelial protein C receptor (EPCR), and thrombin.[54] Once activated, it affects coagulopathy via a dual mechanism. First, it directly proteolytically cleaves and inactivates factors Va and VIIIa, resulting in prevention of clot formation. Second, it derepresses fibrinolysis through actions on PAI-1 mediated through tissue plasminogen activator and plasmin. Indirectly, protein C also functions as a sink for thrombin production, diverting thrombin away from functional clot formation.

Normally, protein C works as serine protease to balance thrombosis in the microvasculature during low flow states. Indeed, recombinant-activated protein C, which was purported to prevent end organ damage and failure in septic shock, was initially believed to function by preventing thrombosis and thereby promoting perfusion in end organs. Newer data has illuminated that activated protein C has direct cytoprotective effects mediated by direct binding through its Gla domain to both PAR-1 and its own receptor, EPCR.[55,56] It functions through multiple downstream signaling mechanisms to stabilize the endothelial membrane, is antiapoptotic, cleaves extracellular histones, and has other inflammamodulatory effects. Why there is a large activation of protein C after trauma, which seems to drive ATC, remains an interesting and important question.

Currently, it is hypothesized that the body is activating a large concentration of directly cytoprotective protease in an attempt to survive after severe injury and shock. Activated protein C release would be protective by stabilizing the endothelium, protecting against cell death, maintaining microvascular flow during low flow states, and counteracting the deleterious proinflammatory milieu produced by large concentrations of thrombin. In especially severe injury and shock, this local biology would be systemically overactivated. ATC would then be the unfortunate sequela of too much of a good thing. Indeed, in the short term, if the activated protein C protected as described, it would also result in a hypocoagulable milieu—which is termed ATC. Later, when the patient survived through the acute phase, there are good data form the sepsis literature to suggest that there is a depletion of protein C stores and activation (too little of a good thing) that predispose to organ failure and infection.[57]

Evolutionarily it would make sense that severe trauma, which was never meant to be survivable, is now rendered so through modern medical care, thereby unmasking a never-before-seen and measured ATC. The mechanism for why this occurs after trauma is another open scientific question. Following severe injury and hypoperfusion, there is a large activation of protein C, which seems to require but is not directly caused by thrombin production. Several groups' data show that when there is significant tissue injury, there is increased thrombin production.[39,47,52] However, there is concomitant tissue hypoperfusion only when there is activation of protein C.[47,53] Whether this is a result of enhanced conversion, increased EPCR, or thrombomodulin expression on the endothelial surface after shock or some other mechanism remains an important area of ongoing study.

Most clinically important for trauma patients is that this combination of tissue injury and shock are necessary to produce activated protein C–driven ATC. More recent work indicates that this same mechanism drives coagulopathy early after traumatic brain injury.[53] Newer data have confirmed these findings and shown more conclusively that activated protein C is associated with factor Va and VIIIa depletion and derepression of fibrinolysis.

These clinical studies have been extended into animal models that have codified these mechanisms. Chesebro and colleagues[58] successfully replicated the human findings in the first animal model of ATC. In these experiments, tissue injury and hypoperfusion (but neither alone) produced coagulopathy in a mouse model of injury and shock. This coagulopathy was associated with protein C activation and, in mechanistic proof, the ATC could be prevented by antibody blockade of activated protein C.

Although protein C is clearly a driver of coagulopathy after trauma, the field remains in its infancy with minimal characterization. Others have suggested alternative mechanisms. Rizoli and colleagues[59] have suggested that critical factor deficiencies exist after trauma. Platelet dysfunction has been suggested, as has enhanced early fibrinolysis via multiple mechanisms.[60] Clearly, there is much work to do to characterize the natural course of coagulation after trauma. Further work continues to complete this characterization and understanding of what are no doubt multiple phenotypes of coagulopathies of trauma.

HEMOSTATIC RESUSCITATION

Along with the discovery and initial characterization of ATC, the second and concurrent discovery that has revolutionized trauma resuscitation is the rediscovery of plasma-based resuscitation. As described, since the late 1970s there has been a move away from whole blood–based resuscitation to large-volume crystalloid and oxygen-carrying, capacity-driven resuscitation.[30] Ultimately these resuscitation practices continued with the addition of the need for damage control surgery. In the last decade, two landmark papers discovered trends in survival after injury and have initiated a paradigm shift in the manner in which both soldiers and civilian injured are resuscitated. Each retrospectively examined the ratio of plasma to PRBC units and/or platelet to red blood cell units received after injury. In each cohort, the ratio was correlated with morbidity and survival rates. The first report of this ratio benefit came from Borgman and colleagues[61] in 2007. They reported that soldiers who received a high ratio of plasma to PRBCs (1:1.4) had markedly increased survival compared with those with either a medium (1:2.5) or low (1:8) ratio. Mortality in the groups ranged from 65% in the low ratio group to 34% in the medium group and 19% in the high group despite similar wounding patterns and injury severities. Echoing this work in severely injured civilian cohort, Holcomb and colleagues[62] examined data from 16 civilian Level I trauma centers in the United States and found that high plasma to PRBC ratios improved both 6-hour and 30-day survival. In addition, the investigators extended the plasma analyses to include platelets and showed that high platelet to PRBC ratios were also significantly protective. The combination of a high plasma and high platelet to PRBC ratio were additively protective and conferred higher 6-hour and 30-day survival, reduced truncal hemorrhage, and reduced ICU and hospital days. Multiple other single and small multicenter, military and civilian, and United States and international reports with similar findings followed and a great deal of discussion and argument transpired.[63,64] Indeed, it is not hyperbole to suggest that this single topic has dominated discussion and investigation at the major national and international meetings since the publication of these initial military and civilian papers.

Other work has studied the effects of high ratio resuscitation on traumatic brain injury. In addition, other work has suggested that the mortality benefits shown after high ratio resuscitation may be independent of the effects of measurable coagulation. Brown and colleagues[65] recently reported that a high FFP to PRBC ratio provides a mortality benefit independent of admission coagulopathy. Mechanistic examination of the effect of plasma has shown that plasma-based resuscitation may result in improved cellular survival and reduced permeability.[66] Together, these new data suggest a potential role for plasma-based resuscitation independent of the correction or attenuation of coagulopathy. Further work continues to elucidate the mechanisms underlying the benefits of balanced ratio, plasma-based resuscitation.

Although the data are overwhelmingly positive, controversy remains regarding the benefits of high ratio plasma and platelet transfusion. The primary issue revolves around the issue of survival bias. As in all retrospective noncontrolled data, the question of whether patients survived because of the high ratio resuscitation or survived long enough to get the high ratio resuscitation remains an important question. However, it is impossible to resolve this question with retrospective data alone in the absence of reliable longitudinal outcome measures. Indeed, despite the plethora of evidence and general acceptance of the benefit of plasma-based resuscitation, there are some conflicting data and alternative viewpoints. The group from Denver Health suggested a U-shaped survival curve with the maximum benefit at 1:2 and increasing mortality with higher ratio.[67] Davenport and colleagues[68] suggested similar data and reported that the ideal resuscitation ratio of plasma to PRBCs was 1:2. Snyder and colleagues,[69] from the University of Alabama, suggested that any purported benefit of high ratio resuscitation was rendered statistically meaningless when controlled for survival bias. The Stanford group suggested that the timing of resuscitation was more predicative of good outcome than ultimate ratio.[70] Scalea and colleagues[71] suggested they could find no benefit to aggressive use of FFP in a prospective cohort of 806 civilian trauma patients.

To address this controversy, the United States Department of Defense funded a trial aimed at capturing real-time prospective data of how it is done at 10 major Level 1 trauma centers in the United States.[72] The Prospective Observational Multicenter Massive Transfusion (PROMMTT) study captured data on over 12,000 patients triaged to trauma centers. Of these 12,000-screened patients, 1245 were transfused and 297 patients received a massive transfusion (MT) as defined by greater than 10 units of product transfusion over 24 hours. In an attempt to eliminate survival bias, data was collected by teams of research assistants who stood in the emergency department, interventional radiology (IR), ICU, and OR and collected real-time data of resuscitation fluid, medications, interventions, and outcome. This data was merged with demographic and long-term outcome data providing a minute-by-minute data set allowing for non-survival biased analysis. In addition, patients' blood was collected and assayed for a wide variety of functional and antigen coagulation and inflammation mediators. Currently, there is great expectation that the results of the PROMMTT study will add clarity to the ideal resuscitation ratio after injury.

Ultimately, despite being embraced by the trauma community, the concept of high ratio or 1:1 resuscitation has never been tested prospectively. To address this, National Institutes of Health and the United States Department of Defense have funded a 15-center, prospective trial of resuscitation after trauma. The Pragmatic, Randomized Optimum Platelet and Plasma Ratios (PROPPR) trial seeks to enroll approximately 580 severely injured patients projected to require MT at 15 major Level

I trauma centers. Patients will be randomized to receive PRBC/platelet/plasma ratios of 1:1:1 versus 1:1:2. Primary endpoints will be 24-hour and 28-day mortality. Of equal importance to the clinical study outcomes, blood will be collected at admission and functionally assayed for a multitude of functional and antigen mediators of coagulation and inflammation. This will represent an unprecedented comprehensive functional description of the natural history of coagulation and inflammation after injury.

NEXT STEPS

Few prospective data regarding changes in trauma resuscitation exist. Notwithstanding, there has been a move toward greater consensus and an increasing lack of disagreement in this area. The trauma community has embraced a resuscitative conduct that seeks to attenuate ATC and limit crystalloid use while aiming for a balanced 1:1 ratio of plasma and PRBCs.

Numerous reports of the advent and modification of MT protocols exist in the trauma literature.[73] From these, and from anecdotal reports and national meeting discussions, it is clear that more and more centers have MT protocols and most embrace the tenants of damage control resuscitation. Further anecdotal reports suggest that there is reduced mortality and significantly reduced rates of ALI, open abdomens, and organ failure.[74]

To codify these changes, considerable insight can come from examining longitudinal data. The largest examination of a cohort of patients from major leading trauma centers comes from the Glue Grant. The Inflammation and the Host Response to Injury is a 10-year prospective project that began in 2002 to examine the genomic response after trauma. To do so, data and samples were collected from 5 Level I trauma centers in the United States. Comprehensive clinical and sampling data exists on almost 2000 patients. Care of patients enrolled into the Glue Grant cohort was not protocolized but, instead, was guided by standard operating procedures (SOPs) that were written and published by the study leadership early during the project.[75]

Although generally adhered to and tracked for compliance, none of the SOPs reflected or addressed early resuscitation ratios or fluid management. Seeking an opportunity to examine the shift of resuscitation practices during the period that the two events (definition of ATC and 1:1 resuscitation), Kautza and colleagues[76] queried the Glue Grant data to discern what changed during the period between 2003 and 2009. Separating the data into two periods, early (2004–2007) and late (2008–2009), this group examined the resuscitation practices, MT rates, and outcomes. Other than a slight increase in injury severity in the later time period (injury severity score [ISS] 38 vs 34), there were no significant demographic differences between time periods. Despite increasing injury severity, the incidence of MT and the median 24-hour PRBC transfusions decreased in the later time period. Transfusion ratios stayed the same between time periods ($\sim$1:1.5).

Overall, the analysis showed that a larger amount of balanced blood products (including plasma) were being aggressively given to sicker patients, resulting in earlier arrest of hemorrhage and more sub-MTs, increased survival, and fewer overall MTs. As expected, eliminating many subjects who would have otherwise received an MT through cessation of bleeding short of the 10 unit MT definition resulted in a sicker cohort of patients who ultimately exceeded the 10 unit MT barrier. Ultimately, the author believes this reflects that, in the modern era, patients who are effectively transfused early with a high ratio hemostatic resuscitation can have their bleeding stopped and survive short of needing an MT. Those patients who do not stop bleeding (and hence enter the MT definition) are often bleeding from massive anatomic injury that is often not survivable and for which resuscitation is rendered irrelevant. Modern medical care and resuscitative conduct allows a period of resuscitation and surgical intervention but, ultimately, many of these patients die as a result of overwhelming injury instead of correctable coagulopathy and inflammatory perturbations.

DAMAGE CONTROL SURGERY PLUS DAMAGE CONTROL RESUSCITATION: THE INTEGRATION OF ATC AND HEMOSTATIC RESUSCITATION

As described, the understanding of shock and the pioneering work that has led to the current understanding of postinjury physiology and restoration of circulating volume no doubt saved countless lives. However, it also resulted in a new group of complications generally related to overresuscitation, including ALI and ARDS, multiple organ failure, and abdominal compartment syndrome. Although most physicians initially believed that the sickest patients were now living long enough to have these complications, many conjectured and began to believe that the resuscitative conduct was contributing to these complications directly. This of course led to the advent of damage control resuscitation.

By attenuating operative conduct, leaving abdomens open, and promoting staged operative repair of injuries, patients were spared the second hit of prolonged operative interventions and physiologic disturbances. As a result, mortality benefits of up to 50% were seen.[29] This damage control surgery became the standard of care in both military and civilian surgery worldwide. However, damage control surgical practice was not without its complications. Open abdomens were complicated by anastomotic leak and enteroatmospheric fistulae.[30] Unfortunately, prolonged ventilator dependence, ALI or ARDS, and long ICU stays were common. Despite greatly improved mortality using damage control principles, significant morbidity persisted. Extending this into the modern era, the concept of damage control surgery concept has been combined with the understandings of ATC and hemostatic resuscitation has evolved into the principle of damage control resuscitation.[24,25] Damage control resuscitation suggests that limited surgical principles should be combined with hemostatic resuscitation and, therefore, achieve the benefits of damage control surgery with the elimination of many of the complications seen when damage control surgical principles were exercised in the context of large-volume PRBC and crystalloid-based resuscitation.[77]

In a landmark 2007 paper, a group of United States military and civilian surgeons presented a concept that the ideals of damage control surgery—namely preventing treatment that would cause additional physiologic insult—should be extended into resuscitative practices.[78] This paper suggested that coagulopathy and acidosis could be identified early after casualty and be primarily treated through targeted resuscitative processes. Duchesne and colleagues[37] published a series of papers suggesting that damage control resuscitation would result in better outcomes. In a before-and-after analysis, patients who received damage control resuscitation received fewer crystalloids and more plasma resulting in an odds ratio of 0.4 for mortality. In addition the surviving damage control resuscitation group had shorter hospital stays and less morbidity.[24,25]

Higa and colleagues,[79] and Makley and colleagues,[80] have extended these analyses to an advanced conclusion and suggest that, with appropriate damage control resuscitation, damage control laparotomy may not be necessary. Indeed, their data showed that the open abdomen rate reduced from 36% to 9% and the mortality rate reduced from 22% to 13%. In addition the reported a $2.2 M reduction in hospital costs resulting from decreased surgery.[79] Combination of damage control resuscitation with damage control surgery resulted in a greater survival benefit.[37]

The concept of damage control surgery correctly rests on the premise that each patient has a limited amount of physiologic or biologic reserve before irreversible inflammatory perturbations, organ damage, and mortality occur. Proper resuscitative conduct seeks to extend this reserve, thereby allowing intervention and repair of injuries without the patient exhausting this physiologic and inflammatory reserve. Without any resuscitation, the time before physiologic exhaustion and death is extremely short. Hence, understanding shock and the importance of initial resuscitation resulted in huge mortality benefits by extending this period, which allowed intervention and survival. The next step was attenuating the surgical interventions through the concept of damage control to avoid accelerating physiologic collapse.

Now, in the modern era of hemostatic resuscitation, physicians are able to extend the period before collapse and avoid proinflammatory sequela, which allows more definitive treatment, and results in improved outcomes. The understanding that there is a short window of time and physiologic reserve that should not be exceeded was extremely important and was the crucial understanding that allowed improved mortality. During the subsequent decade after damage control surgery, the understanding of the coagulation and inflammatory milieu and the effects of resuscitation have shown how resuscitative practices can lower the physiologic and biologic reserve. Essentially better resuscitation practices allow a longer window of time for this physiologic reserve, thereby improving mortality and reducing morbidity.[31,37,81]

SUMMARY

The understanding of the biology and physiology of severely injured patients has changed considerably over the past decade. Concomitant with this new biologic understanding has been a paradigm shift in the resuscitative conduct after injury, which has so far shown significant reduction in morbidity and mortality after injury. That said, the understanding of the coagulation and inflammatory milieu after trauma remains extremely limited. Understanding of the mechanistic drivers of ATC is in its infancy. The understanding of the cross-talk between coagulation and inflammation is an exciting and rapidly evolving field. Although the trauma community has reacted to new understandings of ATC and hemostatic resuscitation, the ideal resuscitative protocol and the mechanisms driving reduced morbidity and mortality remain an open clinical and experimental question. Additional data is needed to comprehensively characterize coagulation and inflammation after injury and to mechanistically track the effect of hemostatic plasma and platelet balanced ratio resuscitation on the coagulation and inflammation milieu. With the huge burden of trauma on military personnel and civilian injured, additional data will go far to guide resuscitative practices even beyond the current practice of hemostatic resuscitation.

REFERENCES

1. Pruitt BA Jr, Wolf SE. An historical perspective on advances in burn care over the past 100 years. Clin Plast Surg 2009;36(4):527–45.
2. Pearce FJ, Lyons WS. Logistics of parenteral fluids in battlefield resuscitation. Mil Med 1999;164(9):653–5.
3. Hess JR, Holcomb JB. Transfusion practice in military trauma. Transfus Med 2008;18(3):143–50.

4. Stansbury LG, Hess JR. Blood transfusion in World War I: the roles of Lawrence Bruce Robertson and Oswald Hope Robertson in the "most important medical advance of the war". Transfus Med Rev 2009;23(3):232–6.
5. Strauss RG. Elmer L. DeGowin, MD: blood transfusions in war and peace. Transfus Med Rev 2006;20(2):165–8.
6. Simmons RL, Heisterkamp CA 3rd, Collins JA, et al. Acute pulmonary edema in battle casualties. J Trauma 1969;9(9):760–75.
7. Murthi SB, Stansbury LG, Dutton RP, et al. Transfusion medicine in trauma patients: an update. Expert Rev Hematol 2011;4(5):527–37.
8. Shoemaker WC, Kvetan V, Fyodorov V, et al. Clinical algorithm for initial fluid resuscitation in disasters. Crit Care Clin 1991;7(2):363–81.
9. Shoemaker WC, Peitzman AB, Bellamy R, et al. Resuscitation from severe hemorrhage. Crit Care Med 1996;24(Suppl 2):S12–23.
10. Ducey JP, Lamiell JM, Gueller GE. Arterial-venous carbon dioxide tension difference during severe hemorrhage and resuscitation. Crit Care Med 1992;20(4): 518–22.
11. Wang P, Ba ZF, Burkhardt J, et al. Measurement of hepatic blood flow after severe hemorrhage: lack of restoration despite adequate resuscitation. Am J Physiol 1992;262(1 Pt 1):G92–8.
12. Wang P, Chaudry IH. Crystalloid resuscitation restores but does not maintain cardiac output following severe hemorrhage. J Surg Res 1991;50(2):163–9.
13. Soucy DM, Rude M, Hsia WC, et al. The effects of varying fluid volume and rate of resuscitation during uncontrolled hemorrhage. J Trauma 1999;46(2):209–15.
14. Shires GT. Pathophysiology and fluid replacement in hypovolemic shock. Ann Clin Res 1977;9(3):144–50.
15. Shires GT, Canizaro PC. Fluid resuscitation in the severely injured. Surg Clin North Am 1973;53(6):1341–66.
16. Giesecke AH Jr, Grande CM, Whitten CW. Fluid therapy and the resuscitation of traumatic shock. Crit Care Clin 1990;6(1):61–72.
17. Hariri RJ, Firlick AD, Shepard SR, et al. Traumatic brain injury, hemorrhagic shock, and fluid resuscitation: effects on intracranial pressure and brain compliance. J Neurosurg 1993;79(3):421–7.
18. Falk JL, O'Brien JF, Kerr R. Fluid resuscitation in traumatic hemorrhagic shock. Crit Care Clin 1992;8(2):323–40.
19. Committee on Trauma, American College of Surgeons. ATLS: Advanced Trauma Life Support Program for Doctors, 8th edition. Chicago: American College of Surgeons; 2008.
20. Murad MH, Stubbs JR, Gandhi MJ, et al. The effect of plasma transfusion on morbidity and mortality: a systematic review and meta-analysis. Transfusion 2010;50(6):1370–83.
21. Gunst MA, Minei JP. Transfusion of blood products and nosocomial infection in surgical patients. Curr Opin Crit Care 2007;13(4):428–32.
22. Johnson JL, Moore EE, Kashuk JL, et al. Effect of blood products transfusion on the development of postinjury multiple organ failure. Arch Surg 2010;145(10): 973–7.
23. Moore FA, Moore EE, Sauaia A. Blood transfusion. An independent risk factor for postinjury multiple organ failure. Arch Surg 1997;132(6):620–4 [discussion: 4–5].
24. Duchesne JC, Kimonis K, Marr AB, et al. Damage control resuscitation in combination with damage control laparotomy: a survival advantage. J Trauma 2010; 69(1):46–52.

25. Duchesne JC, Islam TM, Stuke L, et al. Hemostatic resuscitation during surgery improves survival in patients with traumatic-induced coagulopathy. J Trauma 2009;67(1):33–7 [discussion: 7–9].
26. Stone H, Strom P, Mullins R. Management of the major coagulopathy with onset during laparotomy. Ann Surg 1983;197:532–5.
27. Rotondo MF, Schwab CW, McGonigal MD, et al. 'Damage control': an approach for improved survival in exsanguinating penetrating abdominal injury. J Trauma 1993;35(3):375–82 [discussion: 82–3].
28. Rotondo MF, Zonies DH. The damage control sequence and underlying logic. Surg Clin North Am 1997;77(4):761–77.
29. Shapiro MB, Jenkins DH, Schwab CW, et al. Damage control: collective review. J Trauma 2000;49(5):969–78.
30. Smith BP, Adams RC, Doraiswamy VA, et al. Review of abdominal damage control and open abdomens: focus on gastrointestinal complications. J Gastrointestin Liver Dis 2010;19(4):425–35.
31. Santry HP, Alam HB. Fluid resuscitation: past, present, and the future. Shock 2010;33(3):229–41.
32. Diaz JJ Jr, Dutton WD, Ott MM, et al. Eastern Association for the Surgery of Trauma: a review of the management of the open abdomen–part 2 "Management of the open abdomen". J Trauma 2011;71(2):502–12.
33. Dubose JJ, Lundy JB. Enterocutaneous fistulas in the setting of trauma and critical illness. Clin Colon Rectal Surg 2010;23(3):182–9.
34. Lee JC, Peitzman AB. Damage-control laparotomy. Curr Opin Crit Care 2006; 12(4):346–50.
35. Blackbourne LH. Defining combat damage control surgery. US Army Med Dep J 2008;67–72.
36. Blackbourne LH, McMullin N, Eastridge B, et al. Aggressive proactive combat damage control surgery. US Army Med Dep J 2007;3–6.
37. Duchesne JC, McSwain NE Jr, Cotton BA, et al. Damage control resuscitation: the new face of damage control. J Trauma 2010;69(4):976–90.
38. Bouillon B, Brohi K, Hess JR, et al. Educational initiative on critical bleeding in trauma: Chicago, July 11–13, 2008. J Trauma 2010;68(1):225–30.
39. Brohi K, Cohen MJ, Davenport RA. Acute coagulopathy of trauma: mechanism, identification and effect. Curr Opin Crit Care 2007;13(6):680–5.
40. Hess JR, Brohi K, Dutton RP, et al. The coagulopathy of trauma: a review of mechanisms. J Trauma 2008;65(4):748–54.
41. Kirkpatrick AW, Chun R, Brown R, et al. Hypothermia and the trauma patient. Can J Surg 1999;42(5):333–43.
42. Martini WZ. Coagulopathy by hypothermia and acidosis: mechanisms of thrombin generation and fibrinogen availability. J Trauma 2009;67(1):202–8 [discussion: 8–9].
43. Martini WZ. Fibrinogen availability and coagulation function after hemorrhage and resuscitation in pigs. Molecular Medicine 2011;17(7–8):757–61.
44. Martini WZ, Holcomb JB. Acidosis and coagulopathy: the differential effects on fibrinogen synthesis and breakdown in pigs. Ann Surg 2007;246(5):831–5.
45. Schreiber MA. Coagulopathy in the trauma patient. Curr Opin Crit Care 2005; 11(6):590–7.
46. Waibel BH, Schlitzkus LL, Newell MA, et al. Impact of hypothermia (below 36 degrees C) in the rural trauma patient. J Am Coll Surg 2009;209(5):580–8.
47. Cohen MJ, Call M, Nelson M, et al. Critical role of activated protein C in early coagulopathy and later organ failure, infection and death in trauma patients. Ann Surg 2012;255(2):379–85.

48. Laroche M, Kutcher ME, Huang MC, et al. Coagulopathy following traumatic brain injury. Neurosurgery 2012.
49. Stein S, Smith D. Coagulopathy in traumatic brain injury. Neurocrit Care 2004; 1(4):479–88.
50. Brohi K, Singh J, Heron M, et al. Acute traumatic coagulopathy. J Trauma 2003; 54(6):1127–30.
51. MacLeod JB, Lynn M, McKenney MG, et al. Early coagulopathy predicts mortality in trauma. J Trauma 2003;55(1):39–44.
52. Brohi K, Cohen MJ, Ganter MT, et al. Acute traumatic coagulopathy: initiated by hypoperfusion: modulated through the protein C pathway? Ann Surg 2007; 245(5):812–8.
53. Cohen MJ, Brohi K, Ganter MT, et al. Early coagulopathy after traumatic brain injury: the role of hypoperfusion and the protein C pathway. J Trauma 2007; 63(6):1254–61 [discussion: 61–2].
54. Esmon CT. The protein C pathway. Chest 2003;124(Suppl 3):26S–32S.
55. Esmon CT. Interactions between the innate immune and blood coagulation systems. Trends Immunol 2004;25(10):536–42.
56. Esmon CT. Inflammation and the activated protein C anticoagulant pathway. Semin Thromb Hemost 2006;32(Suppl 1):49–60.
57. Rezaie AR. Regulation of the protein C anticoagulant and antiinflammatory pathways. Curr Med Chem 2010;17(19):2059–69.
58. Chesebro BB, Rahn P, Carles M, et al. Increase in activated protein C mediates acute traumatic coagulopathy in mice. Shock 2009;32(6):659–65.
59. Rizoli SB, Scarpelini S, Callum J, et al. Clotting factor deficiency in early trauma-associated coagulopathy. J Trauma 2011;71(5 Suppl 1):S427–34.
60. Kashuk JL, Moore EE, Sawyer M, et al. Primary fibrinolysis is integral in the pathogenesis of the acute coagulopathy of trauma. Ann Surg 2010;252(3):434–42 [discussion: 43–4].
61. Borgman MA, Spinella PC, Perkins JG, et al. The ratio of blood products transfused affects mortality in patients receiving massive transfusions at a combat support hospital. J Trauma 2007;63(4):805–13.
62. Holcomb JB, Wade CE, Michalek JE, et al. Increased plasma and platelet to red blood cell ratios improves outcome in 466 massively transfused civilian trauma patients. Ann Surg 2008;248(3):447–58.
63. Borgman MA, Spinella PC, Holcomb JB, et al. The effect of FFP: RBC ratio on morbidity and mortality in trauma patients based on transfusion prediction score. Vox Sang 2011;101(1):44–54.
64. Holcomb JB, Zarzabal LA, Michalek JE, et al. Increased platelet:RBC ratios are associated with improved survival after massive transfusion. J Trauma 2011;71: 2(Suppl 3):S318–28.
65. Brown LM, Aro SO, Cohen MJ, et al. A high fresh frozen plasma: packed red blood cell transfusion ratio decreases mortality in all massively transfused trauma patients regardless of admission international normalized ratio. J Trauma 2011; 71:2(Suppl 3):S358–63.
66. Pati S, Matijevic N, Doursout MF, et al. Protective effects of fresh frozen plasma on vascular endothelial permeability, coagulation, and resuscitation after hemorrhagic shock are time dependent and diminish between days 0 and 5 after thaw. J Trauma 2010;69(Suppl 1):S55–63.
67. Kashuk JL, Moore EE, Johnson JL, et al. Postinjury life threatening coagulopathy: is 1:1 fresh frozen plasma:packed red blood cells the answer? J Trauma 2008; 65(2):261–70 [discussion: 70–1].

68. Davenport R, Curry N, Manson J, et al. Hemostatic effects of fresh frozen plasma may be maximal at red cell ratios of 1:2. J Trauma 2011;70(1):90–5 [discussion: 5–6].
69. Snyder CW, Weinberg JA, McGwin G Jr, et al. The relationship of blood product ratio to mortality: survival benefit or survival bias? J Trauma 2009;66(2):358–62 [discussion: 62–4].
70. Riskin DJ, Tsai TC, Riskin L, et al. Massive transfusion protocols: the role of aggressive resuscitation versus product ratio in mortality reduction. J Am Coll Surg 2009;209(2):198–205.
71. Scalea TM, Bochicchio KM, Lumpkins K, et al. Early aggressive use of fresh frozen plasma does not improve outcome in critically injured trauma patients. Ann Surg 2008;248(4):578–84.
72. Rahbar MH, Fox EE, Del Junco DJ, et al. Coordination and management of multi-center clinical studies in trauma: Experience from the PRospective Observational Multicenter Major Trauma Transfusion (PROMMTT) Study. Resuscitation 2012; 83(4):459–64.
73. Schuster KM, Davis KA, Lui FY, et al. The status of massive transfusion protocols in United States trauma centers: massive transfusion or massive confusion? Transfusion 2010;50(7):1545–51.
74. Cotton BA, Au BK, Nunez TC, et al. Predefined massive transfusion protocols are associated with a reduction in organ failure and postinjury complications. J Trauma 2009;66(1):41–8 [discussion: 8–9].
75. Nathens AB, Johnson JL, Minei JP, et al. Inflammation and the Host Response to Injury, a large-scale collaborative project: Patient-Oriented Research Core-standard operating procedures for clinical care. I. Guidelines for mechanical ventilation of the trauma patient. J Trauma 2005;59(3):764–9.
76. Kautza BC, Cohen MJ, Cuschieri J, et al. Changes in massive transfusion over time: an early shift in the right direction? J Trauma 2012;72(1):106–11.
77. Cotton BA, Gunter OL, Isbell J, et al. Damage control hematology: the impact of a trauma exsanguination protocol on survival and blood product utilization. J Trauma 2008;64(5):1177–82 [discussion: 82–3].
78. Holcomb JB, Jenkins D, Rhee P, et al. Damage control resuscitation: directly addressing the early coagulopathy of trauma. J Trauma 2007;62(2):307–10.
79. Higa G, Friese R, O'Keeffe T, et al. Damage control laparotomy: a vital tool once overused. J Trauma 2010;69(1):53–9.
80. Makley AT, Goodman MD, Belizaire RM, et al. Damage control resuscitation decreases systemic inflammation after hemorrhage. J Surg Res 2012;175(2): e75–82.
81. Hatch QM, Osterhout LM, Podbielski J, et al. Impact of closure at the first take back: complication burden and potential overutilization of damage control laparotomy. J Trauma 2011;71(6):1503–11.

Improving Trauma Care in the ICU

Best Practices, Quality Improvement Initiatives, and Organization

Mansoor Khan, MBBS(Lond), MRCS(Eng), FRCS(GenSurg),
Joseph J. DuBose, MD*

KEYWORDS

- Trauma • Intensive care • ICU organization • Best practices • Outcomes

KEY POINTS

- "Best practice" implementation in the intensive care setting, while challenging, has significant potential to improve outcomes.
- The use of quality improvement initiatives to ensure compliance with best practice interventions has been shown to improve patient outcome and decrease cost.
- Current data regarding intensive care unit organization favors a multidisciplinary approach led by a dedicated intensivist when possible, although additional study is required.

INTRODUCTION

Trauma remains a considerable cause of mortality and morbidity worldwide, constituting a tangible public health burden with significant associated social and economic costs. As technological capabilities continue to advance the care of critically injured patients, improvements in patient monitoring, measures to prevent complications, and use of new treatments require coordinated implementation to optimize benefit. The modern trauma intensive care unit (ICU) is an increasingly complex environment of care where best practices involving health care advances must continually be identified and effectively implemented. The performance of these efforts should be repeatedly reassessed using readily identified metrics consistent with the highest quality delivery of care. In addition, ICU health care providers and support personnel must be organized into teams capable of providing the appropriate configuration of expertise required for this unique environment.

Conflicts of Interest: None.
Division of Trauma, Acute Care Surgery and Surgical Critical Care, R Adams Cowley Shock Trauma Center, University of Maryland, Baltimore, MD, USA
* Corresponding author. 22 South Greene Street, Room T5R46, Baltimore, MD 21201.
E-mail address: jdubose@umm.edu

Surg Clin N Am 92 (2012) 893–901
doi:10.1016/j.suc.2012.04.003
0039-6109/12/$ – see front matter Published by Elsevier Inc.

surgical.theclinics.com

Experiences of the past decade suggest that the interplay of three factors will continue to propel advancements in trauma ICU care:

- Establishment of best practices
- Measurement of performance/quality improvement
- Effective ICU organization.

BEST PRACTICES IN THE TRAUMA ICU

The term "best practice" has, in recent years, become ubiquitous in the vernacular of ICU care. Although a precise definition has escaped this term, practically speaking, it implies the systematic implementation of the components of care that have been shown to improve outcomes according to the best available data sources. Ideally, these data sources would consist of well-designed clinical trials. In reality, however, many best practices are established by professional organizations or collections of experts in a respective field who, after carefully scrutinizing the available data on a topic, provide evidence and consensus-based guidelines for the management of clinical problems within the ICU environment.

Given the wide array of care items required for a critically ill patient in the ICU, consisting of hundreds of daily actions performed by health care providers, a wide range of best practice interventions could be introduced to this complex environment. A review of the contemporary medical literature reveals best practice guidelines for a wide range of topics pertinent to daily ICU care, shown in **Box 1**. These best practice interventions have been effectively incorporated into the daily care environment through a variety of means, either as individual components of care or through grouping, or "bundling," of interventions.

In 2002, the Surviving Sepsis Campaign developed by the Society of Critical Care Medicine, the European Society of Critical Care Medicine, and the International Sepsis Forum sponsored by Eli Lilly (Indianapolis, IN) introduced the concept of "care bundles" through which consensus recommendations of several international organizations could be applied to the improvement of outcomes in the management of sepsis. The science supporting the individual practices included in the bundles, although based on levels of evidence varying from randomized prospective control trials to professional consensus, nonetheless represent standard of care practices that individually improve care. When applied together, the collective application of bundled interventions result in an even greater improvement in outcomes. The initial campaign of the Institute for Healthcare Improvement (IHI), with the stated objective of saving 100,000 lives, recommended four primary prophylactic components be included in a Ventilator Associated Pneumonia (VAP) bundle: (1) elevation of the head of the bed between 30° and 45°, (2) daily sedation vacation and assessment

---

Box 1
Available best practice guidelines in modern trauma ICU practice

Sepsis management[1,2]

Nutritional support[3]

Analgesia/sedation[4]

Thromboembolic prophylaxis[5]

Family presence on rounds[6]

Noise reduction in the ICU environment.[7]

of readiness to extubate, (3) peptic ulcer disease prophylaxis, and (4) venous thromboembolic prophylaxis unless contraindicated. Several institutions have shown the application of this bundled approach to be effective for the prevention of VAP and other ICU complications, with excellent results.[8-12]

Berriel-Cass and colleagues,[8] in a study of IHI bundled improvement implementation at two regional hospitals in Michigan, were able to show a VAP reduction of more than 50%. Cocanour and colleagues[9] at The University of Texas Medical School found that VAP bundle implementation, in conjunction with daily audits of compliance and weekly feedback sessions with staff, resulted in lower VAP rates and improved VAP-associated costs. In a third study, DuBose and colleagues,[12] at Los Angeles County + University of Southern California Medical Center (LAC+USC) found that a quality rounds checklist incorporating the VAP bundle measures resulted in a 24% decrease in the number of pneumonias in their trauma ICU, with an estimated cost savings during that same period of approximately $400,000.

Overall, the successes achieved with the 100,000 lives initiative inspired the IHI to build on these efforts through the 5 Million Lives Campaign, designed to protect patients from 5 million incidents of medical harm. In the accomplishment of this task, the IHI enlisted more than 4000 US hospitals in a renewed national commitment to improve patient safety faster than ever before.

MEASURING PERFORMANCE/QUALITY IMPROVEMENT INITIATIVES

Despite emerging evidence supporting the use of bundled measures for VAP prevention and other components of care within the trauma ICU, critical examination of current practices reveals persistent challenges and potential barriers to effective implementation of these strategies[13-17]:

- Need for additional staff education and training
- Inadequate staffing levels to support a dedicated team to implement and monitor
- Concern over cost-effectiveness of these strategies in general.

Acknowledging these challenges, it becomes evident that simply adopting broad, hollow policies of best practice implementation within the trauma ICU environment is not enough. These initiatives simply will not prove successful without effective investment in their adequate conduct. Critical measures of successful implementation must be recorded, critically assessed at regular intervals, and correlated with outcomes and opportunities for improvement. Although this can be accomplished in several ways, recently introduced approaches using principles used in other industries, such as quality improvement initiatives, have shown considerable promise.

Borne out of the revolution in industrial processes that occurred in the United States during the 1920s, quality improvement initiatives have evolved to be incorporated into a variety of different arenas. During this evolution, proponents of quality improvement philosophies have often studied process improvement endeavors found to be successful in one field to innovatively modify them for use in another. One recent example of such an exchange includes the manner in which members of the critical care community have altered a common successful practice used in the aviation industry for application in the realm of trauma critical care. The flight of contemporary airframes is a high-performance, complex endeavor in which overlooked safety measures significantly increase the risk for adverse outcome, including death. These facts were not lost on the B-17 test pilots of Boeing, who in 1935 were confronted with one of the most advanced flying craft their industry had ever seen. Faced with the daunting task of preparing this complex new plane for safe flight, these pioneers developed pilot checklists consisting of consistent and reproducible step-by-step algorithms for takeoff, flight, landing, and taxiing.

Not unlike the B-17 of the 1930s, the modern ICU has become increasingly more advanced than its predecessors. To effectively and safely accomplish the myriad important tasks required for optimal patient care in the ICU, significant manpower and attention to detail are required, often requiring innovative solutions and tools. In 2001, Pronovost and colleagues[18] described their use of an ICU daily goals form, which was associated with a 50% reduction in ICU levels of service (LOS). In conjunction with a nationwide movement for quality improvement in health care, many groups have followed suit in adopting checklists and other tools to help them improve adherence to best practice measures in complex health care settings.

In a recent report, DuBose and colleagues[12] conducted a prospective before-and-after study design to examine the effectiveness of an LAC+USC Quality Rounds Checklist (QRC) tool for promoting compliance with 16 prophylactic measures for ventilator-associated pneumonia, deep vein thrombosis or pulmonary embolism, central line infection, and other trauma ICU complications (**Fig. 1**). The QRC tool was implemented on a daily basis for 1 year, providing the ability to assess monthly compliance rates by a multidisciplinary team for the development of strategies for real-time improvement. Compliance and outcomes were then captured over 1 year of QRC use. The investigators found that QRC use was associated with a sustained improvement of VAP bundle and other compliance measures over a year of use. Ventilator-associated pneumonia rates were significantly lower after QRC introduction, with an adjusted mean difference of −6.65 (per 1000 device days; 95% CI, −9.27 to −4.04; $P = .008$). During the year of QRC use, 3% of patients developed a VAP if all four daily bundle measures were met for the duration of trauma ICU stay, compared with 14% with partial compliance ($P = .04$). The overall VAP rate with full compliance was 5.29 versus 9.23 (per 1000 device days) with partial compliance. Compared with the previous year, a 24% reduction in the number of pneumonias was recorded for the year of QRC use, representing an estimated cost savings of approximately $400,000.

Electronic medical records, which are becoming an increasing presence in the modern trauma ICU, have also been proposed as effective tools of best practice and quality improvement in the intensive care environment. In clinical practice, these types of medical record systems have been espoused to improve the processing of the large amounts of clinical and laboratory data inherent to the care of the critically ill. They can, however, also be used to provide cues for adherence to clinical practice guidelines and evidence-based practices.[19] Although the potential of the electronic medical record is apparent, additional study is required to better link the use of these tools of medical informatics to subsequent patient outcomes.[20]

Regardless of the tool or approach used, the successful implementation of best evidence interventions requires some form of quality improvement initiative to track not only compliance with interventions but also outcomes. In the environment of

Date:	Fellow:										INTUBATED ONLY										
	Age	Gender	ICU Day	PUD Prophylaxis	DVT/PE Prophylaxis	Central Line Day	Sedation Holiday	Glucose Control Type	Low Blood Glucose Level for 24 hr	High Blood Glucose Level for 24 hrs	Vent Day	Intubation Method	Low Tidal Volume	Assessed for Weaning Protocol	Gross Contamination of Respirator Circuit	Continuous Subglottic Suctioning	Code Status	HOB at least 30 degrees	Nutrition Evaluated	Antibiotic need / Culture Evaluation	Invasive Device Need Considered
MR#																					

Fig. 1. *LAC + USC* daily quality rounding checklist.

modern health care, these outcomes must consider both clinical and economic variables. Successful quality improvement initiatives in this regard are often best facilitated through cooperative efforts with specially trained partners from nonmedical fields, or through the advanced training of health care personnel. These partners can contribute to the optimization of care in a team approach that has become the hallmark of modern ICU organization.

TRAUMA ICU ORGANIZATION

The effective implementation of quality improvement initiatives, based on best-evidence practices, requires the cooperative effort of a dedicated multidisciplinary health care team. Given the breadth of knowledge required to provide optimal care in the modern era, this team should consist of health care providers and associated support personnel capable of delivering the appropriate expertise to the bedside on a daily basis. The proposed composition of this team has varied from among facilities experienced with the implementation of the concepts. At the authors' institution, R Adams Cowley Shock Trauma Center, routine daily rounding team members include an intensivist and dedicated team members from infectious disease, nutrition, physical therapy, respiratory therapy, and nursing; pharmacy representatives; and various medical and nursing trainees. Other possible team members are included in **Box 2**. Similar arrangements may not, however, be feasible or realistic at other facilities with different staffing limitations.

Another group of partners increasingly discussed as potentially important to the rounding team process has been the patient family. Although this concept potentially

---

Box 2
Potential multidisciplinary rounding team members

Board certified intensivist

Clinical nursing staff

Respiratory therapy

Nutritional medicine

Infectious disease

Anesthesiology

Physical therapy

Ward nurse manager

Nurse practitioner

Occupational therapy

Clinical pharmacist

Social Worker

Trauma nursing coordinator/administrator

Physicians assistants

Hospital chaplain

Critical care technicians

Residents and fellows

Nursing students

supports more effective communication with family members and better involves them in care, in practice additional research is required to establish the most effective modality through which to accomplish these goals. In a recent study by Jacobowski and colleagues,[21] a team of investigators from Vanderbilt University School of Medicine invited the families of 227 critically ill patients to participate in daily interdisciplinary rounds. These researchers found that although family satisfaction with frequency of communication increased, participation decreased their satisfaction regarding time for decision making, and overall satisfaction scores did not differ between families who attended rounds and those that did not. The investigators concluded that structured interdisciplinary family rounds can improve some families' satisfaction, whereas others feel rushed to make decisions by this involvement. Additional data suggest, however, that family involvement at critical junctures of care, particularly in end-of-life decision making, may have more clear value.[22,23] Although the topic of family involvement in the construct of trauma ICU organization requires further study, effective means of communication using team concepts are advisable.

The leadership of a multidisciplinary team, and the relationship of that team to other services providing care, also continues to be a topic requiring additional study. Several models for ICU organization have been described and are in clinical use, each with their own potential benefits and/or limitations. Existing models include closed, open, or mixed/hybrid alternatives. In the closed model, patients admitted to the intensive care unit are managed exclusively by an intensivist-led team. In this arrangement, the ICU team has primary responsibility for all components of care, using surgical partners and other specialties in a consultant status only. Once the patient is discharged from the ICU, care is then transitioned to the initial admitting surgical or medical service. The open model constitutes a reversal of these roles, with the primary admitting medical or surgical team using intensive care providers as consultants, but retaining primary responsibility for all components of care they do not explicitly delegate to the intensivist or multidisciplinary team. Finally, the mixed/hybrid model provides for the active management of an individual patient by multiple providers from different specialties. This organizational model provides for greater longitudinal involvement of the primary admitting team, but requires close coordination of a potentially large team of disparate providers to optimize outcome. In practice, many open or mixed/hybrid models are highly individualized in their organization to the facility that uses them.

Several recent examinations have suggested that the closed model of ICU organization may be related to improved outcomes in a variety of ICU settings.[24–27] In a study of adult 24 regional ICUs in King County, Washington, Treggiari and colleagues[24] showed that adjusted hospital mortality among ICU patients with acute lung injury (ALI) was improved in ICUs with closed organizational formats. The precise reason for this finding, however, was not elucidated in this or a subsequent examination by the same group reported in 2008.[25] In this second report, the investigators examined clinical treatment variables from the same patient populations, noting that although the patients with ALI treated in closed units received lower tidal volume ventilation, no other differences were seen in measured processes of care. Moreover, the difference in delivered tidal volumes did not completely account for the improved mortality observed in closed-model ICUs.

Even in the austere environment of a combat theater, organizational models featuring critical care physician–led teams have shown the ability to provide sophisticated critical care potentially capable of optimizing outcome.[26,27] Lettieri and colleagues,[27] in a before-and-after study examining the introduction of an intensivist to the ICU of a US military Combat Support Hospital in deployed Afghanistan, found that this initiative resulted in decreases in ICU mortality (6.6% vs 4.0%; $P<.001$), duration of mechanical ventilation (4.7 $\pm$ 3.9 days vs 3.1 $\pm$ 2.7 days; $P<.001$), and ventilator-associated pneumonia (42.5% vs 8.0%; $P<.001$). Although this topic requires further study, these experiences may have important learning applications for civilian medical care systems.

Other studies have supported the mortality benefit associated with management of critically ill patients by a dedicated, intensivist-led team in a closed unit,[28,29] but additional study on this topic is required. Although it seems rationale that a closed organization of ICU care would prove more conducive to the effective implementation of best-evidence practices and quality improvement initiatives, a direct linkage between this organizational construct and these intermediate outcomes has yet to be definitively established.

Although the closed model has several potential attractive benefits, shortfalls in physician staffing and differences in intensivist availability continue to drive regional differences in ICU modeling. In a recent report by Hyzy and colleagues,[30] the investigators examined the organizational models and staffing of 115 ICUs from 72 hospitals in the state of Michigan. They found that only 25% of sites used a closed model of ICU management, and the need for hospitalists to staff attending physician positions correlated strongly with the use of an open ICU model. At only 18 sites (20%) were all ICU staff physicians board certified in ICU care. In the absence of intensivists, alternate models of care, including a hospitalist model, were frequently used.

These regional challenges in ICU staffing have been addressed in many ways. The advent of telemedicine in the ICU, as outlined by Cannon and colleagues elsewhere in this issue, has emerged as a potentially cost-effective means of delivering critical care to understaffed intensive care environments in need of this important expertise. Although the clear benefits of ICU telemedicine systems remain unclear, these systems seem safe and are likely to improve with the inevitable advancement of technology. Undoubtedly, future study will be dedicated to this emerging component of care.[31–33]

In the past decade, the critical care community has continued to investigate the importance of ICU organization on subsequent patient outcome. Although a significant need exists for continued research in this area of investigation,[34] existing data support multidisciplinary approaches and the adoption of a closed construct when feasible. The exploration of alternative options for understaffed regions, including the incorporation of ICU telemedicine, are likely to prove valuable avenues of energy and monetary expenditure.

Additional explorations of care improvement and quality initiatives continue to be driven by several sources, including organizations such as the Leapfrog Group, which is a voluntary program aimed at mobilizing employer purchasing power to alert America's health industry that big leaps in health care safety, quality, and customer value will be recognized and rewarded. Among other initiatives, Leapfrog works with its employer members to reward hospitals that have a proven record of high-quality care. Although the direct impact of these initiatives on individual patient outcome requires additional study, the modern ICU provider must be familiar with these organizations and their objectives to keep pace with the ongoing evolution in quality improvement that both private and federal quality initiatives continue to nurture.

SUMMARY

Optimizing the care of the trauma ICU patient population remains a dynamic evolution. Continued efforts to define best-evidence practices are required. Quality improvement initiatives must be effectively used to track the implementation of these practices.

Finally, ICUs must be organized effectively, using multidisciplinary approaches with intensivist-led direction, to provide the appropriate configuration of expertise to the patient care environment. Experiences of the past decade suggest that the interplay of these three factors is required to optimize patient outcome after injury.

REFERENCES

1. Levy MM, Dellinger RP, Townsend SR, et al. The Surviving Sepsis Campaign: results of an international guideline-based performance improvement program targeting severe sepsis. Intensive Care Med 2010;36(2):222–31.
2. Levinson AT, Casserly BP, Levy MM. Reducing mortality in severe sepsis and septic shock. Semin Respir Crit Care Med 2011;32(2):195–205.
3. Casaer MP, Mesotten D, Hermans G, et al. Early versus late parenteral nutrition in critically ill adults. N Engl J Med 2011;365(6):506–17.
4. Marin J, Heymann A, Basell K, et al. Evidence and consensus-based German guidelines for the management of analgesia, sedation and delirium in intensive care—short version. Ger Med Sci 2010;8:Doc02.
5. Schuerer DJ, Whinney RR, Freeman BD, et al. Evaluation of the applicability, efficacy, and safety of a thromboembolic event prophylaxis guideline designed for quality improvement of the traumatically injured patient. J Trauma 2005;58(4): 731–9.
6. Cypress BS. Family presence on rounds: a systematic review of the literature. Dimens Crit Care Nurs 2012;31(1):53–64.
7. Konkani A, Oakley B. Noise in hospital intensive care units—a critical review of a critical topic. J Crit Care 2011. [Epub ahead of print].
8. Berriel-Cass D, Adkins FW, Jones P, et al. Eliminating nosocomial infections at Ascension Health. Jt Comm J Qual Patient Saf 2006;32:612–20.
9. Cocanour CS, Pininger M, Domonoske BD, et al. Decreasing ventilator-associated pneumonia in a trauma ICU. J Trauma 2006;61:122–9 [discussion: 129–30].
10. Curley MA, Schwalenstocker E, Deshpande JK, et al. Tailoring the Institute for Healthcare Improvement 100,000 Lives Campaign to pediatric settings: the example of ventilator-associated pneumonia. Pediatr Clin North Am 2006;53: 1231–51.
11. 5 Million Lives Campaign. Institute for Healthcare Improvement Web site. Available at: http://www.ihi.org/offerings/Initiatives/PastStrategicInitiatives/5MillionLivesCampaign/Pages/default.aspx. Accessed January 12, 2012.
12. DuBose J, Teixeira PG, Inaba K, et al. Measurable outcomes of quality improvement using a daily rounds checklist: one year analysis in a trauma intensive care unit with sustained ventilator-associated pneumonia reduction. J Trauma 2010; 69(4):855–60.
13. Heyland DK, Cook DJ, Dudek PM. Prevention of ventilator associated pneumonia: current practice in Canadian intensive care units. J Crit Care 2002;17: 161–7.
14. Craven DE. Preventing ventilator-associated pneumonia in adults: sowing seeds of change. Chest 2006;130:251–60.
15. Babcock HM, Zack JE, Garrison T, et al. An educational intervention to reduce ventilator-associated pneumonia in an integrated health system: a comparison of effects. Chest 2004;125:2224–31.
16. Kollef JH. Prevention of hospital-associated pneumonia and ventilator-associated pneumonia. Crit Care Med 2004;32:1396–405.

17. Rello J. Changing physician's behavior in the intensive care unit. Crit Care Med 2002;30:2593–4.
18. Pronovost PJ, Berenholtz SM, Ngo K, et al. Developing and pilot testing quality indicators in the intensive care unit. J Crit Care 2003;18(3):145–55.
19. Hildreth AN, Enniss T, Martin RS, et al. Surgical intensive care unit mobility is increased after institution of a computerized mobility order set and intensive care unit mobility protocol: a prospective cohort analysis. Am Surg 2010;76(8): 818–22.
20. Adhikari N, Lapinsky SE. Medical informatics in the intensive care unit: an overview of technology assessment. J Crit Care 2003;18(1):41–7.
21. Jacobowski NL, Girard TD, Mulder JA, et al. Communication in critical care: family rounds in the intensive care unit. Am J Crit Care 2010;19(5):421–30.
22. Mahcare Delgado E, Callahan A, Paganelli G, et al. Multidisciplinary family meetings in the ICU facilitate end-of-life decision making. Am J Hosp Palliat Care 2009;26(4):295–302.
23. Pronovost PJ, Holzmueller CG, Clattenburg L, et al. Team care: beyond open and closed care units. Curr Opin Crit Care 2006;12(6):604–8.
24. Treggiari MM, Martin DP, Yanez ND, et al. Effect of intensive care unit organizational model and structure on outcomes in patients with acute lung injury. Am J Respir Crit Care Med 2007;176(7):685–90.
25. Cooke CR, Watkins TR, Kahn JM, et al. The effect of intensive care unit staffing model on tidal volume in patients with acute lung injury. Crit Care 2008;12(6): R134.
26. Grathwohl KW, Venticinque SG. Organizational characteristics of the austere intensive care unit: the evolution of military trauma and critical care medicine; applications for civilian medical care systems. Crit Care Med 2008;36(Suppl 7): S275–83.
27. Lettieri CJ, Shah AA, Greenburg DL. An intensivist-directed intensive care unit improves clinical outcomes in a combat zone. Crit Care Med 2009;37(4): 1256–60.
28. Van der Sluis FJ, Slagt C, Liebman B, et al. The impact of open versus closed format ICU admission practices on the outcome of high risk surgical patients: a cohort analysis. BMC Surg 2011;11:18.
29. Chittawatanarat K, Pamorsinlapathum T. The impact of closed ICU model on mortality in general surgical intensive care unit. J Med Assoc Thai 2009;92(12): 1627–34.
30. Hyzy RC, Flanders SA, Pronovost PJ, et al. Characteristics of intensive care units in Michigan: not an open and closed case. J Hosp Med 2010;5(1):4–9.
31. Boots RJ, Singh S, Terblanch M, et al. Remote care by telemedicine in the ICU: many models of care can be effective. Curr Opin Crit Care 2011;17(6):634–40.
32. Groves RH Jr, Holcomb BW Jr, Smith ML. Intensive care telemedicine: evaluating a model for proactive remote monitoring and intervention in the critical care setting. Stud Health Technol Inform 2008;131:131–46.
33. Smith AC, Armfield NR. A systematic review and meta-analysis of ICU telemedicine reinforces the need for further controlled investigations to assess the impact of telemedicine on patient outcomes. Evid Based Nurs 2011;14(4):102–3.
34. Murphy DJ, Fan E, Needham DM. ICU staffing and patient outcomes: more work remains. Crit Care 2009;13(1):101.

Advanced Technologies in Trauma Critical Care Management

Jeremy W. Cannon, MD, SM[a,b,*], Kevin K. Chung, MD[c],
David R. King, MD[d]

KEYWORDS

- Innovation • Trauma critical care • Ultrasound • Hemodynamic monitoring
- Extracorporeal therapy • Wound management

KEY POINTS

- Bedside ultrasonography is now universal in the trauma intensive care unit (ICU) for rapid diagnosis in patients with unstable hemodynamics, for assessment of volume status, and for performing invasive procedures in the ICU.
- ICU monitors are becoming progressively more advanced and less invasive. Examples of modern monitoring technology include waveform analysis, complexity analysis, electrical velocimetry, smart monitoring, and telemonitoring.
- Advanced therapies now employed to improve patient outcomes in modern critical care include active thermoregulation, extracorporeal gas exchange, and extracorporeal blood purification.
- Trauma ICU patients commonly have large open wounds related to their injury or body cavities that require temporary closure. Negative pressure wound management has been widely used in the management of these large wounds and open body cavities.
- Novel technologies and therapies in critical care should be systematically evaluated by applying the recently defined Innovation Development Exploration Assessment Long-term study (IDEAL) criteria. Revisions to the US Food and Drug Administration approval system should also be considered to assure continued innovation in this field.

The opinions expressed in this document are solely those of the authors and do not represent an endorsement by or the views of the United States Air Force, the United States Army, the Department of Defense, or the United States Government.
This work was supported by a grant from the Defense Medical Research and Development Program.
The authors have nothing to disclose.
[a] Division of Trauma and Acute Care Surgery, San Antonio Military Medical Center, 3551 Roger Brooke Drive, Fort Sam Houston, San Antonio, TX 78234, USA; [b] Department of Surgery, Uniformed Services University of the Health Sciences, Bethesda, MD 20814, USA; [c] Clinical Division, US Army Institute of Surgical Research, 3698 Chambers Pass, Fort Sam Houston, San Antonio, TX 78234, USA; [d] Division of Trauma, Emergency Surgery and Surgical Critical Care, Massachusetts General Hospital and Harvard Medical School, 165 Cambridge Street, Suite 810, Boston, MA 02114, USA
* Corresponding author. Division of Trauma and Acute Care Surgery, San Antonio Military Medical Center, 3551 Roger Brooke Drive, Fort Sam Houston, San Antonio, TX 78234.
E-mail address: jcannon@massmed.org

INTRODUCTION

Postoperative surgical and trauma patients in the mid-1900s benefitted from the nexus of several concepts that led to the establishment of intensive care units (ICUs) in major medical centers across the country:

- Cohorting critically ill patients in a specialized unit
- Use of mechanical ventilation to support patients with respiratory failure
- Use of both non-nvasive and invasive hemodynamic monitors
- Frequent measurement of blood gas values and other laboratory parameters.

The history of these advances and their application in modern critical care has been thoroughly reviewed by multiple expert authors.[1–5] What sets the trauma ICU apart from other critical care environments is the frequent need for ongoing massive resuscitation and the periodic use of the ICU as an extension of the operating room for invasive procedures.[6] In the trauma ICU, particular emphasis is placed on frequent reassessment of patients with severe injuries, on continuing the damage control therapy initiated in the emergency department or the operating room, and on providing an environment for the application of standardized treatment protocols for managing a range of clinical problems from traumatic brain injury to thromboprophylaxis in the acutely injured patient.[7,8]

This care environment is characterized by a high degree of specialization and the use of advanced technologies; however, recent studies have also highlighted the importance of simple practices such as hand hygiene and a daily rounds checklist for improving outcomes.[9,10] Furthermore, the benefits of ICU-based therapies are widely recognized as beneficial in both the developed and developing world, which should push researchers to continue to explore novel therapies that are both cost-conscious and scalable.[11]

The following paragraphs describe a range of technologies that have transformed the care of trauma patients in the ICU in recent years. Although in some instances, the technology is not specific to a trauma population, the authors have chosen to discuss these particular applications, because they represent recent advances that have either advanced or revolutionized the care provided in the trauma ICU.

ULTRASOUND-BASED APPLICATIONS

Surgeon-performed ultrasound was first introduced as a real-time diagnostic tool in the early 1990s. Since that time, there has been a steady rise in the use of ultrasound for a range of applications in critically ill patients, to the point where ultrasound systems are ubiquitous in ICUs today. Surgeons and other intensivists caring for trauma patients use the various types of ultrasound equipment shown in **Table 1** on nearly a daily basis.[12]

Several reviews on surgeon and intensivist-performed ultrasound provide a comprehensive overview of this broad topic.[13–18] The following sections focus on the most common and emerging uses for ultrasound as a diagnostic, monitoring, and therapeutic tool in critically ill trauma patients.

Ultrasound for Diagnosis and Monitoring

Focused assessment with sonography for trauma examination

The Focused Assessment with Sonography for Trauma (FAST) examination was first promoted by Rozycki and colleagues.[19] This study is performed in the trauma bay, where a low-frequency ultrasound probe is used to assess for fluid in the right upper quadrant, left upper quadrant, pericardium, and pelvis.[20] This examination has been adopted by trauma surgeons across the world and has also been used to good effect in combat casualty triage.[21]

Table 1
Types of ultrasound transducers commonly used in the ICU

Probe Type	Frequency Range[a]	Features	ICU Applications
Linear array	13–5 MHz	Higher frequency range High resolution Shallow penetration Variable footprint depending on the probe design	CVL insertion PICC/PIV insertion A-line insertion Evaluation for DVT
Small curved array	8–5 MHz	Intermediate frequency range Medium resolution Moderate penetration Small footprint	Follow-up FAST IVC evaluation Drain placement Thoracic imaging
Large curved array	5–2 MHz	Lower frequency range Lower resolution Deeper penetration Wide footprint	Follow-up FAST IVC evaluation Drain placement
Phased array	8–1 MHz	Wide frequency range Variable resolution Variable penetration Small footprint	Follow-up FAST IVC evaluation Drain placement Thoracic imaging Cardiac imaging

Abbreviations: CVL, central venous line; DVT, deep venous thrombosis; FAST, focused assessment with sonography for trauma; IVC, inferior vena cava; PIV, peripheral intravenous line.
[a] By convention frequency ranges are listed from high to low frequency.
Photos courtesy of Sonosite, Inc., Bothell, WA; with permission.

Over time, the FAST examination has largely replaced diagnostic peritoneal lavage for identifying intra-abdominal fluid in trauma patients. Furthermore, with the addition of chest windows, the extended FAST can also rapidly diagnose a pneumothorax or hemothorax. By consensus, the learning curve for this examination has been defined as 200 examinations, of which at least half of these examinations should have positive findings.[22,23] The sensitivity and specificity of this study for identifying intraperitoneal fluid in a blunt trauma patient range from 62% to 89% and 95% to 100%, respectively, depending on the patient population being evaluated, the experience of the sonographer, and the comparative gold standard study.[20]

The role of the FAST examination in penetrating abdominal trauma remains unclear, as neither a positive nor negative result appears to reliably predict the need for operative intervention.[24] In contrast, in patients with penetrating anterior thoracoabdominal trauma, the subxyphoid window is very useful for identifying pericardial fluid warranting operative exploration. This examination has a sensitivity of up to 100% and specificity of 97%[25] with false-negatives primarily arising when pericardial blood decompresses into the pleural space.[26]

At the authors' institutions, the FAST examination is typically performed during the trauma evaluation by emergency medicine and general surgery residents, with staff oversight. All images are saved for quality control review using subsequent computed tomography (CT) imaging or operative findings for determination of false-negative and false-positive examinations. Management decisions based on the FAST findings are directly supervised by the staff trauma surgeon, who views the FAST images in real time.

In the ICU, follow-up FAST examinations can detect interval development of significant hemoperitoneum[27] and can identify complications of nonoperative management of solid organ injuries.[28] Thus, repeated FAST examinations can be an important diagnostic adjunct early in the ICU management of trauma patients.

Intensivist-diagnosed deep venous thrombosis

Trauma patients are at high risk for developing thromboembolic complications. At the same time, obtaining timely diagnostic ultrasound evaluation of the extremities is not always possible. Recent evidence suggests that intensivists trained in basic ultrasound can diagnose deep venous thrombosis (DVTs) with a high degree of accuracy thereby accelerating the treatment of this complication.[29]

Thoracic ultrasound

Thoracic ultrasound has gained increased acceptance in the ICU as a diagnostic tool.[30] To minimize rib interference, a phased array or curved array probe with a small footprint is typically used for these examinations. The authors use chest ultrasound in the following manner:

- To identify a pneumothorax or hemothorax that needs to be drained acutely
- To differentiate a finding of consolidation versus effusion on radiograph.

Ultrasound to assess hypotension/fluid status

Both comprehensive and focused ultrasound examinations have been described as an adjunct to hemodynamic monitoring in trauma patients in the ICU. In particular, ultrasound can be useful in 2 scenarios:

- Hypotensive trauma patients in the ICU without an obvious source of hemodynamic instability
- Critically ill polytrauma patients with end-organ dysfunction and an unclear intravascular volume status.

In an acutely hypotensive trauma patient in the ICU, both transthoracic and transesophageal ultrasound examinations have been advocated. Using a subxyphoid approach, inferior vena cava (IVC) diameter measurement with ultrasound can discriminate patients responsive to volume resuscitation as compared with nonresponders.[31] Alternatively, a more comprehensive transesophageal echocardiography (TEE) examination can more specifically pinpoint the etiology of the hypotension and can guide both therapeutic interventions and ongoing resuscitation.[18] The downside of the latter approach is the extensive additional training required to gain proficiency and the need for specialized equipment. However, as experience with ultrasound among intensivists broadens, use of TEE in the ICU will likely increase with time. In addition, relatively inexpensive disposable TEE probes such as the ClariTEE (ImaCor, Incorporated, Garden City, NY, USA) may lower barriers to using this approach.

In the more chronic trauma ICU patient, ultrasound imaging can be used to assess the patient's cardiac function and volume status. Two groups have advocated similar approaches using portable ultrasound technology in which several cardiac and IVC views are obtained to assess the patient's current physiologic state (**Fig. 1**).[32–34] No patient outcomes are provided by either group; so further study in this area is required to guide future practice.

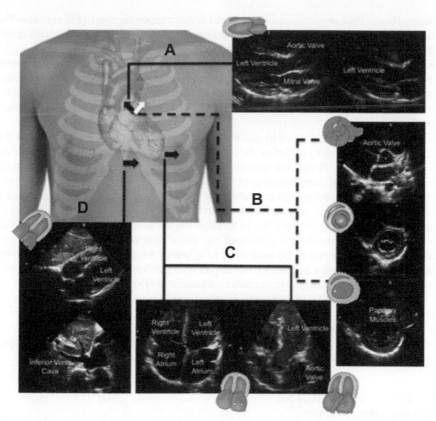

Fig. 1. Ultrasound assessment of volume status and cardiac function in the ICU uses a number of different sonographic windows. *(A)* Left parasternal long axis view. *(B)* Parasternal short axis view. *(C)* Apical 4-chamber view. *(D)* Subxyphoid view; caliber can be measured from the subxyphoid view through the liver. Arrowhead indicates the position of the marker on the ultrasound transducer. *(Adapted from* Ferrada P, Murthi S, Anand RJ, et al. Transthoracic focused rapid echocardiographic examination: real-time evaluation of fluid status in critically ill trauma patients. J Trauma 2011;70:57, with permission; and Kirk CR. Thumbnail guide to congenital heart disease. Available at: http://www.crkirk.com/thumbnail/index.htm; with permission. Accessed December 3, 2011.)

ULTRASOUND-GUIDED INTERVENTIONS

Among trauma ICU patients, the most common ultrasound-guided interventions are vascular access and drain placement.[35] Ultrasound-guided placement of internal jugular lines has become the standard of care.[36] A high-frequency linear array probe is typically used either for a 1-time view of the target vein or in real time using a 1- or 2-person technique. Recently, ultrasound-guided subclavian central venous catheter placement has also been described.[37] However, the reliability of the landmark approach and the steep learning curve for the image-guided approach make ready adoption of this technique unlikely.

If the femoral vein is being considered for short-term access, an ultrasound examination for patency should be considered, especially in trauma patients in the ICU. In addition, the relationship of the vein to the artery can be variable, especially in younger patients, which becomes readily apparent with a quick ultrasound assessment.[38]

Ultrasound can also be used for positioning peripherally inserted central catheters (PICC). This technique was recently described when a survey of the jugular vein ipsilateral to the PICC insertion quickly ruled in or out malpositioning of the catheter.[39] If a malpositioned catheter was identified, ultrasound guidance permitted repositioning of the catheter without procedural interruption.

Arterial cannulation is also facilitated by ultrasound guidance. Radial artery catheter insertion is made more reliable with this technique using a high-frequency probe. Cannulation of the femoral artery can also be guided with ultrasound imaging whether for arterial line placement or insertion of an access sheath for diagnostic studies or therapeutic interventions.

Ultrasound can also be used to guide fluid aspiration and drain placement in the ICU. This most commonly includes ultrasound-guided thoracentesis and paracentesis. In both instances, ultrasound can be used to mark out the optimal needle insertion site and to evaluate for completeness of fluid evacuation. In the case of thoracentesis, ultrasound guidance reduces procedure time, increases the likelihood of accessing fluid on the first attempt, and reduces complications.[40,41] For paracentesis, a low-frequency probe (eg, 2 MHz) is used to localize the intra-abdominal fluid, after which the abdominal wall should be assessed by either adjusting the image depth on a broad-bandwidth probe or by switching to a higher frequency probe (eg, 5 MHz). This technique facilitates access to the target fluid pocket while minimizing the risk of injury to the inferior epigastric vessels or abdominal wall varices.[35]

Over the past 20 years, use of bedside ultrasound by surgeons for both diagnosis and management in critically ill trauma patients has grown dramatically. Consequently, surgeons should continue to take a leading role in defining standards for quality assurance and certification while also continuing to explore new and varied applications for this technology.

ADVANCES IN ICU MONITORING
Pulmonary Artery Catheter

The pulmonary artery catheter (PAC), once regarded as the gold standard of all hemodynamic monitors for extremely ill patients, has seen a dramatic decline in use over the past decade. Multiple well-designed clinical trials have failed to demonstrate any clinical advantage to its routine use in many populations including general ICU patients, septic patients, complex postsurgical patients, and those with severe respiratory dysfunction.[42–46] Likely, this failure to demonstrate any morbidity or mortality benefit is related to the common error of assuming a pressure measurement is equivalent to volume or flow.[47] Clinicians are also well known to misinterpret the data provided by the PAC.[48–51] Additionally, there are risks to the patient associated with placement and residence of a catheter within the pulmonary artery, including an increased risk of pulmonary embolism, bloodstream infections, a catheter-induced hypercoagulable state, and other technical complications.[52–55] Finally, most data generated by the PAC can now be acquired through other less invasive technologies such as bedside echocardiography, central venous pressure monitoring, and cardiac electrical velocimetry.

These limitations aside, it is difficult to condemn an entire monitoring modality based on this evidence. There remain certain patients in whom multiple clinical conditions often generate an array of conflicting information, leaving the clinician with a confusing clinical impression. For these situations, an algorithm for the application of the PAC and interpretation of the data obtained may provide some insight to the patient's physiology[56]; however, this approach has not been systematically evaluated. Another potential advantage to the PAC is that it lends itself to continuous waveform interpretation, which the authors use extensively in their preclinical laboratory studies, although no data currently exist to support this practice in the ICU.

Waveform Analysis

Multiple physiologic measurements taken in the ICU are acquired with relatively high sampling rates. These high sampling rates produce data that are far greater in volume and complexity than the human brain can adequately process and interpret in real time. Consequently, automated waveform analysis of those physiologic parameters captured in high granularity has the potential to increase understanding of the patient's physiology without adding additional invasive monitors. For example, instead of examining just the systolic and diastolic blood pressure on the arterial line tracing, waveform analysis allows interpretation of the change in slopes of the arterial line tracing, providing far more insight than the raw pressure values alone.

With the exception of fetal heart monitoring in the laboring mother, waveform variability and complexity analysis technologies have not matured enough to make their way into routine clinical practice; however, in time, these new technologies will very likely have a role in triage of trauma patients, prediction of ICU decompensation, and as tools to assess occult physiologic abnormalities that routinely go undetected with current monitoring paradigms.[57–60] Monitoring approaches currently under active investigation in the ICU include plethysmography variability, arterial pressure and heart rate complexity analysis, continuous noninvasive hemoglobin determination, cardiac electrical velocimetry, and multiple vital sign integration with automated interpretation. **Fig. 2** illustrates the

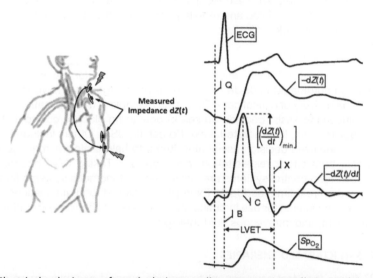

Fig. 2. Electrical velocimetry for calculating cardiac output. A small sinusoidal current is passed between a pair of electrodes, and the impedence to electrical flow conducted by the red cell mass within the thoracic cavity is measured (*left*). Shown are a representative electrocardiogram (ECG) tracing, ECG impedance waveform –dZ(t), first derivative of the impedance waveform dZ(t)/dt, and pulse oximetry waveform SpO_2. The first derivative of the impedance waveform (dZ(t)/dt) is used with an ECG to determine the beginning of electrical systole (Q), aortic valve opening (B), maximal deflection of the dZ(t)/dt waveform (C), and the closing of the aortic valve (X). Stroke volume and cardiac output are calculated from these reference points. A high degree of correlation between cardiac output measured by Doppler and electrical velocimetry has been demonstrated. *Abbreviation:* LVET, left ventricular ejection time. (*Modified from* Schmidt C, Theilmeier G, Van Aken H, et al. Comparison of electrical velocimetry and transoesophageal Doppler echocardiography for measuring stroke volume and cardiac output. Br J Anaesth 2005;95:606; with permission.)

principles of electrical velocimetry for measuring cardiac output noninvasively as an example of the advanced monitoring devices that will be available for use in the ICU in the near future.

Smart Monitoring, Telemonitoring, and Telepresence

A smart monitor is any monitoring device that provides more information than simply the measured data. This can include waveform analysis as described previously, spectral interpretation, integration of multiple inputs, and decision support. This technology likely has emerged, in part, as a necessity to enable the clinician to integrate far more data than would otherwise be possible by simply examining an ICU flow sheet or the bedside monitors. One of the most practical applications of smart monitoring is automated decision support, which has been used for the resuscitation of burn patients and combat casualties.[61] Additionally, multiple parameter inputs have already been successfully used in some ICUs,[62] while others have demonstrated the utility of automated integration of existing vital sign data for triaging trauma patients.[63]

Telemonitoring is another example of information integration and oversight that is gaining interest in modern ICU care. These systems stream all monitoring data including alarms, imaging studies, electronic medical record data, and often video images of the patient to an intensivist tasked with evaluating multiple patients. Recent results suggest this approach improves survival while decreasing cost,[64,65] although others have not corroborated these results.[66] This concept can also be extended to telepresence using various fixed and mobile platforms that virtually bring the intensivist to the patient's bedside.[67–70]

Decision Assist and Support

By leveraging biomedical engineering expertise and computer technology, various algorithms and automated bedside protocols have emerged that have the potential to optimize the delivery of critical care. One such example is the application of various software solutions to assist bedside nurses in optimizing glucose control in the ICU (eg, EndoTool, Hospira, Incorporated, Lake Forest, IL, USA). Others include the application of computerized decision assist algorithms to help clinicians manage hemorrhagic shock, burn shock resuscitation, and sepsis.[71] Taking this concept 1 step further, closed-loop control systems are completely autonomous systems that adjust therapy based on real-time feedback. Examples of closed loop applications that are under active investigation for use in critical care include mechanical ventilation, sedation management, and intravenous fluid therapy.[72–75]

ADVANCES IN ICU-BASED THERAPIES

The ICU affords the ideal environment to provide support or replacement of failing organ systems. Gas exchange support through mechanical ventilation has been the hallmark of ICU care for decades. Now even more advanced and novel therapies are appearing in ICUs with great regularity. This section focuses on some of these emerging therapeutic modalities.

Cooling for Neuroprotection

Cerebral anoxia represents the greatest cause of late mortality in patients who initially survive cardiopulmonary arrest. Consequently, adjuncts to neuroprotection during the vulnerable postresuscitation period have been the subject of numerous preclinical and clinical investigations. Following 2 positive prospective, randomized trials demonstrating a mortality benefit to systemic cooling in comatose survivors of a ventricular tachycardia or ventricular fibrillation cardiac arrest, there has been great interest in this therapeutic modality.[76,77] In the trauma population, extensions of this evidence have been applied to traumatic brain injury with refractory intracranial hypertension, anoxic brain injury from near-hanging, and both cold- and warm-water drownings.[78–80]

The use of deep hypothermia after traumatic arrest is another example of this concept. Animal data suggest a significant survival benefit to this immediate cooling approach,[81–83] and the first clinical trial is expected to begin shortly.[84]

Therapeutic hypothermia in an ICU setting is best performed with the aid of a treatment algorithm to ensure the rate of cooling, the target temperature, the duration of cooling, the rate of rewarming, shivering control, and the frequency of laboratory draws are standardized. Equipment for performing therapeutic hypothermia consists of either an invasive or noninvasive thermoregulation device and a temperature probe, preferably in the esophagus or bladder (**Fig. 3**). Options for cooling range from ice packs to gel pads to catheters that fill with temperature-controlled saline. The authors' preference is to use a cooling catheter that produces very reliable temperature control during all phases of therapy, reduces the burden of nursing care especially during the rewarming phase, and minimizes contact with the patient's vulnerable skin. The catheter should be discontinued after completion of therapy due to a theoretical risk of thromboembolic complications.

Gas Exchange

Support of both oxygenation and ventilation with a mechanical ventilator has been a constant in critical care from the very beginning. Although this technology has evolved from negative pressure ventilators to microprocessor-based equipment with digital displays, the core concept of using the lungs for gas exchange has never changed. Advances in the use of this technology include the current standard of lung-protective ventilation, which has reduced mortality from respiratory failure,[85] and new ventilator modes such as airway pressure release ventilation (APRV).[86] However, in patients with severe respiratory failure, even with optimal ventilator management, up to one-third still die with their disease. Recent clinical evidence and technological improvements have led to a renewed interest in using extracorporeal gas exchange in

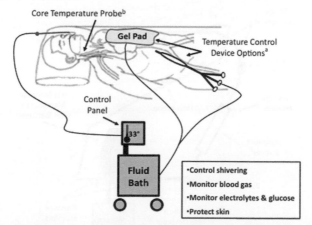

Fig. 3. Setup for therapeutic hypothermia or active thermoregulation. [a] Shown are a cooling gel pad and an invasive thermoregulation catheter as 2 temperature control options. [b] Core temperature can be measured by a pulmonary artery catheter, esophageal probe, bladder probe, or rectal probe.

this patient population to avoid barotrauma, volutrauma, and biotrauma while also permitting early physical therapy.[87]

The components of an extracorporeal life support (ECLS) circuit include a mechanical pump, a gas exchange membrane, a heat exchanger, and pressure monitors (**Fig. 4**). Venovenous ECLS (vvECLS) is used in most cases of adult respiratory failure, as it can provide all of the gas exchange needs of most adult patients using modern membranes made of polymethylpentene (PMP). In select cases of isolated hypercapnic respiratory failure, a low-flow arteriovenous pumpless gas exchange circuit can rapidly normalize the $PaCO_2$. If circulatory support is required, venoarterial ECLS (vaECLS) becomes necessary.

ECLS can be safely used in adult trauma patients. This advanced therapy should be done in an experienced center with clearly defined indications for initiating ECLS, established treatment protocols, and a staff well versed in ECLS circuit management.[88] In such centers, this therapy can be applied in patients with high-grade air leaks from tracheobronchial injuries, large pulmonary emboli with hemodynamic compromise, and in cases of right heart failure and hypoxemia following lung resection or pneumonectomy for trauma. In cases of severe accidental hypothermia, vvECLS can rapidly restore normothermia due to the high blood flow rates and the efficiency of the integrated heat exchanger in modern gas exchange membranes.[89]

Extracorporeal Blood Purification

Renal replacement therapy is the most common extracorporeal blood purification modality used in modern ICUs for the purposes of metabolic and volume management in the setting of acute kidney injury. Intermittent renal replacement strategies in the ICU include intermittent hemodialysis (IHD) for hemodynamically stable patients and sustained low-efficiency dialysis (SLED), a hybrid technique that extends IHD over a longer period of time, for those who are hemodynamically unstable. Continuous renal replacement modalities include continuous venovenous hemofiltration (CVVH), hemodialysis (CVVHD) and hemodiafiltration (CVVHDF). At comparable doses, studies have failed to demonstrate an advantage of IHD over continuous modalities.[90]

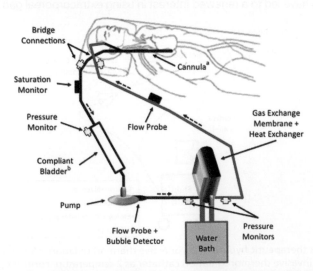

Fig. 4. Schematic of a vvECLS circuit. [a] A double lumen venous cannula (27–31 Fr) for single-site vvECLS is illustrated. [b] Optional with a centrifugal pump.

However, it has become evident that a minimum acceptable dose of therapy exists and likely needs to be achieved for optimal care. Trying to achieve a higher dose of therapy with daily IHD and SLED or higher dose CVVHDF has not improved outcomes.[91] Future areas of investigation include patient selection and timing of renal replacement therapy, identifying alternative and more sensitive biomarkers of renal injury, and timing of renal replacement therapy termination.

Recently, there has been a paradigm shift among the nephrology and critical care communities toward broadening the scope of blood purification toward various extra-renal therapies. Extracorporeal blood purification for the purpose of immune modulation in sepsis and other types of shock, liver support, and combining various extracorporeal organ support modalities such as lung, kidney and liver into 1 comprehensive multiple organ support therapy (MOST) have all been described.[92]

WOUND MANAGEMENT

No discussion of paradigm shifts and technological breakthroughs in trauma critical care would be complete without mention of negative pressure wound therapy. From open body cavities to fasciotomy incisions, this therapy has transformed both acute and chronic wound care over the past decade. This approach has been applied to almost every conceivable wound[93] and has proven beneficial in even the austere environment of combat casualty care.[94]

Damage Control Closure

Temporary closure techniques of the open abdomen have evolved significantly since the introduction of damage control surgery.[95,96] When considering an approach to temporary closure of the abdominal cavity, the following criteria must be met:

- Can be fashioned quickly with readily available supplies
- Underlying organs (eg, bowel, liver), wound edges, and fascial layers are protected
- A sterile dressing is maintained for hours to days
- Effluent from the wound is collected so that it does not macerate the tissues.

Vacuum-assisted closure readily meets all of these principles, and variations on this approach have been used in a variety of practice settings from resource-limited trauma centers[97] and austere combat environments[98] to high-volume urban academic centers.[99,100]

Vacuum-assisted damage control closure of the abdomen can be applied using either a commercially available product or an expedient setup with supplies commonly used in the operating room. Two commercially available body cavity closure devices include the ABThera (Kinetic Concepts, Incorporated, San Antonio, TX, USA) and the RENASYS-F/AB Abdominal Dressing Kit (Smith & Nephew, Incorporated, St. Petersburg, FL, USA). Alternatively, an expedient temporary closure approach for the abdominal cavity is illustrated in **Fig. 5**. If definitive closure is contraindicated or impossible, to avoid loosing abdominal domain, the authors often combine a vacuum-assisted closure method with some form of low level fascial tension such as a Wittmann Patch (Starsurgical, Incorporated, Burlington, WI, USA) or a sheet of mesh that can be serially tightened. In these cases, the authors are careful to maintain a nonadherent barrier between the bowel and these adjunctive closure devices to minimize bowel trauma and the risk of developing an enteroatmospheric fistula.

The concept of temporary thoracotomy closure has been recently described and may become more widely accepted in time.[101] Rather than packing the chest, the authors prefer to use a modified negative pressure wound closure. In these situations,

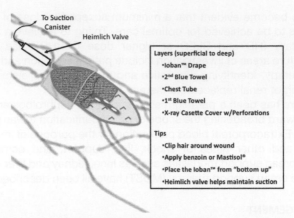

To Suction Canister

Heimlich Valve

Layers (superficial to deep)
•Ioban™ Drape
•2nd Blue Towel
•Chest Tube
•1st Blue Towel
•X-ray Casette Cover w/Perforations

Tips
•Clip hair around wound
•Apply benzoin or Mastisol®
•Place the Ioban™ from "bottom up"
•Heimlich valve helps maintain suction

Fig. 5. Damage control temporary abdominal closure, which protects the bowel, the fascia, and the skin while controlling and monitoring fluid output. This technique is referred to as a vacuum pack (VP).

the authors first insert 2 or 3 chest tubes and position them as usual. A sterile nonadherent layer such as a single ply radiography cassette cover (without fenestrations) is then placed over the lung and the chest tubes to partition the intrathoracic space from the superficial wound space. A negative pressure wound sponge, operating room towel, or laparotomy pad is then placed in the wound, and suction is applied to this with either a commercial vacuum system or low-level continuous wall suction (eg, 75–125 mm Hg).

Negative Pressure Wound Therapy

Severely injured patients who require ongoing management in the ICU often have large wounds. These include fasciotomy wounds, degloving injuries, open fractures, traumatic amputation sites, and large torso or perineal wounds. After thorough debridement of devitalized tissue, removal of contamination, and confirming hemostasis, a vacuum-assisted dressing can be applied to the wound bed. For burn wounds or abrasions adjacent to wound, the authors apply a layer of XEROFORM petrolatum gauze (Covidien, Mansfield, MA, USA) to the area and place it in continuity with the negative pressure dressing. If the wound is significantly contaminated, an active fungal or mold infection is suspected, or soft tissue viability is questionable, the authors do not apply a vacuum-assisted dressing at the index procedure and use gauze dressings instead. In these cases, the authors moisten the gauze with saline, mafenide acetate (Sulfamylon), or a Sulfamylon/amphotericin mixture depending on the level of suspicion for infection in the wound.

As with temporary closure of body cavities, a vacuum-assisted dressing is an interim management strategy that allows stabilization of the wound bed and wound edges between serial washouts. During this interim period, patients experience less pain as bedside dressing changes are no longer necessary, and nursing staff can direct time and attention to other aspects of the patient's care.

For large wounds or previously contaminated wounds, the authors' approach is to return the patient to the operating room in 24 to 72 hours (depending on the appearance of the wound at the last evaluation) for re-examination of the wound, assessment of muscle and soft tissue viability, additional debridement, and thorough irrigation. This can also be done in the ICU under sedation, particularly if the patient is tenuous from a hemodynamic or respiratory standpoint.

There are several pitfalls with using such a dressing for a large wound:

- Suction failure leading to accumulation of infected fluid in the wound bed
- Bleeding into the sponge or canister
- Delayed re-evaluation of the wound, leading to regression of the wound bed.

Manufacturers have attempted to incorporate safety alarms that disable the pump and alert the care team to a problem if the previously mentioned issues arise. However, vigilance with frequent reassessment of the dressing and surrounding tissues and aggressive attention to alarms is always required to ensure safe and effective negative pressure wound management strategy.[93]

The timing of definitive wound closure with either sutures or skin grafting is a matter of ongoing debate and investigation.[102] In some instances, wound closure by secondary intention using serial vacuum-assisted dressing changes is deemed optimal. However, the authors' approach is more often to close these wounds once the patient's nutritional status is optimized, and the wound has healthy edges with no evidence of infection. Following delayed closure, the authors typically apply a vacuum-assisted incisional dressing. This can be done with a conventional vacuum dressing or with premade commercial products for this application (eg, Prevena Incision Management System, Kinetic Concepts, Incorporated, San Antonio, TX, USA). These dressings consist of an occlusive dressing placed directly on the wound with small fenestrations for fluid evacuation. A negative pressure sponge or gauze dressing is then applied over this layer. The authors remove this dressing in 3 to 5 days and typically transition to no dressing so long as there is no ongoing drainage from the wound.

EVALUATION AND IMPLEMENTATION OF NOVEL TECHNOLOGIES AND THERAPIES

The evolutionary and revolutionary concepts presented in this article have radically transformed the overall paradigm of critical care and the trauma ICU environment over the past decade. In some instances, these changes have occurred after careful consideration with a relative abundance of clinical evidence (eg, adult ECLS and therapeutic hypothermia for neuroprotection). In others, practical expedience drove the paradigm shift with very little evidence to support such a radical transition (eg, vacuum-assisted wound management). Going forward, as new concepts and ideas emerge, how should the trauma and surgical communities find balance between these 2 extremes? On the 1 hand, introducing unproven technologies on an unsuspecting public can have disastrous consequences, while on the other, stifling innovation or burying good ideas in a mire of red tape is counter to the very nature of the specialty of critical care. The following paragraphs suggest an approach to this dilemma with regards to evaluating current novel therapies and future innovations in the ICU.

IDEAL Criteria and US Food and Drug Administration Considerations

In 2009, a multidisciplinary commission met at Oxford University to discuss innovation and advancement in the surgical specialties.[103–105] The objective of this commission was to promote surgical innovation while preventing future technological breakthroughs or innovative therapies from getting beyond a so-called tipping point of use before being reasonably evaluated. The quintessential example where the latter occurred was the widespread adoption of laparoscopic cholecystectomy prior to a careful evaluation of the risks and benefits of this surgical approach. The conclusion of this commission was that new ideas or evolutionary therapies need to be evaluated using an IDEAL framework as illustrated in **Box 1**. Using this approach, ideas that fill a capability gap or address a clinical need, such as smart monitors or negative

Box 1
IDEAL Steps for evaluating novel technologies or therapies

Innovation (stages 0–1)

    Initial procedures or early application of therapy

    Animal studies (stage 0) and human studies (stage 1) explore proof of concept and safety

    Informed consent including alternatives (from patient or legally authorized representative [LAR])

    If time permits, inform hospital leadership

    Report new procedure or therapy regardless of outcome

    Need to develop infrastructure and systems for such reporting

    Recent example: pyloric transposition[106]

Development (Stage 2a)

    Pilot study for innovation refinement (typically no more than 30 patients)

    Protocols should be registered (eg, www.clinicaltrials.gov)

    Approval by institutional review board (IRB) and possibly an ethics committee

    Informed consent including alternatives (from patient or LAR)

    Establish a risk minimization review process (eg, data safety monitoring board)

    Report consecutive series of patients without omission

    Include selection criteria, denominator of patients potentially eligible, and refinements

    Recent example: ileostomy for fulminant *Clostridium difficile* colitis[107]

Exploration (stage 2b)

    Larger possibly multicenter study (typically hundreds of patients in total)

    Uniformity of physician implementation across centers is essential

    IRB approval and informed consent including alternatives (from patient or LAR)

    Learning curve data will become available

    Collect data prospectively in a systematic fashion

    Report a range of outcomes including technical, clinical, and patient-reported

    Report quality control measures applied to ensure uniformity of practice and use of therapy

    Report numbers of patients seeking the new therapy if possible

    Recent example: minimally invasive esophagectomy[108]

Assessment (stage 3)

    Randomized trial to assess effectiveness versus standard therapy

    Consider alternative designs if randomized control trial not feasible or ethical (eg, case-control study)

    Recent example: Conventional ventilatory support versus Extracorporeal membrane oxygenation for Severe Adult Respiratory failure (CESAR) trial for adult ECLS[88]

Long-term study (Stage 4)

    Assessment of long-term outcomes and surveillance for rare complications

    Best accomplished through establishment of a registry

    Recent example: endovascular management of blunt aortic injuries[109]

pressure wound therapy, can be vetted in a systematic fashion without unduly delaying clinical availability if a benefit is demonstrated.

A related matter in the area of technology development that at once hinders the introduction of safe technology in this country while also permitting the introduction of unproven devices is the Food and Drug Administration (FDA) approval process. At present, device approval by the FDA for some devices is based on the arcane concept of legacy approval.[110,111] This process allows the introduction of technology into the medical community without first demonstrating safety, much less benefit. In contrast, if a device is not felt to be substantially equivalent to some already approved device, it must be evaluated through the premarket approval (PMA) process, which may swing too far in the other direction of an exorbitantly expensive overevaluation in some cases. There must be a better, more balanced approach to this process in the future that the surgical community should demand to ensure new technology is evaluated in a safe, timely, cost-effective fashion going forward.

Examples

Some of the emerging concepts where the IDEAL framework can be applied are apparent in the current surgical literature (see **Box 1**). Examples in trauma management include novel resuscitation strategies for exsanguination shock,[112] balloon aortic occlusion for pelvic or torso trauma with hemodynamic instability,[113,114] whole blood transfusion for trauma resuscitation,[115] and rib fracture stabilization.[116]

In each instance, an evolutionary or revolutionary idea is being promoted to treat a high-risk clinical problem with relatively few viable options at present. The challenge is to responsibly evaluate these concepts with individualized levels of clinical study, often with the support and oversight of an appropriate national organization. Funding for these evaluations should consist of a balance of local institutional funds, funds from private foundations, support from national research institutes, and in some cases industry partners that can and should shoulder some of the burden of expense as is done in the area of pharmaceutical development. By following the IDEAL approach, innovation can continue at an appropriate and safe pace with less risk of finding that costly interventions have no clinical utility or even worse cause harm only after their widespread implementation.

SUMMARY

This article illustrated the transformation that has occurred in the critical care of the most severely injured trauma patients. The universal application of bedside ultrasound imaging has greatly enhanced the ICU toolkit for diagnosis, monitoring, and interventional procedural guidance. Today's monitors are becoming more focused on derivative information while also becoming generally less invasive. Temperature regulation is becoming widely recognized as a valuable treatment strategy, and the ability to target and maintain a specific temperature or rate of cooling/rewarming has been enhanced by new technology. Extracorporeal organ support or replacement for gas exchange and blood purification is becoming more commonplace in ICUs as clinical evidence for the merits of this approach builds. Finally, the management of open body cavities and large wounds has been transformed through the application of negative pressure. As these ideas advance and other ideas emerge, it is imperative that surgeons balance rapid development with circumspect evaluation of these ideas. Adoption of the IDEAL framework should make the process of innovation both more systematic and more streamlined, although significant changes to the FDA approval system are needed to ensure The United States' continued place on the cutting edge of critical care trauma therapy.

ACKNOWLEDGMENTS

The authors gratefully acknowledge input given to this article by LTC Tim Nunez, MD, and MAJ Scott Marshall, MD.

REFERENCES

1. Grenvik A, Pinsky MR. Evolution of the intensive care unit as a clinical center and critical care medicine as a discipline. Crit Care Clin 2009;25(1):239–50.
2. Puri N, Puri V, Dellinger RP. History of technology in the intensive care unit. Crit Care Clin 2009;25(1):185–200.
3. Rosengart MR. Critical care medicine: landmarks and legends. Surg Clin North Am 2006;86(6):1305–21.
4. Weil MH, Shoemaker WC. Pioneering contributions of Peter Safar to intensive care and the founding of the Society of Critical Care Medicine. Crit Care Med 2004;32(Suppl 2):S8–10.
5. Weil MH, Tang W. From intensive care to critical care medicine: a historical perspective. Am J Respir Crit Care Med 2011;183(11):1451–3.
6. Barba CA. The intensive care unit as an operating room. Surg Clin North Am 2000;80(3):957–73.
7. Brain Trauma Foundation Guidelines. Available at: https://www.braintrauma.org/coma-guidelines/. Accessed December 7, 2011.
8. EAST Practice Management Guidelines. Available at: http://www.east.org/research/treatment-guidelines. Accessed December 7, 2011.
9. Dubose J, Teixeira PG, Inaba K, et al. Measurable outcomes of quality improvement using a daily quality rounds checklist: one-year analysis in a trauma intensive care unit with sustained ventilator-associated pneumonia reduction. J Trauma 2010;69(4):855–60.
10. Zingg W, Imhof A, Maggiorini M, et al. Impact of a prevention strategy targeting hand hygiene and catheter care on the incidence of catheter-related bloodstream infections. Crit Care Med 2009;37(7):2167–73.
11. Adhikari NK, Fowler RA, Bhagwanjee S, et al. Critical care and the global burden of critical illness in adults. Lancet 2010;376:1339–46.
12. Smith RS, Fry WR. Ultrasound instrumentation. Surg Clin North Am 2004;84(4):953–71.
13. Ballard RB, Rozycki GS, Knudson MM, et al. The surgeon's use of ultrasound in the acute setting. Surg Clin North Am 1998;78(2):337–64.
14. Lee SY, Frankel HL. Ultrasound and other imaging technologies in the intensive care unit. Surg Clin North Am 2000;80(3):975–1003.
15. Habib FA, McKenney MG. Surgeon-performed ultrasound in the ICU setting. Surg Clin North Am 2004;84(4):1151–79.
16. Beaulieu Y, Marik PE. Bedside ultrasonography in the ICU: part 2. Chest 2005;128(3):1766–81.
17. Beaulieu Y, Marik PE. Bedside ultrasonography in the ICU: part 1. Chest 2005;128(2):881–95.
18. Subramaniam B, Talmor D. Echocardiography for management of hypotension in the intensive care unit. Crit Care Med 2007;35(Suppl 8):S401–7.
19. Rozycki GS, Ochsner MG, Schmidt JA, et al. A prospective study of surgeon-performed ultrasound as the primary adjuvant modality for injured patient assessment. J Trauma 1995;39(3):492–8.
20. Patel NY, Riherd JM. Focused assessment with sonography for trauma: methods, accuracy, and indications. Surg Clin North Am 2011;91(1):195–207.

21. Beekley AC, Blackbourne LH, Sebesta JA, et al. Selective nonoperative management of penetrating torso injury from combat fragmentation wounds. J Trauma 2008;64(Suppl 2):S108–16.
22. Scalea TM, Rodriguez A, Chiu WC, et al. Focused Assessment with Sonography for Trauma (FAST): results from an international consensus conference. J Trauma 1999;46(3):466–72.
23. American College of Emergency Physicians. Use of ultrasound imaging by emergency physicians. Ann Emerg Med 2001;38(4):469–70.
24. Biffl WL, Kaups KL, Cothren CC, et al. Management of patients with anterior abdominal stab wounds: a Western Trauma Association multicenter trial. J Trauma 2009;66(5):1294–301.
25. Rozycki GS, Feliciano DV, Ochsner MG, et al. The role of ultrasound in patients with possible penetrating cardiac wounds: a prospective multicenter study. J Trauma 1999;46(4):543–51.
26. Ball CG, Williams BH, Wyrzykowski AD, et al. A caveat to the performance of pericardial ultrasound in patients with penetrating cardiac wounds. J Trauma 2009;67(5):1123–4.
27. Blackbourne LH, Soffer D, McKenney M, et al. Secondary ultrasound examination increases the sensitivity of the FAST exam in blunt trauma. J Trauma 2004; 57(5):934–8.
28. Rozycki GS, Knudson MM, Shackford SR, et al. Surgeon-performed Bedside Organ Assessment with Sonography after Trauma (BOAST): a pilot study from the WTA Multicenter Group. J Trauma 2005;59(6):1356–64.
29. Kory PD, Pellecchia CM, Shiloh AL, et al. Accuracy of ultrasonography performed by critical care physicians for the diagnosis of DVT. Chest 2011; 139(3):538–42.
30. Reissig A, Copetti R, Kroegel C. Current role of emergency ultrasound of the chest. Crit Care Med 2011;39(4):839–45.
31. Yanagawa Y, Sakamoto T, Okada Y. Hypovolemic shock evaluated by sonographic measurement of the inferior vena cava during resuscitation in trauma patients. J Trauma 2007;63(6):1245–8.
32. Gunst M, Ghaemmaghami V, Sperry J, et al. Accuracy of cardiac function and volume status estimates using the bedside echocardiographic assessment in trauma/critical care. J Trauma 2008;65(3):509–16.
33. Gunst M, Sperry J, Ghaemmaghami V, et al. Bedside echocardiographic assessment for trauma/critical care: the BEAT exam. J Am Coll Surg 2008; 207(3):e1–3.
34. Ferrada P, Murthi S, Anand RJ, et al. Transthoracic focused rapid echocardiographic examination: real-time evaluation of fluid status in critically ill trauma patients. J Trauma 2011;70(1):56–62.
35. Nicolaou S, Talsky A, Khashoggi K, et al. Ultrasound-guided interventional radiology in critical care. Crit Care Med 2007;35(Suppl 5):S186–97.
36. Feller-Kopman D. Ultrasound-guided central venous catheter placement: the new standard of care? Crit Care Med 2005;33(8):1875–7.
37. Fragou M, Gravvanis A, Dimitriou V, et al. Real-time ultrasound-guided subclavian vein cannulation versus the landmark method in critical care patients: a prospective randomized study. Crit Care Med 2011;39(7):1607–12.
38. Warkentine FH, Clyde Pierce M, Lorenz D, et al. The anatomic relationship of femoral vein to femoral artery in euvolemic pediatric patients by ultrasonography: implications for pediatric femoral central venous access. Acad Emerg Med 2008;15(5):426–30.

39. Schweickert WD, Herlitz J, Pohlman AS, et al. A randomized, controlled trial evaluating postinsertion neck ultrasound in peripherally inserted central catheter procedures. Crit Care Med 2009;37(4):1217–21.

40. Doelken P, Strange C. Chest ultrasound for "dummies." Chest 2003;123(2): 332–3.

41. Gordon CE, Feller-Kopman D, Balk EM, et al. Pneumothorax following thoracentesis: a systematic review and meta-analysis. Arch Intern Med 2010;170(4): 332–9.

42. Sandham JD, Hull RD, Brant RF, et al. A randomized, controlled trial of the use of pulmonary-artery catheters in high-risk surgical patients. N Engl J Med 2003; 348(1):5–14.

43. Harvey S, Young D, Brampton W, et al. Pulmonary artery catheters for adult patients in intensive care. Cochrane Database Syst Rev 2006;3:CD003408.

44. Wheeler AP, Bernard GR, Thompson BT, et al. Pulmonary-artery versus central venous catheter to guide treatment of acute lung injury. N Engl J Med 2006; 354(21):2213–24.

45. Richard C, Warszawski J, Anguel N, et al. Early use of the pulmonary artery catheter and outcomes in patients with shock and acute respiratory distress syndrome: a randomized controlled trial. JAMA 2003;290(20):2713–20.

46. Polanczyk CA, Rohde LE, Goldman L, et al. Right heart catheterization and cardiac complications in patients undergoing noncardiac surgery: an observational study. JAMA 2001;286(3):309–14.

47. Vincent JL, Weil MH. Fluid challenge revisited. Crit Care Med 2006;34(5): 1333–7.

48. Chang J, Thompson T, Lavieri M, et al. Improving pulmonary artery catheter waveform interpretation. AMIA Annu Symp Proc 2006;876.

49. Johnston IG, Jane R, Fraser JF, et al. Survey of intensive care nurses' knowledge relating to the pulmonary artery catheter. Anaesth Intensive Care 2004;32(4): 564–8.

50. Trottier SJ, Taylor RW. Physicians' attitudes toward and knowledge of the pulmonary artery catheter: Society of Critical Care Medicine membership survey. New Horiz 1997;5(3):201–6.

51. Gnaegi A, Feihl F, Perret C. Intensive care physicians' insufficient knowledge of right-heart catheterization at the bedside: time to act? Crit Care Med 1997;25(2): 213–20.

52. King DR, Cohn SM, Feinstein AJ, et al. Systemic coagulation changes caused by pulmonary artery catheters: laboratory findings and clinical correlation. J Trauma 2005;59(4):853–7.

53. Chen YY, Yen DH, Yang YG, et al. Comparison between replacement at 4 days and 7 days of the infection rate for pulmonary artery catheters in an intensive care unit. Crit Care Med 2003;31(5):1353–8.

54. Rello J, Coll P, Net A, et al. Infection of pulmonary artery catheters. Epidemiologic characteristics and multivariate analysis of risk factors. Chest 1993;103(1):132–6.

55. Evans DC, Doraiswamy VA, Prosciak MP, et al. Complications associated with pulmonary artery catheters: a comprehensive clinical review. Scand J Surg 2009;98(4):199–208.

56. Pinsky MR, Vincent JL. Let us use the pulmonary artery catheter correctly and only when we need it. Crit Care Med 2005;33(5):1119–22.

57. King DR, Ogilvie MP, Pereira BM, et al. Heart rate variability as a triage tool in patients with trauma during prehospital helicopter transport. J Trauma 2009; 67(3):436–40.

58. Ryan ML, Ogilvie MP, Pereira BM, et al. Heart rate variability is an independent predictor of morbidity and mortality in hemodynamically stable trauma patients. J Trauma 2011;70(6):1371–80.

59. Cooke WH, Salinas J, Convertino VA, et al. Heart rate variability and its association with mortality in prehospital trauma patients. J Trauma 2006;60(2):363–70.

60. Cancio LC, Batchinsky AI, Salinas J, et al. Heart-rate complexity for prediction of prehospital lifesaving interventions in trauma patients. J Trauma 2008;65(4):813–9.

61. Salinas J, Chung KK, Mann EA, et al. Computerized decision support system improves fluid resuscitation following severe burns: an original study. Crit Care Med 2011;39(9):2031–8.

62. Saeed M, Villarroel M, Reisner AT, et al. Multiparameter Intelligent Monitoring in Intensive Care II: a public-access intensive care unit database. Crit Care Med 2011;39(5):952–60.

63. Chen L, Reisner AT, Gribok A, et al. Exploration of prehospital vital sign trends for the prediction of trauma outcomes. J Spec Oper Med 2010;10(3):55–62.

64. Breslow MJ, Rosenfeld BA, Doerfler M, et al. Effect of a multiple-site intensive care unit telemedicine program on clinical and economic outcomes: an alternative paradigm for intensivist staffing. Crit Care Med 2004;32(1):31–8.

65. Lilly CM, Cody S, Zhao H, et al. Hospital mortality, length of stay, and preventable complications among critically ill patients before and after tele-ICU reengineering of critical care processes. JAMA 2011;305(21):2175–83.

66. Morrison JL, Cai Q, Davis N, et al. Clinical and economic outcomes of the electronic intensive care unit: results from two community hospitals. Crit Care Med 2010;38(1):2–8.

67. Latifi R, Hadeed GJ, Rhee P, et al. Initial experiences and outcomes of telepresence in the management of trauma and emergency surgical patients. Am J Surg 2009;198(6):905–10.

68. Rogers FB, Ricci M, Caputo M, et al. The use of telemedicine for real-time video consultation between trauma center and community hospital in a rural setting improves early trauma care: preliminary results. J Trauma 2001;51(6):1037–41.

69. Saffle JR, Edelman L, Theurer L, et al. Telemedicine evaluation of acute burns is accurate and cost-effective. J Trauma 2009;67(2):358–65.

70. Chung KK, Grathwohl KW, Poropatich RK, et al. Robotic telepresence: past, present, and future. J Cardiothorac Vasc Anesth 2007;21(4):593–6.

71. Salinas J, Nguyen R, Darrah MI, et al. Advanced monitoring and decision support for battlefield critical care environment. US Army Med Dep J 2011; APR-JUN:73–81.

72. Fields AM, Fields KM, Cannon JW. Closed-loop systems for drug delivery. Curr Opin Anaesthesiol 2008;21(4):446–51.

73. Haddad WM, Bailey JM. Closed-loop control for intensive care unit sedation. Best Pract Res Clin Anaesthesiol 2009;23(1):95–114.

74. Kacmarek RM. The mechanical ventilator: past, present, and future. Respir Care 2011;56(8):1170–80.

75. Kramer GC, Kinsky MP, Prough DS, et al. Closed-loop control of fluid therapy for treatment of hypovolemia. J Trauma 2008;64(Suppl 4):S333–41.

76. Hypothermia after Cardiac Arrest Study Group. Mild therapeutic hypothermia to improve the neurologic outcome after cardiac arrest. N Engl J Med 2002;346(8): 549–56.

77. Bernard SA, Gray TW, Buist MD, et al. Treatment of comatose survivors of out-of-hospital cardiac arrest with induced hypothermia. N Engl J Med 2002;346(8): 557–63.

78. Borgquist O, Friberg H. Therapeutic hypothermia for comatose survivors after near-hanging—a retrospective analysis. Resuscitation 2009;80(2):210–2.
79. Polderman KH. Induced hypothermia and fever control for prevention and treatment of neurological injuries. Lancet 2008;371:1955–69.
80. Varon J, Acosta P. Therapeutic hypothermia: past, present, and future. Chest 2008;133(5):1267–74.
81. Alam HB, Duggan M, Li Y, et al. Putting life on hold—for how long? Profound hypothermic cardiopulmonary bypass in a swine model of complex vascular injuries. J Trauma 2008;64(4):912–22.
82. Sailhamer EA, Chen Z, Ahuja N, et al. Profound hypothermic cardiopulmonary bypass facilitates survival without a high complication rate in a swine model of complex vascular, splenic, and colon injuries. J Am Coll Surg 2007;204(4):642–53.
83. Tisherman SA, Safar P, Radovsky A, et al. Profound hypothermia (less than 10 degrees C) compared with deep hypothermia (15 degrees C) improves neurologic outcome in dogs after two hours' circulatory arrest induced to enable resuscitative surgery. J Trauma 1991;31(8):1051–61.
84. Emergency preservation and resuscitation (EPR) for cardiac arrest from trauma (EPR-CAT). Available at: http://clinicaltrials.gov/ct2/show/NCT01042015. Accessed December 15, 2011.
85. Ventilation with lower tidal volumes as compared with traditional tidal volumes for acute lung injury and the acute respiratory distress syndrome. The Acute Respiratory Distress Syndrome Network. N Engl J Med 2000;342(18):1301–8.
86. Habashi NM. Other approaches to open-lung ventilation: airway pressure release ventilation. Crit Care Med 2005;33(Suppl 3):S228–40.
87. Brodie D, Bacchetta M. Extracorporeal membrane oxygenation for ARDS in adults. N Engl J Med 2011;365(20):1905–14.
88. Peek GJ, Mugford M, Tiruvoipati R, et al. Efficacy and economic assessment of conventional ventilatory support versus extracorporeal membrane oxygenation for severe adult respiratory failure (CESAR): a multicentre randomised controlled trial. Lancet 2009;374:1351–63.
89. Ruttmann E, Weissenbacher A, Ulmer H, et al. Prolonged extracorporeal membrane oxygenation-assisted support provides improved survival in hypothermic patients with cardiocirculatory arrest. J Thorac Cardiovasc Surg 2007;134(3):594–600.
90. John S, Eckardt KU. Renal replacement strategies in the ICU. Chest 2007;132(4):1379–88.
91. Palevsky PM, Zhang JH, O'Connor TZ, et al. Intensity of renal support in critically ill patients with acute kidney injury. N Engl J Med 2008;359(1):7–20.
92. Cruz D, Bellomo R, Kellum JA, et al. The future of extracorporeal support. Crit Care Med 2008;36(Suppl 4):S243–52.
93. Orgill DP, Bayer LR. Update on negative-pressure wound therapy. Plast Reconstr Surg 2011;127(Suppl 1):105S–15S.
94. Leininger BE, Rasmussen TE, Smith DL, et al. Experience with wound VAC and delayed primary closure of contaminated soft tissue injuries in Iraq. J Trauma 2006;61(5):1207–11.
95. Fabian TC. Damage control in trauma: laparotomy wound management acute to chronic. Surg Clin North Am 2007;87(1):73–93.
96. Diaz JJ Jr, Cullinane DC, Dutton WD, et al. The management of the open abdomen in trauma and emergency general surgery: part 1—damage control. J Trauma 2010;68(6):1425–38.

97. Campbell AM, Kuhn WP, Barker P. Vacuum-assisted closure of the open abdomen in a resource-limited setting. S Afr J Surg 2010;48(4):114–5.
98. Vertrees A, Greer L, Pickett C, et al. Modern management of complex open abdominal wounds of war: a 5-year experience. J Am Coll Surg 2008;207(6): 801–9.
99. Bee TK, Croce MA, Magnotti LJ, et al. Temporary abdominal closure techniques: a prospective randomized trial comparing polyglactin 910 mesh and vacuum-assisted closure. J Trauma 2008;65(2):337–42.
100. Hatch QM, Osterhout LM, Ashraf A, et al. Current use of damage-control laparotomy, closure rates, and predictors of early fascial closure at the first take-back. J Trauma 2011;70(6):1429–36.
101. Lang JL, Gonzalez RP, Aldy KN, et al. Does temporary chest wall closure with or without chest packing improve survival for trauma patients in shock after emergent thoracotomy? J Trauma 2011;70(3):705–9.
102. Utz ER, Elster EA, Tadaki DK, et al. Metalloproteinase expression is associated with traumatic wound failure. J Surg Res 2010;159(2):633–9.
103. Barkun JS, Aronson JK, Feldman LS, et al. Evaluation and stages of surgical innovations. Lancet 2009;374:1089–96.
104. Ergina PL, Cook JA, Blazeby JM, et al. Challenges in evaluating surgical innovation. Lancet 2009;374:1097–104.
105. McCulloch P, Altman DG, Campbell WB, et al. No surgical innovation without evaluation: the IDEAL recommendations. Lancet 2009;374:1105–12.
106. Goldsmith HS, Chandra A. Pyloric valve transposition as substitute for a colostomy in humans: a preliminary report. Am J Surg 2011;202(4):409–16.
107. Neal MD, Alverdy JC, Hall DE, et al. Diverting loop ileostomy and colonic lavage: an alternative to total abdominal colectomy for the treatment of severe, complicated Clostridium difficile associated disease. Ann Surg 2011;254(3):423–7.
108. Blazeby JM, Blencowe NS, Titcomb DR, et al. Demonstration of the IDEAL recommendations for evaluating and reporting surgical innovation in minimally invasive oesophagectomy. Br J Surg 2011;98(4):544–51.
109. Demetriades D, Velmahos GC, Scalea TM, et al. Diagnosis and treatment of blunt thoracic aortic injuries: changing perspectives. J Trauma 2008;64(6): 1415–8.
110. Curfman GD, Redberg RF. Medical devices–balancing regulation and innovation. N Engl J Med 2011;365(11):975–7.
111. Challoner DR, Vodra WW. Medical devices and health—creating a new regulatory framework for moderate-risk devices. N Engl J Med 2011;365(11):977–9.
112. Blackbourne LH, Baer DG, Cestero RF, et al. Exsanguination shock: the next frontier in prevention of battlefield mortality. J Trauma 2011;71(Suppl 1):S1–3.
113. White JM, Cannon JW, Stannard A, et al. Endovascular balloon occlusion of the aorta is superior to resuscitative thoracotomy with aortic clamping in a porcine model of hemorrhagic shock. Surgery 2011;150(3):400–9.
114. Martinelli T, Thony F, Declety P, et al. Intra-aortic balloon occlusion to salvage patients with life-threatening hemorrhagic shocks from pelvic fractures. J Trauma 2010;68(4):942–8.
115. Spinella PC, Perkins JG, Grathwohl KW, et al. Warm fresh whole blood is independently associated with improved survival for patients with combat-related traumatic injuries. J Trauma 2009;66(Suppl 4):S69–76.
116. Mayberry JC, Ham LB, Schipper PH, et al. Surveyed opinion of American trauma, orthopedic, and thoracic surgeons on rib and sternal fracture repair. J Trauma 2009;66(3):875–9.

Long-Range Critical Care Evacuation and Reoperative Surgery

David Zonies, MD, MPH[a,b],*

KEYWORDS

- Military medicine • Aeromedical transport • Critical care air transport
- Damage control • Extracorporeal membrane oxygenation

KEY POINTS

- Advanced long-range critical care transport has significantly reduced evacuation times during recent military conflict.
- Flight physiology increases the complexity of critical care transport during long-range patient movement. Special consideration must be given to trauma care during en-route resuscitation.
- Specialized transport teams are evolving to provide rescue therapies such as adult extracorporeal membrane oxygenation and specialized burn care.
- The military critical care transport team may serve as a model for civilian practice. Joint military-civilian programs may provide improved capability for national disaster planning.
- Protocol-based follow-on care during evacuation optimizes patient outcome.

INTRODUCTION

Staged evacuation through multiple echelons of care has been the hallmark of medical treatment during the current conflicts in Iraq and Afghanistan. The development and maturation of the US Air Force Critical Care Air Transport Team (CCATT) has been key in the rapid movement of critically injured service members, providing a survival advantage. Aggressive early surgery, hemostatic resuscitation, and ongoing surgical management throughout the continuum of care have been major successes in recent combat operations.

In previous conflicts, movement of patients out of the theater of operations ranged from weeks to months.[1] During Vietnam, the average length of stay before patients

The views and opinions expressed in this article are those of the author and do not reflect the official policy or position of the US Air Force, US Department of Defense, or the US Government.
[a] Department of Trauma & Critical Care, Landstuhl Regional Medical Center, CMR 402, Box 1824, APO, AE 09180, Germany; [b] 86th MDS Acute Lung Rescue Team, Ramstein AB, Germany
* Corresponding author. Department of Trauma & Critical Care, Landstuhl Regional Medical Center, CMR 402, Box 1824, APO, AE 09180.
E-mail address: david.zonies@amedd.army.mil

Surg Clin N Am 92 (2012) 925–937
doi:10.1016/j.suc.2012.05.001
0039-6109/12/$ – see front matter Published by Elsevier Inc.

were moved to the continental United States (CONUS) was 45 days. The current military structure of evacuation holds a dictum that patients must continue to move along the system of care as early as physiologically possible. As a result of this enhanced capability, rapid aeromedical transport of patients from point of injury to their final destination outside the theater of operations now occurs in 4 to 5 days.

The long-range transport of trauma patients in a mobile intensive care unit (ICU) has evolved over the past 2 decades. Rapid evacuation with interval reoperative surgery in a damage-control fashion continues to improve outcome for patients. Such lessons learned from current military conflicts will be important for future conflicts, and may be a model for civilian practice in natural disasters and humanitarian response.

HISTORY

The United States aeromedical evacuation (AE) system started in 1943 when the Army Air Corps (pre–United States Air Force [USAF]) began training medical crews at Bowman Field, Kentucky. The Corps developed a multipurpose airframe that provided large cargo space for transporting equipment and troops to the combat zone. On the return trip, the cabin compartment was reconfigured to carry patients. This modification provided combatant commanders the ability to rapidly transport wounded warriors to medical facilities for specialized care.

Throughout World War II, more than 1 million patients were moved by air transport. By the early 1950s, the newly established USAF committed assets such that during peacetime or conflict, the movement of combat casualties would primarily occur by airlift. This policy has stood for more than 50 years and remains the primary mode of casualty evacuation from theaters of conflict.

During the cold war, military operations became smaller and more mobile (**Fig. 1**). A new requirement was identified to develop a deployable medical asset scaled to fit the smaller operation. With movement away from the traditional fixed combat support hospital, a mobile forward surgical team (FST) was developed. The FST comprises general and orthopedic surgeons, anesthesia, and operating-room nursing, which permits early resuscitation and surgery closer to combat operations in a far-forward

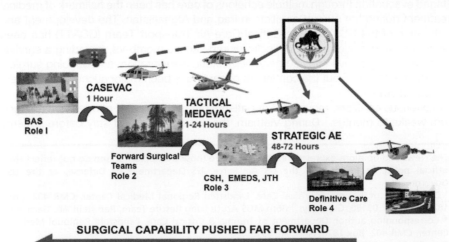

Fig. 1. Route from injury to definitive care. AE, aeromedical evacuation; BAS, battalion aid station; CASEVAC, casualty evacuation; CSH, combat support hospital; EMEDS, expeditionary medical system; JTH, joint theater hospital; MEDEVAC, medical evacuation.

location. Coincident with the development of the smaller team concept, damage-control surgery was emerging as a new management paradigm that had clear applications for the management of combat injuries and fit well with the FST doctrine. The FST would treat acute injury for several hours and might perform initial surgery, but did not have long-term holding capacity for the critically ill patient in the immediate postoperative period.

With a change in the paradigm of surgical care, a gap existed in the transfer of ICU-level care among those who may be stabilized but not appropriate for standard AE by medical attendants or flight nurses. Movement within the theater to the next echelon without decrement in quality of care required evacuation by a more advanced team. The USAF identified this need and developed the advanced-care CCATT in the mid-1990s. With advances in critical care and the miniaturization of equipment (ventilators, transport monitors, suction devices), the types of patients qualifying for urgent transport transitioned from stable casualties to some of the most critically ill polytrauma patients only hours or days postinjury.

TEAM COMPOSITION

CCATT is a 3-person specialized team that augments the AE system. Each CCATT comprises 3 members:

- Physician trained in a high-acuity specialty
- ICU-level nurse
- Cardiopulmonary respiratory therapist.

Physicians include those from the fields of surgical critical care, pulmonary critical care, emergency medicine, anesthesia, and cardiology. Nurses are experienced in surgical ICU care and typically have been deployed previously as ground-based ICU nurses. Similarly, cardiopulmonary respiratory therapists must be adept in ventilator management and typically have previously been deployed as ground-based technicians. Each team member is specially selected for the mission and must maintain proficiency within their respective field. In addition, all members must complete an initial didactic course at the USAF School of Aerospace Medicine (Wright-Patterson AFB, Dayton, OH, USA) where key principles of flight physiology, austere care, crew resource management, and familiarization with equipment is covered. In addition, all members must qualify in an altitude chamber and master evacuation procedures during potential mid-air emergencies.

Before each deployment cycle, all members must validate their proficiency at a specially designated CCATT training center in Cincinnati, Ohio. Based at a level-I trauma clinical site, this 2-week course focuses on current clinical updates and reviews lessons learned from previous CCATT deployments. Team building is a major focus of validation, with complex patient scenarios presented in a realistic flight simulator. Once each team member passes the validation phase, they are assigned to a CCATT.

To optimize both patient safety and casualty throughput, each CCATT may care for a maximum of 6 critically ill patients including up to 3 on a ventilator. In the event of additional casualties requiring urgent evacuation, additional CCATTs are added to the aircraft.

In years past, specific aircraft were designated for medical evacuation. The C-9 Nightingale, a modified McDonnell Douglas C-9, was used from 1968 to 2005. During the current conflicts, CCATTs use aircraft of opportunity: airframes designed primarily for cargo transport are reconfigured for patient movement. This environment presents multiple environmental challenges beyond clinical care. Noise levels in certain aircraft may exceed 90 dB, requiring all crewmembers to wear ear protection. Loss of audible patient evaluation requires constant visual vigilance of the patient and monitoring systems. To mitigate some sensory loss, noise-reduction communication headsets permit intrateam dialog that may be invaluable. An additional environmental consideration for patient movement is vibration. Although the patient is secured to litter stanchions, considerable vibration and turbulence may be accentuated during missions, requiring steep ascent or descent when altitude must be rapidly achieved or lost during combat operations.

CCATTs must be cognizant of the hypobaric environment in this mobile ICU, where the typical cabin pressure is set to 8000 ft. General considerations include interval monitoring of endotracheal cuffs to prevent overdistention or rupture. Any possible or potential gas-filled space must be evaluated and monitored for expansion. Chest drains must be properly vented and the stomach decompressed, and injuries placing a patient at potential risk require preflight evaluation and en-route vigilance. Such injuries include occult pneumothoraces, progression of pneumocephalus in severe traumatic brain injury, and ocular gas expansion. Without x-ray capability mid air, teams are now being trained to use portable ultrasound to aid in mid-air diagnosis of these potential complications.

Flight times may be as long as 12 hours from the combat zone to the regional medical center in Europe. Typical en-route evacuation from the combat zone to Landstuhl Medical Center, Germany, occurs on the Globemaster III C-17 (**Fig. 2**). This aircraft is the primary AE aircraft for long-range transport. With on-board oxygen supply, ambient lighting, and temperature control, this aircraft has assumed the primary responsibility for AE/CCATT patient movement.

LONG-RANGE EN-ROUTE CARE

Successful long-range ICU missions at 36,000 ft are predicated on detailed preparation using principles of crew resource management.[2] Checklists and transparent communication among all team members are key to uncomplicated movement of patients. Any potential contingency needs to be addressed before transportation to include needs for ongoing administration of blood products. Using principles of damage-control resuscitation, teams may transport patients with packed red blood cells, fresh frozen plasma, and occasionally fresh whole blood available from downrange facilities.[3] Clinically relevant thrombocytopenia must be addressed preflight, as platelets cannot logistically be flown because of the need for continuous agitation.

Oxygen consumption requirements, battery life for units, and medication requirements are planned for a 72-hour contingency. This factor is built in to the mission should there be a mechanical diversion or tactical reason for delayed transport of patients. For

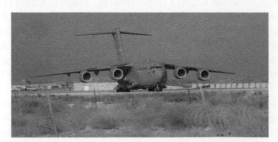

Fig. 2. C-17 Globemaster, which serves as the primary CCATT platform for long-range patient transport.

aircraft without on-board oxygen, CCATTs travel with portable compressed liquid oxygen. Ventilator adjustments may be made as the patient transitions from the ground-based ventilator to a transport ventilator. The currently approved system for use aboard USAF airframes is the Uni-Vent Eagle Impact 754 (Impact Instrumentation, West Caldwell, NJ, USA). This internal compressor system permits volume-controlled (VC) ventilation with flow rates up to 60 L/min. For patients intolerant of VC ventilation or those requiring higher gas flow, the Pulmonetics LTV 1000 (Pulmonetics Systems, Minneapolis, MN, USA) is an alternative ventilator that provides pressure control and intermittent ventilation, with flows of up to 100 L/min. Next-generation ventilators that produce additional alternative modes are currently under investigation for airworthiness.

Given the complex nature of single teams transporting multiple critically injured patients over long distances, there has been a movement toward automating many of the current provider functions. Moreover, weight limitations may exist in tactical environments requiring conservation of resources. Johannigman and colleagues[4] have recently demonstrated the value of autonomous control of oxygen delivery during mechanical ventilation. A control algorithm was used to adjust oxygen delivery intermittently targeting an Spo_2 above 94% $\pm$ 2%. A 44% reduction in oxygen use was observed, allowing the opportunity for conservation of resources.

Future research initiatives may extend beyond autonomous ventilators, to include targeted closed-loop feedback resuscitation devices. With the use of noninvasive devices such as peripheral tissue oxygen monitors, such technologies would permit precise upregulation or downregulation of fluids and vasopressor support in a more rapid fashion than human control. Several Department of Defense (DoD) research centers are continuing to develop such technologies in an effort to augment the CCATT and potentially improve patients' outcome.

Many en-route clinical practices are an extension of the Joint Theater Trauma System's Clinical Practice Guideline (CPG) program.[5] As many of these patients are still in the early resuscitation phase, it is paramount that the high-level support be maintained throughout the chain of care. For example, early in the Iraq war it was identified that burn resuscitation was inconsistent with both underresuscitation and overresuscitation. In 2006, the burn CPG was established, and fluid resuscitation is now consistently documented and reviewed throughout all echelons of care.[6] CCATTs play a critical role during resuscitation, as many of these patients are moved within 24 hours of thermal injury.

One of the most difficult casualties to transport is the patient with severe traumatic brain injury (TBI). In attempts to mitigate a "second hit" of hypoxia or hypotension, there have been legitimate concerns over the process of AE itself. Between the physiologic stress of flight and the evolution of brain injury, the timing of transport remains controversial. A potential increased risk of intracranial pressure, reduction of cerebral blood flow, and worsening cerebral edema during the first few days after primary injury gives pause as to the proper timing of the patient's movement.[7] Neuroinflammatory cytokines and chemokines modulate the neurotropic response to injury, and it remains unclear whether the physiologic changes at altitude modulate this response. As a surrogate marker, patients with a Glasgow Coma Score of 8 or worse will routinely be monitored by an intracranial pressure (ICP) monitor or ventriculostomy.[8] Teams may continue to manage patients with hyperosmolar therapy during the immediate postoperative phase or even as part of a nonoperative management strategy. Between January 2007 and June 2008, 12% of patients had the diagnosis of TBI, the majority (80%) ventilated, with a third requiring invasive neural monitoring. Even though it is one of the signature injuries of the current conflict, no data exist on the physiologic effects of long-range transport of patients who sustain a mild TBI. Ongoing research efforts are examining the relationships between g-force, altitude change, and ICP.

LONG-RANGE TRANSPORT LOGISTICS

With patients moving through various time zones, Zulu time (Greenwich Mean Time, GMT + 0) is used for mission planning and in-flight documentation. This global standard used by the flying community reduces the risk of missed medication doses and permits both sending and receiving facilities to be clear about the timing of procedures and operations. Furthermore, on all transport medical records, significant clinical events are dated using the Julian calendar system for uniform reference.

The CCATT equipment package weighs approximately 700 lb (317.5 kg). Each piece of medical equipment must be certified as airworthy for use aboard all transport-capable military aircraft. Because of the special nature of military operations, the process of airworthiness certification exceeds that of the civilian Federal Aviation Administration. Each piece of equipment must pass baseline testing of environmental extremes (aircraft vibration, temperatures from −40° to 140°C, humidity ∼95%), endure acceleration up to 9 g-forces in multiple directions, function at an unpressurized altitude of 18,000 ft, and tolerate emergent rapid decompression (rapid altitude change from 8000 to 45,000 ft). The equipment must not produce or be affected by electromagnetic interference and cannot risk fire during gaseous vapor testing. Once the equipment meets standard, it must validate properly on a patient in flight. In cases where equipment may be critically required but has not undergone formal testing, a waiver for flight may be obtained, which is performed on a case-by-case basis through the USAF Air Mobility Command.

A recent example of the airworthiness process was approval of a negative pressure wound therapy (NPWT) system for open soft-tissue wounds and management of the open abdomen. Although this equipment had been used both in theater and at fixed facilities since 2003, NPWT was not approved for flight. Consequently, patients were routinely converted to wet-to-dry dressings preevacuation. Ultimately in 2006, an commercial system approved by the Food and Drug Administration was certified as airworthy (Vac Freedom System; Kinetic Concept, Inc, San Antonio, TX, USA), permitting the routine use of NPWT during aeromedical transport. An observational study of combat casualties confirmed the feasibility and logistics surrounding such equipment, allaying fears of in-flight equipment failure.[9]

Any piece of medical equipment placed at the time of transfer will follow the patient throughout the evacuation chain. All such patient movement items (PMI) are tracked through the Patient Movement Items Tracking System, a bar-code–based tracking database. PMI is serviced and recycled at various hubs throughout the evacuation chain, ultimately returning to facilities in theater.

SPECIALIZED LONG-RANGE TRANSPORT TEAMS

Since the early 1950s, the US Army Burn Flight Team (BFT) has been transporting severely burned patients to definitive care in the DoD Burn Center in San Antonio, Texas. In the current conflict, the BFT transports patients from Europe back to the United States. Over a 4-year period (2003–2007), 540 burned military casualties were transferred to the US Burn Center. Two hundred six (38%) patients were transported on 57 missions by the BFT and 174 (32%) were transported by a standard CCATT.[10] More than 94% of transferred patients survived their injuries. As an augmentation team to the CCATT package, the BFT brings additional expertise of burn-wound management and specialized ventilator management to the patient with inhalation injury. Approximately 12% of transferred patients have direct evidence of inhalation injury, and the BFT equipment complement includes fiberoptic bronchoscopy and alternative modes of ventilation to include the high-frequency percussive ventilation. As a hospital-based team, the lead physician of the burn team provides continuity of care as he or she becomes the patient's attending surgeon.

Approximately 12% of trauma patients will develop an acute lung injury.[11,12] Among those who progress to acute respiratory distress syndrome (ARDS), 16% will fail conventional ventilation. Further, ARDS has been shown to be independently associated with in-hospital mortality.[11] Early during combat operations, a cohort of patients with ARDS exceeding standard CCATT capability for en-route pulmonary support began to emerge. These patients were not supported by the standard transport ventilators or exceeded the clinical expertise of CCATT personnel. This cohort of patients identified at the combat support hospital precluded safe CCATT transport, requiring rescue therapy. Patients either improved slowly over time to meet criteria for AE (CCATT) or died of severe respiratory failure in theater.

Physicians at the receiving facility in Landstuhl, Germany identified this capability gap. A dedicated team of medical and surgical intensivists instituted specialized therapies unavailable to the standard CCATT mission. In 2005, the Acute Lung Rescue Team (ALRT) was developed to augment the CCATT mission. All team members are based at Landstuhl's ICU and are experienced in the care of polytrauma patients with severe ARDS. The team consists of 2 physicians, critical care nurses, and respiratory therapists. Redundancy at each position is required because of high-stress mission times that exceed 24 continuous duty hours. In addition to competence in standard CCATT requirements, all are skillful in the use of advanced ventilator modes and extracorporeal membrane oxygenation (ECMO).

The ALRT team carries an expanded medication supply to support a critically ill patient with severe ARDS. In addition to vasopressor support, inhaled epoprostenol (iPGI$_2$, Flolan; GlaxoSmith-Kline, Triangle Park, NC, USA) is available as adjuvant therapy in life-threatening hypoxic pulmonary failure. A nitric oxide analogue delivered via inhalation, epoprostenol preferentially vasodilates well-ventilated areas of the pulmonary vasculature and improves arterial oxygenation.[13] An additional adjunct used by the team for controlling CO_2 during lung protective permissive hypercapnea and severe respiratory acidosis is Tris-hydroxymethyl aminomethane (THAM). In the presence of multiorgan failure, THAM may effectively control acidosis and contribute to the reversal of cellular dysfunction.[14]

Alternative ventilator modes used by ALRT include bilevel and high-frequency percussive ventilation. As both a hospital-based and transport-capable ventilator, the volumetric diffusive respirator (VDR-4; Percussionaire Corp., Sandpoint, ID, USA) is an attractive option for rescue ventilation (**Fig. 3**). This salvage instrument is a pressure-limited, subtidal volume, high-frequency mode.[15] The VDR has been associated

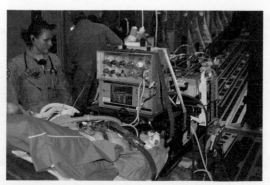

Fig. 3. VDR-4 applied to a patient with refractory hypoxic ARDS.

with improved clearance of particulate matter resulting from inhalation injury, and is an alternative mode when low-volume, lung-protective strategies fail. One logistic limitation for transport is that the unit requires an external compressor for conversion to 50 psi, and one has been waived for special air transport.

Several technological advances for rescue therapy have occurred primarily within Europe and principally with the aid of clinical expertise at the University Hospital in Regensburg, Germany. The clinical expertise at this regional referral ECMO center was leveraged with the operational requirement to rescue the most severely injured patients. In addition, the miniaturization and advanced technology of arteriovenous and venovenous lung assistance made it possible to apply these therapies for long-range casualty transport. Initial transportation of patients in combined hypoxic and hypercarbic ARDS-associated respiratory failure was managed on a percutaneous arteriovenous extracorporeal CO_2-removal lung-assist device (NovaLung iLA, Hechingen, Germany). Recently, the team acquired a transport-capable ECMO unit (Rotaflow; Maquet Corp., Rastatt, Germany), replacing the primary requirement for the NovaLung device. With minimal priming and a favorable hemodynamic profile, the venovenous system is ideal for patients requiring evacuation who are too unstable for alternative ventilator options. Percutaneous cannulation is achieved using the Seldinger technique either at 2 sites (typically right internal jugular and femoral veins) or a single site using a dual-lumen bicaval catheter (Avalon Laboratories, Rancho Dominguez, CA). Several combat casualties have already been evacuated from the combat zone using venovenous ECMO, with a 100% survival rate (**Fig. 4**A, B).[16]

The decision to activate the ALRT is based on several factors and involves a dialog between the team director and the ground personnel. A retrospective review of lung-team patients identified average Fio_2 requirements of 0.92 ± 0.11 versus 0.53 ± 0.14 among CCATT patients. Likewise, positive end-expiratory pressure support was higher (19.0 ± 2.2 vs 6.5 ± 2.4 cm H_2O).[17] Although the ALRT team capability is currently based in Europe, future plans include expansion to multiple teams permitting worldwide transport.

IMPLICATIONS FOR CIVILIAN PRACTICE

CCATT, including the standard package and specialty teams (BFT and ALRT), has application to civilian practice.

Many hospitals prepare for natural and man-made disasters by focusing on internal infrastructure and prehospital coordination.[18,19] In general, hospitals may surge their critical care capability 20% to 50% without significant impact on services.[20] However, when patient load exceeds critical care capacity, hospitals will have to either divert,

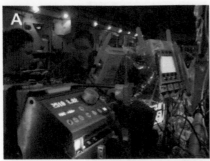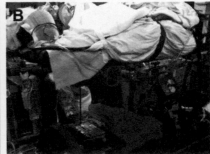

Fig. 4. (*A*) ECMO drive unit (foreground) during tactical maneuvers. (*B*) Patient on venovenous ECMO circuit with LTV-1000 transport ventilator.

retriage, or transfer patients to participating centers within a disaster-plan network. CCATT serves as an autonomous mobile ICU team that may augment hospital-based care, seamlessly transfer critically ill patients to disaster-plan hospitals, or transfer patients to accepting facilities hundreds of miles away. Because CCATT doctrine stipulates care for patients of up to 3 days, CCATT may act as a force multiplier.

Examples whereby CCATT could have augmented or provided rapid evacuation of multiple critically ill patients include the New York attacks in 2001, Hurricane Katrina in 2005, and more recently the 2011 Japanese Tohoku earthquake and tsunami. Occasionally, CCATT support has been requested during joint military-civilian operations.[21,22] After the Haiti earthquake in 2010, CCATTs were activated during Operation Unified Response, transporting critically ill patients from Port-au-Prince to South Florida.[23]

On request, the BFT may serve as a regional resource for homeland defense. With a limited number of verified burn centers throughout the United States, the BFT may serve as an extension of burn/critical care in resource-limited locations and transport large numbers of casualties to any location after a burn disaster. Similarly, the ALRT may serve as a long-range transport option for patients with severe pulmonary compromise requiring alternative modes of ventilation or extracorporeal lung support. Possible utility of ALRT was seen as recently as the global influenza A (H1N1) outbreak in 2009. Over a short period (3 months), 68 patients underwent ECMO support for refractory hypoxia in Australia and New Zealand.[24] Should a similar event occur on the West Coast of the United States or another location thus overwhelming critical care resources, The ALRT could serve as an adult transport team.

At present, many pediatric hospitals and some adult hospitals offer critical care ground transport within their catchment area.[25,26] Using a CCATT model and additional national infrastructure, these teams could be used to respond to regional disasters along with military CCATT. Such a response would permit the appropriate distribution of patients throughout a given region.

REOPERATIVE SURGERY AND CRITICAL CARE AT THE FIXED FACILITY

Patients undergoing strategic AE from the area of combat operations transit through the regional resource trauma center in Landstuhl, Germany. Landstuhl Regional Medical Center (LRMC) is the only American College of Surgeons level-I verified trauma center outside of CONUS, and 1 of 2 verified centers in the DoD. LRMC is staffed with more than 3000 personnel and offers care in more than 40 specialties. As the sole regional medical center, catchment includes patients from Europe, Africa, and Southwest Asia.

Patients transported aboard the Globemaster III C-17 arrive at the nearby Ramstein Air Force Base and are then transferred to a modified ambulance bus for a 40-minute transit to LRMC ICU (**Fig. 5**). At the time of patient transfer, the casualty is typically 72 to 96 hours after injury.

Before arrival, a patient-movement record is electronically transmitted from the sending facility to LRMC. The package includes a description of injuries and previous interventions, operative notes, current medication infusions, used equipment, and recent laboratory values. In addition, all previously performed radiographs and computed tomography (CT) scans are "pushed" forward to the picture-archiving communication system. The receiving team will typically be alerted to incoming patients 8 hours before arrival. All reports and images are reviewed to assist in planning the operative day and movement of patients.

On arrival, care is transferred to the Trauma/ICU service following a formal handoff from the CCATT team leader to the ICU staff physician. The LRMC trauma critical care

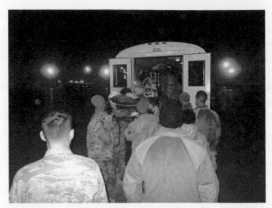

Fig. 5. Transfer of a CCATT patient from the ambulance bus to the aircraft.

team is a multidisciplinary, intensivist-based service. Initial concerns during transfer of care include stabilization after long-range transport and detailed reevaluation. As patients may be arriving during the second phase of damage control (see the article by Chovanes and colleagues elsewhere in this issue), the CCATT is met by a trauma surgeon and intensivist at the bedside.[27]

On arrival at the ICU, all patients undergo the following:

- Replacement of all invasive vascular catheters
- Full-body scrub with 4% chlorhexidine
- Screening culture assessment
- Institution of contact precautions with environmental isolation.

Patients are cleared from isolation once screening cultures return negative. This practice has evolved to mitigate the risk of gram-negative multidrug-resistant infections observed during the earlier years of the Iraq conflict. With patients developing severe multidrug-resistant *Acinetobacter baumanii* infection, these early practices have resulted in the near complete eradication of this organism from this ICU.[28]

After meeting established end points of resuscitation, patients are brought to the operating theater for wound evaluation and serial debridement when indicated. Among United States casualties, definitive extremity wound management is typically deferred because of the short stay in Europe. Patients presenting with an open abdomen may undergo serial washout, restoration of gastrointestinal continuity, or fascial closure when appropriate. At the time of abdominal closure, a distal feeding catheter is placed. In the case of abdominal and thoracic cases that may have had multiple operative teams in multiple facilities, plain radiographs are obtained to rule out retained sponges or instruments.

The hallmark injury pattern in this patient population has been extensive extremity soft-tissue trauma with multiple amputations. Initial wound management is performed in the combat zone with the placement of a negative pressure dressing. These patients then undergo serial and often aggressive wound debridement when areas of necrosis are identified. Some patients with high-level (proximal) extremity amputations have developed invasive fungal infection, likely due to soil inoculation from the initial high-energy blast. Currently under intensive investigation, a blast tissue protocol has been instituted in high-risk patients to identify these organisms for targeted antifungal therapy.

With an average length of stay of 3.3 days, the focus of the Landstuhl Trauma/ICU mission is patient optimization for trans-Atlantic transport to the United States. The critical care interventions performed during a patient's course at LRMC are listed in **Table 1**. A few of these practices bear special mention. Cervical spine clearance is attempted after evaluation of the patient and all radiographs. In the case of the obtunded patient, magnetic resonance imaging in addition to reformatted CT images may be used to clear a cervical spine. A screening lower extremity duplex is performed on all ICU patients, as the risk of deep vein thrombosis and pulmonary embolus is increased in this population.[29] With large injury burden, these catabolic patients receive critical care nutrition consultation. An endoscopically placed nasojejunal feeding catheter is inserted within 24 hours of arrival if one was not previously placed at the time of surgery. This action prevents nutrition from being held during operative cases, and lessens the risk of aspiration during the hypobaric environment of future intercontinental transport whereby hollow viscous distention is a concern. Finally, for patients with renal insufficiency, the Trauma/ICU service provides intensivist-led continuous renal replacement therapy until the patient is physiologically safe for transfer to the United States.

On the morning of departure, the outbound CCATT rounds as part of the multidisciplinary service and receives clearance for patient movement by the attending trauma surgeon. Combat casualties from coalition allies are either repatriated to their home country or receive their definitive care at LRMC. Over the last 5 years (2007–2011), LRMC has cared for more than 8000 trauma patients, 29% requiring ICU-level management. With a mean ICU injury severity score (ISS) of 19, 21% of LRMC trauma patients have an ISS of 16 or greater. Patients capable of returning to theater within 30 days remain at LRMC for their care and rehabilitation. Since 2004 approximately 14,000 patients (21%) have returned to combat from LRMC, which has proved invaluable in terms of preserving our fighting force.

Surgeons at LRMC have the unique perspective of observing all combat casualties evacuated from theaters of combat operations. As part of a robust performance-improvement program, several observations have led to improvements throughout the continuum of care. A review of patients in the period 2005 to 2006 identified 17% of 336 patients who required extremity fasciotomy revision. At the time of follow-on surgery, 35% required additional muscle excision.[30] It was observed that the anterior and deep compartments were most commonly missed or inadequately extended. Such observations led to improvements in predeployment training that now includes 4-compartment fasciotomy training on human cadavers.

Table 1	
Critical care interventions performed at LRMC	
General	Formal tertiary survey
	Attempt to clear the cervical spine
	Ultrasound screen for occult deep venous thrombosis
Neurologic	Invasive monitoring for severe TBI
	Neuroprotective measures
Pulmonary	Alternative ventilator support options (HFPV, HFOV)
	VV-ECMO, VA-ECMO
Nutrition	Endoscopic placement of NJ feeding catheter
Renal	Intensivist-run CRRT

Abbreviations: CRRT, continuous renal replacement therapy; HFOV, High-frequency oscillatory ventilation; HFPV, high-frequency percussive ventilation; NJ, nasal-jejunal; TBI, traumatic brain injury; VA-ECMO, venoarterial extracorporeal membrane oxygenation; VV-ECMO, venovenous extracorporeal membrane oxygenation.

SUMMARY

Despite the complexity associated with critical care evacuation in the austere environment, the USAF CCATT program has transported more than 8000 critically injured casualties since 2001. The associated mortality rate has consistently remained below 1%, a testament to the high standards required for this unique mission. In recent years, improvements in technology and clinical expertise have brought advanced care to wounded warriors never seen previously.

En-route critical care has dramatically changed the chances of survival with a good functional outcome. The maturation of the military trauma system will continue to codify this experience and may provide structural examples to improve civilian trauma system practices. En-route critical care, specialty teams, and military trauma centers remain on alert to support the movement of the most critically ill and injured patients in a dedicated effort to give every soldier, airman, sailor, and marine a chance to return home from their service.

REFERENCES

1. Morris MJ. Acute respiratory distress syndrome in combat casualties: military medicine and advances in mechanical ventilation. Mil Med 2006;171(11): 1039–44.
2. Eisen LA, Savel RH. What went right: lessons for the intensivist from the crew of US airways flight 1549. Chest 2009;136(3):910–7.
3. Holcomb JB. Damage control resuscitation. J Trauma 2007;62(Suppl 6):S36–7.
4. Johannigman JA, Branson R, Lecroy D, et al. Autonomous control of inspired oxygen concentration during mechanical ventilation of the critically injured trauma patient. J Trauma 2009;66(2):386–92.
5. Joint trauma system clinical practice guidelines. 2012; CPGs. Available at: http://www.usaisr.amedd.army.mil/clinical_practice_guidelines.html. Accessed June 14, 2012.
6. JTS burn clinical practice guidelines. 2012; CPGs. Available at: http://www.usaisr.amedd.army.mil/assets/cpgs/Burn_Care_21_Nov_2008.pdf. Accessed June 14, 2012.
7. Goodman MD, Makley AT, Lentsch AB, et al. Traumatic brain injury and aeromedical evacuation: when is the brain fit to fly? J Surg Res 2010;164(2):286–93.
8. JTS neurotrauma clinical practice guidelines. 2012; CPGs. Available at: http://www.usaisr.amedd.army.mil/assets/cpgs/Mgmt_of_Patients_with_%20Severe_Head_Trauma_7_Mar_12.pdf. Accessed June 14, 2012.
9. Fang R, Dorlac WC, Flaherty SF, et al. Feasibility of negative pressure wound therapy during intercontinental aeromedical evacuation of combat casualties. J Trauma 2010;69(Suppl 1):S140–5.
10. Renz EM, Cancio LC, Barillo DJ, et al. Long range transport of war-related burn casualties. J Trauma 2008;64(Suppl 2):S136–44 [discussion: S144–35].
11. Shah CV, Localio AR, Lanken PN, et al. The impact of development of acute lung injury on hospital mortality in critically ill trauma patients. Crit Care Med 2008; 36(8):2309–15.
12. Treggiari MM, Hudson LD, Martin DP, et al. Effect of acute lung injury and acute respiratory distress syndrome on outcome in critically ill trauma patients. Crit Care Med 2004;32(2):327–31.
13. Reily DJ, Tollok E, Mallitz K, et al. Successful aeromedical transport using inhaled prostacyclin for a patient with life-threatening hypoxemia. Chest 2004;125(4): 1579–81.

14. Kallet RH, Jasmer RM, Luce JM, et al. The treatment of acidosis in acute lung injury with tris-hydroxymethyl aminomethane (THAM). Am J Respir Crit Care Med 2000;161(4 Pt 1):1149–53.
15. Allan PF, Osborn EC, Chung KK, et al. High-frequency percussive ventilation revisited. J Burn Care Res 2010;31(4):510–20.
16. Cannon JW, Zonies DH, Benfield RJ, et al. Advanced en-route critical care during combat operations. Bull Am Coll Surg 2011;96(5):21–9.
17. Dorlac GR, Fang R, Pruitt VM, et al. Air transport of patients with severe lung injury: development and utilization of the acute lung rescue team. J Trauma 2009;66(Suppl 4):S164–71.
18. Hick JL, Christian MD, Sprung CL. Chapter 2. Surge capacity and infrastructure considerations for mass critical care. Recommendations and standard operating procedures for intensive care unit and hospital preparations for an influenza epidemic or mass disaster. Intensive Care Med 2010;36(Suppl 1):S11–20.
19. Sprung CL, Kesecioglu J. Chapter 5. Essential equipment, pharmaceuticals and supplies. Recommendations and standard operating procedures for intensive care unit and hospital preparations for an influenza epidemic or mass disaster. Intensive Care Med 2010;36(Suppl 1):S38–44.
20. Rubinson L, Nuzzo JB, Talmor DS, et al. Augmentation of hospital critical care capacity after bioterrorist attacks or epidemics: recommendations of the Working Group on emergency mass critical care. Crit Care Med 2005;33(10):2393–403.
21. Alkins SA, Reynolds AJ. Long-distance air evacuation of blast-injured sailors from the U.S.S. Cole. Aviat Space Environ Med 2002;73(7):677–80.
22. Cancio LC. Airplane crash in Guam, August 6, 1997: the aeromedical evacuation response. J Burn Care Res 2006;27(5):642–8.
23. Kaufman D. Air foce medics evacuating critically ill from Haiti. 2010. Available at: http://www.afmc.af.mil/news/story.asp?id=123187478. Accessed March 1, 2012.
24. Davies A, Jones D, Bailey M, et al. Extracorporeal membrane oxygenation for 2009 influenza A(H1N1) acute respiratory distress syndrome. JAMA 2009; 302(17):1888–95.
25. Orr RA, Felmet KA, Han Y, et al. Pediatric specialized transport teams are associated with improved outcomes. Pediatrics 2009;124(1):40–8.
26. Gebremichael M, Borg U, Habashi NM, et al. Interhospital transport of the extremely ill patient: the mobile intensive care unit. Crit Care Med 2000;28(1): 79–85.
27. Rotondo MF, Zonies DH. The damage control sequence and underlying logic. Surg Clin North Am 1997;77(4):761–77.
28. Hospenthal DR, Crouch HK, English JF, et al. Multidrug-resistant bacterial colonization of combat-injured personnel at admission to medical centers after evacuation from Afghanistan and Iraq. J Trauma 2011;71(Suppl 1):S52–7.
29. Gillern SM, Sheppard FR, Evans KN, et al. Incidence of pulmonary embolus in combat casualties with extremity amputations and fractures. J Trauma 2011; 71(3):607–12 [discussion: 612–3].
30. Ritenour AE, Dorlac WC, Fang R, et al. Complications after fasciotomy revision and delayed compartment release in combat patients. J Trauma 2008;64(Suppl 2): S153–61 [discussion: S161–52].

14. Rosenthal RE, Teirner RM, Noye JM, et al. The treatment of acidosis in acute lung injury with tromethamine (THAM). Ann N Y Acad Sci 2000;916:383–5.

15. Allen PR, Osborn FO, Chung IKK, et al. High-frequency percussive ventilation revisited. J Burn Care Res 2010;31:510–20.

16. Camporota L, Fortes DH, george H Hewett. Advanced airway care during combat operations. Bull Am Coll Surg 2014;99:312–5.

17. Pelosi GH, Fang P, Philis VM, et al. the deployment of critical care air transport teams. J Trauma Acute Care Surg 201;77:S81–87.

18. Holt JK, Crippen DW, Spencer J, Owens Z, Styner. anxiety and infrastructure considerations in mass critical care. Recommendations and standard operating procedures for intensive care unit and hospital preparations for an influenza epidemic or mass disaster. Intensive Care Med 2010;36(Suppl 1):S59–S79.

19. Spring CL, Kesecioglu J. Chapter 5. Essential equipment, pharmaceuticals and supplies. Recommendations and standard operating procedures for intensive care unit and hospital preparations for an influenza epidemic or mass disaster. Intensive Care Med 2010;36(Suppl 1):S38–S44.

20. Ranney ML, Nation Ds, et al. Augmentation of hospital critical care pharmacy services to epidemic. Recommendations of the Working Group on emergency mass critical care. Crit Care Med 2008;36(7):S99–S404.

21. Nichols DA, Reynolds HL. Long-distance air evacuation of Israeli injured soldiers from the Gulf. J Intensive Care Trauma Med 2012;23:S279–85.

22. Camporota L. Airborne sepsis in Gulen. August 1997. the aeromedical evacuation disorders. J Burn Care Res 2004;21(3):S78.

23. Kumbamu D. Airforce medics expanding critical air lift from Iran Med. 20 November. Available at: http://www.airforce.mil/news/story.asp?id=12318743. Accessed March 13, 2017.

24. Davies Z, Jones C, Bellis M, et al. Extracorporeal membrane oxygenation for 2009 influenza A(H1N1) acute respiratory distress syndrome. JAMA 2009;302(17):1888–95.

25. Do RA, Lumes HA, Her Y, et al. Patients supported using mobile extracorporeal with improved outcomes. Crit Care 2015;19(4):1140–8.

26. Gerromasal M, Borg U, Hobbel J, et al. Interhospital transport of the extremely ill patient: the mobile intensive care unit. Crit Care Med 2000;28(1):79–88.

27. Heronus ME, Zohus DH. The damage control sequence and underlying logic. Surg Clin North Am 1997;77:761–77.

28. Rosenthal DR, Crouch GH, Pullan SR, et al. Matching recent protracted extraction of combat-injured personnel at a distance to medical centers after evacuation from Afghanistan and Iran. J Trauma 2012;73(suppl 2):S35–S40.

29. Wilson SM, Sheppard SR, Lewis MH, et al. Incidence of pulmonary embolism in combat casualties with extremity amputations and fractures. J Trauma 2012;73(6):1410–8(discussion 1418–9).

30. Mangram AJ, Dalton WC, Pong P, et al. Complication after prehospital transfusion and massive transfusion for trauma in combat casualties. J Trauma 2005;58(Suppl 2):S51–S21.

Spectrum of Traumatic Brain Injury from Mild to Severe

Michael DeCuypere, MD, PhD[a], Paul Klimo Jr, MD, MPH[a,b,c],*

KEYWORDS

- Traumatic brain injury • Neurotrauma • Cerebral edema
- Intracranial pressure monitoring • Craniectomy

KEY POINTS

- Traumatic brain injury (TBI) is a leading cause of morbidity and mortality after trauma. It is beneficial for all physicians involved in the care of the trauma patient to have a thorough understanding of TBI and current management approaches.
- Nearly 80% of patients with mild to moderate TBI have evidence of residual symptoms 3 months after injury, and survivors typically require some form of long-term rehabilitation. Loss of employment and economic hardship are common among TBI patients.
- Mortality from TBI has seen a significant improvement over the past 2 decades because of improved neurocritical and neurosurgical care, public safety interventions, and avoidance of serious inpatient medical comorbidities.
- Specialized neuroscience critical care centers are equipped to deliver a full array of treatment options, with therapy guided by intracranial pressure monitoring. Nevertheless, initial diagnosis and rapid stabilization by acute care physicians and surgeons remains vital to the survival and care of the TBI patient.

INTRODUCTION

Traumatic brain injury (TBI) is the foremost cause of death in children and young adults and is a key socioeconomic concern for modernized and developing countries alike. The medical and surgical interventions for TBI can be complex and far reaching, often requiring a multidisciplinary approach involving critical care, trauma, and neurosurgical specialists. The management of severe TBI in adults is derived primarily from the Guidelines for the Management of Severe Traumatic Brain Injury, published by

The authors have nothing to disclose.

[a] Department of Neurosurgery, University of Tennessee Health Science Center, 847 Monroe Avenue, Suite 427, Memphis, TN, USA; [b] Semmes-Murphey Neurologic and Spine Institute, 6325 Humphreys Boulevard, Memphis, TN 38120, USA; [c] Department of Neurosurgery, LeBonheur Children's Hospital, 50 North Dunlap Street, Memphis, TN 38103, USA

* Corresponding author. Semmes-Murphey Neurologic and Spine Institute, 6325 Humphreys Boulevard, Memphis, TN 38120.

E-mail address: pklimo@semmes-murphey.com

Surg Clin N Am 92 (2012) 939–957
doi:10.1016/j.suc.2012.04.005
0039-6109/12/$ – see front matter © 2012 Elsevier Inc. All rights reserved.

surgical.theclinics.com

a joint effort of the Brain Trauma Foundation (BTF), the American Association of Neurological Surgeons, and the Congress of Neurological Surgeons.[1] The primary objectives in the management of TBI are the prevention and treatment of elevated intracranial pressure and secondary brain injury, preservation of cerebral perfusion pressure, and maintenance of cerebral oxygenation. In this review the definitions, critical care management, and prognosis of mild, moderate, and severe TBI are discussed, with a focus on current principles of medical and surgical intervention.

EPIDEMIOLOGY OF TRAUMATIC BRAIN INJURY

TBI is a leading cause of traumatic death and disability with substantial socioeconomic burden. Each year in the United States there are an estimated 235,000 hospitalizations for nonfatal TBI. It has been estimated that a TBI occurs every 7 seconds and results in death every 5 minutes. Every year, approximately 1.1 million Americans are treated and released from an emergency department (ED) and 50,000 die as a result of TBI,[2,3] accounting for almost one-third of all trauma-related deaths. The overall annual incidence of TBI in the United States is 506.4 per 100,000 population. When the overall incidence is divided by source, the incidence rate of TBI is 403 ED visits, 85 hospital discharges, and 18 deaths per 100,000 population.[2] Furthermore, approximately 43% of persons discharged with TBI from acute hospitalizations develop TBI-related long-term disability. In 2003, the overall expense for direct TBI medical care was estimated at more than $56 billion per year.[4,5]

Rates of TBI in the United States are highest among American Indian/Alaska Natives and African Americans.[6] The major risk factors for TBI in the United States are age, gender, and low socioeconomic status. Persons younger than 10 years and those older than 74 years have the highest incidence rates, 900 and 659 per 100,000, respectively.[3] The rate among men is nearly twice that of women.[7] For fatal TBI, the rate among males was 3.4 times higher than that for females.[6] The propensity for men to incur TBI is likely attributable to risk-taking behavior and high-risk activities. Hospital discharge and ED visit surveillance data from South Carolina for TBI using primary payer as a surrogate for socioeconomic status indicated that although the uninsured comprise 16% of the state population, they represented 26% of persons with TBI. Furthermore, the risk of acquiring TBI in uninsured patients was nearly twice that of persons who held private insurance.[8]

For hospital discharges, ED visits, and deaths combined, falls were the leading cause of TBI in the United States, accounting for 28% of cases, followed by motor-vehicle collisions (20%), being struck by a motor vehicle (19%), and assaults (11%).[2] Analysis of surveillance data for 7 states indicated transportation-related crashes accounted for 49% of all TBIs while falls accounted for an additional 26%.[9] The leading causes of TBI varied by age. Falls were by far the leading cause of TBI-related hospital discharges among persons 75 years and older, whereas transportation-related crashes was most prominent for persons aged 15 to 24 years.

Penetrating trauma to the brain is less common than blunt injury, but far more severe, with intracranial gunshot wounds associated with very high mortality (**Fig. 1**). Over a 10-year period in the United States, firearm-related TBI disproportionately affected African Americans and was the cause of nearly half of TBI-related deaths in this group. Males were 6 times more likely than females to die from firearm-related TBI. Nearly two-thirds of firearm-related TBIs were classified as suicidal in intent.[6]

A significant improvement in overall TBI mortality has been observed over the past 2 decades, largely attributable to improvements in neurocritical and surgical care. A recent retrospective review of severely injured TBI patients over a 10-year period noted an overall decrease in mortality, which remained significant despite adjustment

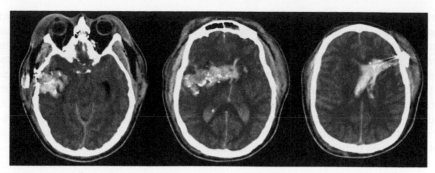

Fig. 1. Intracranial gunshot wound. Consecutive axial noncontrast CT images (*left to right*) demonstrate a gunshot wound to the head with transventricular trajectory proceeding from the right temporal region to the left frontotemporal region.

for age, motor score, and pupillary reaction (27% mortality in 1996 vs 39% mortality in 1984).[10] Advances in neuromonitoring, neuroimaging, and early neurosurgical interventions, as well as specialized neurointensive care units, are likely significant contributors to improved TBI outcomes.

Much attention has been paid to battlefield TBI over the last 10 years with the conflicts in Iraq and Afghanistan. Epidemiologic evidence to date suggests that up to 20% of injuries sustained in modern battle involve the head.[11,12] Data obtained during Operation Iraqi Freedom demonstrated that body armor and combat helmets reduced the incidence of injuries to the head, chest, and abdomen, as well as overall injury severity.[13] Thus, as a result of these improvements, many of the current battlefield fatalities are thought to be nonsurvivable under of the best of circumstances.[14] Modern combat hospitals provide trauma care by specialty physicians and nurses and provide advanced imaging, emergency medical services, early surgical intervention, and intensive care. Furthermore, the US military has implemented the Joint Theater Trauma System (JTTS), an organized effort across all branches to deliver trauma and critical care services in specific geographic regions during battle. This system has led to the development of data-driven clinical practice guidelines (CPGs) for the systematic delivery of care to trauma patients based on injury or injuries (ie, TBI, amputation, burn, and so forth). As a result, the experience and lessons learned in combat with respect to evacuation and stabilization procedures have been used as a model for the delivery of emergent critical care in civilian settings.[15,16]

CLASSIFICATION OF TRAUMATIC BRAIN INJURY

TBI begins with high-energy acceleration or deceleration of the brain within the cranium or with penetration of the brain. In more severe forms of TBI, primary cellular injury is followed by a secondary response that includes changes in cerebral blood flow, local and systemic inflammation, alterations in oxygen delivery and metabolism, and both ischemic and apoptotic death of neural cells. Intravascular clot formation is common in severe TBI and contributes to local ischemia. In this regard, consumption of clotting factors may lead to a systemic coagulopathy.[17] A principal goal of neurocritical care is to intervene in time to prevent and disrupt secondary injury mechanisms.

In general, TBI may be classified as either focal or diffuse. Focal injuries tend to occur at the site of impact, with focal neurologic deficits referable to those areas. The orbitofrontal and anterior temporal lobes are characteristic and are most commonly affected because of the location of the brain in relation to the irregular surface of the skull base. As cranial trauma tends to occur in an anteroposterior direction, the brain moves in a similar fashion and is injured as it traverses over the skull base. Vigilance must be maintained to identify delayed focal contusions and hematomas, which may develop several days after trauma.[18] By contrast, the diffuse shearing of axons as a result of sudden deceleration or rotational forces may occur in the cerebral white matter, gray-white junction, corpus callosum, and brainstem, causing nonlateralizing neurologic deficits such as encephalopathy, or focal deficits such as cranial neuropathies. The consequences of this type of injury can be delayed by up to 12 hours after the initial trauma.[19] Diffuse axonal injury (DAI) appears as subtle petechial white matter hemorrhages on neuroimaging studies.

Mild Traumatic Brain Injury

Mild head trauma is defined as isolated head injury producing a Glasgow Coma Scale (GCS) score of 13 or greater (**Tables 1** and **2**).[20] It represents the most common degree of head injury in patients who present to the ED for evaluation (approximately 80% of all TBI). Most episodes of mild head trauma occur in the context of sports or recreational activities, and patients are usually asymptomatic on presentation. When symptoms are present, headache is the most common complaint; however, nausea and emesis are also common. Patients may occasionally experience brief and transient disorientation, confusion, or amnesia immediately or shortly after the injury.

After a thorough neurologic and mental status examination, additional diagnostic workup and subsequent management may depend on stratification of risk. For instance, approximately 3% of all patients with mild head trauma sustain a sudden, unexpected neurologic deterioration, whereas less than 1% have surgically significant lesions.[21] Determining which patients who have experienced a mild head trauma are at risk for an intracranial lesion and, therefore, require acute neuroimaging has proved difficult in research studies. Results have been conflicting, likely because of the use of different methods, definitions, and outcomes of minor TBI.

As such, a key management decision is whether head computed tomography (CT) scans should be obtained on patients who have sustained mild head trauma. In most adult patients, skull radiographs are not recommended if the patient is deemed to require neuroimaging. CT is the preferred study, as it yields information about both the skull and the brain. In rare instances, skull radiographs may be useful in patients who cannot undergo CT.

Table 1
Glasgow Coma Scale

Motor Response (M)		Verbal Response (V)		Eye Opening (E)	
Follows commands	6				
Localizes to stimulus	5	Oriented	5		
Withdrawal to stimulus	4	Confused, appropriate	4	Spontaneous	4
Flexor posturing	3	Disoriented, inappropriate	3	Opens to voice	3
Extensor posturing	2	Incomprehensible	2	Opens to stimulus	2
No response	1	No response	1	No response	1

The Glasgow Coma Scale (GCS) is a cumulative score of all 3 components. Thus, it ranges from 3 to 15. If intubated, the patient is given a designation of "T" for verbal response. The initial posttrauma GCS score should be given once the patient is adequately stabilized and, if needed, resuscitated.

Table 2			
Indices of severity of traumatic brain injury			
Index	Mild Injury	Moderate Injury	Severe Injury
Glasgow Coma Scale score	13–15	9–12	4–6
Loss of consciousness	<30 min	30 min–24 h	>24 h
Posttraumatic amnesia	0–1 d	>1–<7 d	>7 d

Some studies advocate CT in all patients who have sustained mild head trauma who have a history of loss of consciousness or amnesia for the event.[22,23] Others recommend inpatient or prolonged ED observation to allow rapid identification of those patients whose conditions suddenly deteriorate after mild TBI. Prolonged observation may be of value in some circumstances, such as in intoxicated patients who have sustained a mild head injury and who need to regain sobriety before proper evaluation for a delayed complication of mild TBI. In general, criteria for adult patients who have sustained a mild head trauma that correlate with an increased likelihood of intracranial lesions include[21,24]:

- Headache
- Vomiting
- Age older than 60 years
- Short-term memory deficits
- External signs of trauma above the clavicles
- Posttraumatic seizures.

In addition to these risk factors, warfarin anticoagulation has received considerable attention in the literature. Several studies have failed to demonstrate that therapeutic warfarin anticoagulation elevates risk of intracranial hemorrhage and requires urgent CT imaging in mild TBI patients.[21,25,26] However, it has been demonstrated that pre-injury supratherapeutic warfarin anticoagulation has a significant effect on the outcome of mild TBI.[27,28] As such, generally accepted guidelines regarding the management of the heparin or warfarin anticoagulated TBI patient do not exist in the trauma literature and are left to the discretion of the individual physician. Several trauma centers have recently initiated efforts to define the indications for obtaining an initial head CT as well as subsequent interval imaging, even if the initial scan is normal.

Several studies have sought to define the relationship between antiplatelet therapy and risk of hemorrhage in TBI. Few have demonstrated that antiplatelet or anticoagulation therapy increased the risk of death in TBI patients suffering intracranial hemorrhage.[29,30] A recent analysis of TBI patients taking aspirin or clopidogrel demonstrated an increased risk of mortality with antiplatelet therapy.[31] Jones and colleagues[32] concluded that TBI patients on clopidogrel therapy have an increased risk of morbidity and blood transfusion. However, another recent report found no increased mortality in patients taking warfarin, clopidogrel, or aspirin who suffer TBI with intracranial hemorrhage.[33] Furthermore, Spektor and colleagues[34] found no significant increase in intracranial hemorrhage in patients taking low-dose aspirin who suffered mild to moderate TBI. Once again, generally accepted guidelines for the diagnosis and management of TBI in patients on antiplatelet therapy are nonexistent and vary between institutions and physicians.

At present, there is no standardized assessment used in civilian trauma centers for the initial neurocognitive evaluation of patients with mild TBI. The Military Acute Concussion Evaluation (MACE) is a standardized mental status examination used to evaluate concussion in battle situations. This screening tool was developed to evaluate patients with suspected mild TBI within the first 24 hours after injury, and allows for identification of clinically relevant neurocognitive impairment. This score is then later used, if necessary, to determine whether a cognitive decline or improvement has occurred. A similar assessment in civilian centers could prove useful, especially in the setting of 12- to 24-hour observation periods during which the decision to discharge a patient based on cognitive improvement is in question.

Recent studies using diffusion tensor imaging (DTI) have shed new light on ultrastructural abnormalities in mild TBI. Unlike CT or conventional magnetic resonance imaging (MRI), DTI is sensitive to microstructural axonal injury, the pathologic condition that may be responsible for the persistent cognitive and behavioral impairments that often persist after mild TBI. DTI analysis techniques such as automated region-of-interest analysis, tract-based voxel-wise analysis, and quantitative tractography have demonstrated that frontal and temporal association white matter pathways are most frequently damaged in mild TBI and that the microstructural integrity of these tracts correlates with behavioral and cognitive measures.[35–37]

Most patients who have sustained a mild TBI can be discharged safely from the ED after a normal examination, but observation of 4 to 6 hours is advised.[38] Patients with minor TBI who are discharged should have an appropriate early follow-up arranged. Furthermore, all patients should be educated on the signs and symptoms of delayed complications of head injury. If there are any concerns about the safety of the discharged patient with mild injury, a brief inpatient observation period of 12 to 24 hours is advisable. A second ED visit by the patient who has sustained a mild head injury is common because of persistence of symptoms or the development of new concerns. At this time, a careful neurologic examination to determine the presence of delayed complications (such as delayed cerebral edema) is of utmost importance. At present, there are no data to support a repeat head CT in the presence of a nonfocal neurologic examination if an initial study at the time of the presentation was within normal limits, but this is frequently performed. The US Centers for Disease Control and Prevention have published an online pamphlet detailing discharge instructions for patients following mild TBI (http://www.cdc.gov/concussion/pdf/TBI_Patient_Instructions-a.pdf). In addition to home care guidelines, these instructions detail reasons for a TBI patient to return to the ED:

- Repeated vomiting
- Worsening headache that does not resolve
- Loss of consciousness
- Confusion or agitation
- Seizure
- Difficulty walking or balance difficulties
- Weakness or numbness
- Change in vision.

Moderate Traumatic Brain Injury

Patients with moderate TBI have a GCS score of 9 to 12 (see **Table 2**). These patients comprise approximately 10% of all cases of TBI, and clinical presentation can vary widely. Patients may have had loss of consciousness or a brief posttraumatic seizure and may be confused; however, most patients with moderate TBI can follow commands on arrival to the ED. Facial and other multisystem trauma is often present. Patients may complain of a worsening headache and nausea, and focal neurologic deficits may be present on examination. Moderate TBI is associated with a greater likelihood of abnormal findings on neuroimaging studies.

A unique subset of patients with moderate TBI may present with a lucid interval. During this interval, the patient is able to speak initially but deteriorates to a GCS score consistent with severe TBI within 48 hours.[39] Approximately 75% of these patients have an extra-axial hematoma, either subdural or epidural. If the extra-axial hematomas are detected early and treated rapidly, these patients may have excellent clinical outcomes. The key to the successful management of patients who have sustained moderate TBI involves close clinical observation for subtle changes in mental status or focal neurologic findings, liberal use of CT, and early neurosurgical intervention. A patient presenting with moderate TBI who actively deteriorates in the ED should be immediately stabilized using standard Advanced Trauma Life Support (ATLS) protocol (ie, airway, breathing, circulation, and so forth), receive brief hyperventilation once intubated, and intravenous osmotic therapy (see Medical Intervention for Elevated Intracranial Pressure). The patient should then promptly undergo a CT scan while neurosurgical consultation is obtained.

All patients with moderate TBI should undergo immediate head CT and receive inpatient hospital observation in a critical care setting, even if the initial head CT appears normal. Most patients who have sustained moderate TBI improve significantly over a period of several days.[40] Neurologic examinations should be performed frequently during the inpatient observation. A repeat CT should be performed within 6 to 12 hours if a patient's condition fails to improve.

Severe Traumatic Brain Injury

Severe TBI is defined as a patient who presents acutely with a GCS score of 8 or less (see **Table 2**). Moreover, any intracranial contusion, hematoma, or brain laceration falls within the category of severe TBI. This category comprises approximately 10% of all patients who have sustained TBI and who arrive alive at the ED.[38] Patients typically have abnormal neuroimaging (skull fracture or intracranial hemorrhage), require rapid airway control, and need neurosurgical evaluation with typically either surgical intervention or continuous intracranial pressure (ICP) monitoring. Recovery is prolonged and usually incomplete.[41] A significant percentage of severe TBI patients do not survive to 1 year after injury.[42] Pupillary reactivity, patient age, comorbid medical conditions, initial motor examination, and the presence of prolonged secondary brain or systemic insult affect the patient's overall prognosis.[43,44] Approximately 25% of all patients who sustain severe TBI have lesions that eventually require neurosurgical intervention, and the overall mortality of adult patients who sustain severe TBI is approximately 60%.[38] By contrast, the mortality for children who sustain severe TBI is considerably lower (approximately 20%).[43] Furthermore, whereas most adult survivors of severe TBI suffer from severe long-term disability, children older than 1 year have better neurologic outcomes after severe TBI.[43]

Cushing phenomenon is an acute clinical entity that may occur during the resuscitation of the patient who has sustained severe TBI. This phenomenon includes 3 clinical signs: severe progressive hypertension, bradycardia, and diminished or irregular respiratory effort. The Cushing reflex is associated with significant increases in ICP and impending brain herniation; however, the full triad of clinical signs is seen in only 30% of cases of life-threatening increased ICP.[45] The presence of Cushing phenomenon should prompt immediate aggressive ICP management, including hyperventilation, maximal osmotic therapy, and immediate neurosurgical evaluation. In general, the acute management of severe TBI is directed at reducing secondary injuries, and expediting a definitive diagnosis and management strategy.

CLINICAL MANAGEMENT OF MODERATE AND SEVERE BRAIN INJURY

In 1995, the BTF developed the first TBI guidelines in an effort to develop evidence-based protocols that would improve the survival and outcomes in TBI patients. The most recent iteration was published in 2007 in the *Journal of Neurotrauma*.[1] Similar guidelines for pediatric TBI have been developed.[46] The guidelines for adult TBI are summarized in the following sections.

Acute Evaluation and Management

As with any trauma/critical care situation, an organized team approach is essential to proper clinical evaluation and management. In this setting, ATLS considerations are forefront. The initial goals of care should be immediate attention to airway and cardiopulmonary function, the early identification of the potential for TBI in any trauma victim, and minimization of secondary insults, such as hypoxic-ischemic injury. The GCS is important in categorizing TBI patients and provides a quantifiable measure of impairment, which can help delineate early management sequences.

Optimizing perfusion and oxygenation is of paramount importance in the early phases of resuscitation, as the duration and severity of hypoxia and hypotension in this period has dramatic consequences on overall clinical outcome.[47] Avoidance of hypotension (systolic blood pressure >90 mm Hg) and maintenance of adequate oxygen saturation (>90%) are level II and level III recommendations from the BTF, respectively.[1,48] It is of great importance to note that intravenous fluids and blood products will not increase ICP in a hypotensive patient who has sustained TBI. Approximately 60% of patients with severe TBI have sustained multiple traumatic injuries, and vigilance must be maintained to search for other systematic injuries that may be responsible for observed hypotension.[44] To date, few data exist to support or refute the utility of neurosurgical intervention (intracranial pressure monitoring, craniotomy, and so forth) without cranial imaging in the multitrauma patient requiring emergent laparotomy. Neurologic examination findings were of no independent value in predicting the need for craniotomy in a series of 800 patients with severe injuries to both the head and abdomen.[49] The authors recommend diagnostic abdominal paracentesis in stable patients with potential injuries to both the head and abdomen before imaging of the head. In the hemodynamically unstable patient, emergent laparotomy should proceed first. The decision to place an intracranial pressure monitor in these patients during laparotomy varies between neurosurgeons and is purely anecdotal.

In many patients with moderate TBI and all patients with severe TBI, airway-protective mechanisms are impaired, and tracheal intubation should be performed.

The cervical spine should be immobilized with a rigid cervical collar and the head placed in midline position. The cervical collar not only serves to protect the cervical spine but also keeps the head in the midline to avoid compromising venous drainage, which can increase ICP.

After the airway is secured, acute hyperventilation is a life-saving intervention that can prevent or delay herniation in the patient who has experienced a severe TBI. Reduction of the Pco_2 into the range of 30 to 35 mm Hg is optimal in this scenario. Hyperventilation acts to reduce ICP by up to 25% via initiation of cerebral vasoconstriction.[50] Prolonged hyperventilation below 30 mm Hg is generally not recommended because it may lead to ischemia. Hyperventilation should be viewed only as a short-term life-saving intervention and should be used only when a patient who has sustained severe TBI experiences a sudden neurologic decline and/or demonstrates signs consistent with cerebral herniation.

A detailed neurologic examination should commence immediately after correction of any obvious abnormality in the primary trauma survey. Ideally this should occur before chemical paralysis or sedation for intubation or other bedside procedure. After stabilization of the TBI patient, a CT scan without contrast enhancement should be completed as soon as possible to identify lesions amenable to operative neurosurgical intervention.

Posttraumatic seizures (PTS) occur in as many as 12% of patients who sustain blunt head trauma and in up to 50% of those with penetrating head injury.[1,48] Early PTS can worsen secondary brain injury by causing hypoxia, hypercarbia, release of excitatory neurotransmitters, and an increase in ICP. The prophylactic use of antiepileptic drugs in acute TBI may reduce the risk for early seizures by 66%, but does not prevent late posttraumatic seizures.[51] The goal of emergency antiepileptic therapy is to prevent additional insult to the damaged brain caused by seizures. Benzodiazepines are rapid-acting, first-line anticonvulsants used in the acute setting. Lorazepam (0.05–0.15 mg/kg intravenously, every 5 minutes to a total of 4 mg) is most effective at terminating status epilepticus.[52] Phenytoin (13–18 mg/kg intravenously) or fosphenytoin (13–18 phenytoin equivalents/kg) is typically used for long-term prophylaxis; however, emerging evidence suggests that intravenous dosing of levetiracetam (500–1000 mg intravenously or by mouth twice daily) may be neuroprotective in animal models of closed head injury and subarachnoid hemorrhage.[53] Routine seizure prophylaxis longer than 1 week following TBI is generally not recommended, as evidence to date does not support the use of the prophylactic anticonvulsants for the prevention of late PTS. If late PTS should occur, patients are to be managed in accordance with standard approaches to patients with new-onset seizures.

After initial emergent care, patients with severe TBI require admission to a critical care setting. Available data suggest that outcomes may be improved when specialized neurologic intensive care teams are present to guide management.[54,55] Furthermore, the presence of other traumatic injuries may require a multidisciplinary approach, including input from trauma, orthopedic, craniofacial, ophthalmologic, and other specialty physicians.

Intracranial Pressure Monitoring

If the patient has a GCS of 8 or less, any acute abnormality on CT, or a systolic pressure of less than 90 mm Hg, an ICP monitoring device should be placed. The external ventricular drain (EVD) provides the most accurate and reliable ICP data and also provides a means to control ICP by cerebrospinal fluid removal. Other monitoring options, which do not have this treatment advantage but are less invasive, include the subdural bolt and fiberoptic catheter. Parenchymal ICP monitors typically have negligible drift of ICP during use but cannot be recalibrated while in situ. An EVD is typically the best choice for ICP monitoring in patients with severe head injury and ventricles that are not excessively small, but it does come with a higher risk of hemorrhage during placement.[56] Although no class I data exist for the use of ICP monitoring in severe TBI, it has become standard of care, and a meta-analysis demonstrated improved outcomes in patients with ICP monitoring compared with those without monitoring.[57]

Invasive ICP monitoring provides the most reliable data on ICP, albeit at the cost of a small craniotomy. Some emerging noninvasive technologies for estimation of ICP include transcranial Doppler sonography (TCD) and ultrasound measurement of optic nerve sheath diameter (ONSD).[58–60]

Unfortunately, TCD requires trained operators and cannot be performed in up to 10% of patients because of the lack of acoustic windows. Furthermore, although the modifications of TCD waves that occur during intracranial hypertension have been shown to correlate well with cerebral perfusion pressure, they are unable to differentiate between perfusion-pressure effects caused by ICP and those produced by an increase in cerebrovascular resistance.[59–62]

The optic nerve and its sheath can be visualized by means of ultrasonography, and several studies have reported a good ONSD-ICP correlation.[63–65] However, this modality is compromised by intraorbital disorders such as neoplasms, inflammatory diseases, sarcoidosis, pseudotumor cerebri, Graves disease, and extrinsic compression of the optic nerve. Furthermore, traumatic optic neuropathy and ocular trauma may make interpretation difficult. To date, no general consensus exists on the clinical application of the ultrasonographic measurement of ONSD; however, this has been proposed as a promising noninvasive method of ICP measurement.

Tissue Oxygenation and Metabolic Monitoring

The goal of metabolic monitoring is the measurement of oxygen delivery to the brain with jugular venous saturation (Sjo_2) monitors, brain tissue oxygenation monitors (Licox; Integra LifeSciences Corp., Plainsboro, NJ, USA), and near-infrared spectroscopy. Alternatively, the metabolic state of the brain can be assessed using microdialysis catheters. Sjo_2 monitoring provides an estimate of oxygen delivery to the brain with goal mean values of 56% to 74%. Alternatively, arteriojugular differences of oxygen content ($Ajdo_2$) as an indicator of oxygen extraction of the brain may offer valuable prognostic information, with higher mean extraction values being more desirable in a TBI setting.[66] Furthermore, recent data indicate that periods of low brain tissue oxygen tension ($Pbro_2$) may correlate with poor outcome or death in pediatric TBI.[67] Based on current level III recommendations from the BTF, Sjo_2 less than 50% or $Pbro_2$ less than 15 mm Hg are indications for treatment if these values are being monitored.[48] These devices have not become standard of care and require further study.

Medical Intervention for Elevated Intracranial Pressure

Current BTF guidelines support maintaining ICP at less than 25 mm Hg and cerebral perfusion pressure at greater than 60 mm Hg. Increased ICP, particularly when compartmentalized, compresses structures such as the brain and blood vessels, leading to ischemia and eventual herniation. General medical management of elevated ICP includes control of the airway, strict avoidance of hypotension or hypoxia, elevation of the patient's head to 30°, and administration of intravenous mannitol, 0.5 to 1 g/kg over 10 minutes. Administration of hypertonic saline is another alternative. A recent retrospective study demonstrated that an intravenous bolus of 23.4% saline, 30 mL, given over 10 to 15 minutes, may effectively reverse herniation and decrease ICP, with only transient hemodynamic repercussions.[68] There is also recent evidence to suggest that this is as effective in lowering ICP as mannitol, and may have a longer duration of effect.[69] As a low-volume infusion, this concentration of saline may be beneficial in cases where the volume status of the patient dictates caution with large infusions. Hypertonic saline aids in maintaining high serum sodium concentration and thereby promotes water movement from the intracranial compartment into the vasculature. When used clinically, 2% saline solutions can be given by a peripheral line; however, 3% and higher concentrations of saline should be administered through a central venous catheter to minimize phlebitis. Swan-Ganz catheters (pulmonary artery catheters) are still used in some trauma centers for measurement of intravascular volume status. However, transduction of central venous pressure via central venous catheter has largely supplanted this modality, as Swan-Ganz catheter use in trauma patients has been associated with significantly higher complication rate and overall mortality.[70] Other less invasive (and less common) modalities for measuring volume status in the critical care setting include the Vigileo monitor (Edwards Lifesciences, Irvine, CA, USA) and ultrasound-based assessment such as bedside echocardiography. As a continuous infusion, hypertonic saline solutions are commonly prepared as a 1:1 ratio of sodium acetate to sodium chloride to minimize the development of hyperchloremic metabolic acidosis. The use of hypertonic saline, interestingly, has not received a level III or better recommendation by the BTF for use in trauma-induced increased ICP.[71,72] Because of the complexity of this therapy and the need for precise temperature regulation to achieve benefit, a treatment protocol should be used in these instances, as discussed by Cannon and colleagues elsewhere in this issue.

Induced hypothermia for TBI remains controversial, in large part because of the lack of compelling outcome-benefit data from randomized clinical trials.[47,51] Recent animal studies, however, show potential for induced hypothermia with improved neurophysiologic outcomes in nontraumatic brain injury.[52] Nevertheless, based on a level III recommendation from the BTF, the use of prophylactic hypothermia for severe TBI is not warranted.[48] It may be used, however, for a short period of time (2–3 days) for refractory intracranial hypertension.[73]

If other medical methods of lowering elevated ICP prove unsuccessful, pharmacologic coma should be afforded consideration. The postulated effect of pharmacologic coma on ICP is via reduction of cerebral metabolism with concomitant reductions in cerebral blood flow and tissue oxygen demand. The most commonly used agent, pentobarbital, can be administered intravenously at a loading dose of 5 mg/kg, followed by an infusion of 1 to 3 mg/kg/h. A high-dose regimen may also be used with an intravenous bolus dose of 10 mg/kg over 30 minutes followed by a 5 mg/kg/h infusion for 3 hours, followed by 1 mg/kg/h titrated to burst suppression on continuous electroencephalogram monitoring. Another option for pharmacologic coma is propofol, which is given in an intravenous loading dose of 2 mg/kg, followed by a titrated infusion of up to 200 mg/kg/min.[74] If these efforts fail to control ICP, surgical intervention should be considered; however, should the patient be unsuitable for surgery and ICP elevation remains intractable, the patient's condition is likely terminal.[48,74,75]

Surgical Intervention for Elevated Intracranial Pressure

Surgical management may be beneficial in selected patients with severe TBI and refractory intracranial hypertension; however, there are several injuries that do not warrant surgical intervention. For instance, diffuse or disseminated injuries, such as DAI and contusional injury, are typically managed with medical means.

Conditions in which neurosurgery is warranted are those related to breach of the calvaria or presence of expanding intracranial hematoma or malignant cerebral edema. Depressed skull fractures often require debridement and elevation. Symptomatic or expanding subdural and epidural hematomas usually require evacuation.

Epidural hematoma (EDH; **Fig. 2**) is primarily a disease of the young and accounts for 0.5% to 1% of all patients who experience TBI.[2] EDHs are most often unilateral, and the deterioration of a patient who has an EDH from arterial bleeding can be rapid and dramatic. EDHs are rare in older adults and children younger than 2 years because of the close attachment of the dura to the skull in both populations. EDHs larger than 30 cm³ in volume should be evacuated surgically, regardless of the patient's GCS score. Furthermore, comatose patients with an acute EDH and unilateral anisocoria on papillary examination should undergo immediate surgical evacuation.[76]

Subdural hematoma (SDH; **Fig. 3**) is much more common than EDH and is present in 12% to 30% of patients who have sustained a severe TBI.[77] SDH is common in older

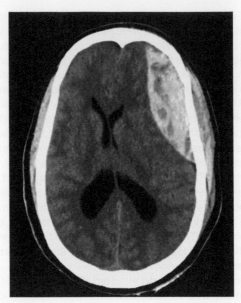

Fig. 2. Epidural hematoma. Axial noncontrast CT image demonstrates a large left frontal epidural hematoma.

adults, most often as the result of a fall. The overall mortality of patients who have an SDH and require surgical intervention is between 40% and 60%.[77] Because of associated brain injury caused by the SDH, the potential for delay in clinical signs and symptoms and the more advanced mean age of the at-risk population, the mortality associated with SDH is much higher than that associated with EDH.

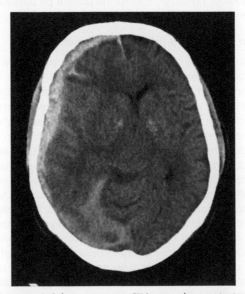

Fig. 3. Subdural hematoma. Axial noncontrast CT image demonstrates a large right fronto-temporoparietal subdural hematoma with right-to-left shift of midline structures.

Decompressive craniectomy for malignant cerebral edema is a relatively new clinical approach in the intervention and management of severe TBI; however, it remains unclear whether craniectomy improves the functional outcome in patients with refractory elevated ICP. For instance, in a study of 57 patients with severe TBI, early decompressive craniectomy was associated with a good outcome in 58% of patients, along with a relatively low mortality (<20%).[78] By contrast, a retrospective study from France was able to show a favorable outcome in only 25% of severe TBI patients who received craniectomy.[79] More recently, Rosenfeld and colleagues[80] demonstrated that patients who underwent decompressive craniectomy for uncontrolled ICP had significant improvement in ICP control and better clinical outcomes than controls. In addition, military neurosurgeons from the United States report favorable outcomes in blast-related TBI patients who undergo early decompressive craniectomy.[81,82] A retrospective study of the Trauma Coma Data Bank, on the other hand, suggested there was no significant improvement with craniectomy.[83] Most recently, a large multicenter trial in Australia and New Zealand demonstrated that early bilateral decompressive craniectomy for diffuse cerebral injury decreased ICP and the length of stay in the intensive care unit, but was associated with more unfavorable outcomes.[84] However, this study has been heavily criticized as being methodologically flawed and fundamentally assessing the wrong operation (ie, bifrontotemporoparietal craniectomy) in a patient population who would not typically be managed with surgical intervention (ie, diffuse bilateral cerebral injury).[85–87] Despite the conflicting evidence, decompressive craniectomy for refractory elevated ICP is increasingly performed in many trauma centers internationally. Perhaps the most difficult component of interpreting available data is the lack of agreement regarding surgical technique for craniectomy (bilateral vs unilateral, release of dura, timing of surgery, surgical cutoff age, and TBI severity on presentation).[88]

OUTCOME AND PROGNOSIS IN TRAUMATIC BRAIN INJURY

The oldest and most widely implemented outcome measure in TBI is the Glasgow Outcome Scale (GOS; **Table 3**).[89] The GOS is determined by a clinician at some point during the patient's recovery. Common time points used to evaluate the GOS include 3 months, 6 months, and 12 months after injury. Vegetative state (GOS 2) refers to a patient who is alive but unresponsive. A patient who is severely disabled (GOS 3) is conscious but requires others for daily support because of their disability. A moderately disabled patient (GOS 4) suffers some degree of disability but is independent for daily activities. A TBI patient who has attained a good recovery score (GOS 5) has resumed most normal daily activities but may have minor residual problems. From a practical standpoint, the GOS can be reduced to two categories: favorable (good recovery and moderate disability) versus unfavorable (severe disability, vegetative

Table 3	
Glasgow Outcome Scale	
Score	**Outcome**
1	Dead
2	Vegetative state
3	Severe disability
4	Moderate disability
5	Good recovery

Table 4 Glasgow Outcome Scale—Extended	
Score	Outcome
1	Dead
2	Vegetative state
3	Lower severe disability
4	Upper severe disability
5	Lower moderate disability
6	Upper moderate disability
7	Lower good recovery
8	Upper good recovery

state, and death). The majority of patients (approximately 70%) with a severe TBI will fall into the two extremes of the GOS: those with good recovery and those who die.

Although the GOS has been used extensively, it has been criticized as being insufficiently sensitive to subtle deficits in cognition, mood, and behavior. These limitations in the GOS create uncertainty in the assessment of patients who have achieved a good recovery but have not returned to preinjury status. To address these shortcomings, the GOS was modified and a structured interview was proposed to accurately categorize a patient's disability.[90,91] This version has been termed the GOS—Extended (GOS-E; **Table 4**). This 8-point scale uses additional categories to further stratify the middle and upper end of the GOS. In addition, the implementation of a structured interview has resulted in improved interrater reliability.[91–93]

From a purely clinical standpoint, the most useful prognostic indicators in TBI are the neurologic examination and GCS at presentation. The Medical Research Council CRASH trial is the largest and most sophisticated study of TBI outcome, and has associated 6-month outcomes with age, GCS score, pupil reactivity, and the presence of extracranial injury, in addition to radiographic and other data collected from more than 8500 TBI patients in several countries. Of note, advancing age was most associated with poor outcome in high-income countries, and low GCS score was most associated with poor outcome in low-income to middle-income countries. The absence of pupil reactivity was the third strongest predictor of poor outcome in high-income and low-income countries. Radiographically, obliteration of the third ventricle and midline shift was most likely to be associated with mortality within 14 days, and nonevacuated hematoma was most likely to be associated with poor outcome at 6 months.[94] Recent studies using DTI and diffusion-weighted MRI correlated well with GCS score at 6 to 12 months after trauma, and may aid in future TBI prognostication.[95,96]

SUMMARY

TBI is both a common and a costly traumatic disease entity. Victims of TBI are characteristically young, and injury often results in loss of employment and economic hardship. Societal expense includes cost of long-term care of the TBI patient as well as diminished productivity. Nearly 80% of patients with mild to moderate TBI have evidence of residual symptoms 3 months after injury, and survivors typically require some form of long-term rehabilitation. The prominence of TBI during the United States war on terrorism in recent years has served to increase public awareness and has affected the treatment of this injury.

Mortality from TBI has seen a significant improvement over the past 2 decades. This decrease is multifactorial in nature and involves improved neurocritical and neurosurgical care, public safety interventions, and avoidance of serious medical comorbidities (venous thromboembolism, gastric stress ulceration, and so forth). Furthermore, specialized neuroscience critical care centers are equipped to deliver a full array of treatment options, with therapy guided by ICP and monitoring of cerebral perfusion pressure. Nevertheless, initial diagnosis and rapid stabilization by acute care physicians and surgeons remains vital to the survival and care of the TBI patient.

Research in neurotrauma is advancing rapidly. Novel physiologic monitoring devices may elucidate more efficacious therapies for TBI, and advanced imaging modalities may lead to more accurate anatomic diagnosis of brain injury. With this in mind, further improvement in morbidity and mortality from TBI as well as improvement in functional outcome is on the horizon.

REFERENCES

1. Bullock MR, Povlishock JT. Guidelines for the management of severe traumatic brain injury. Editor's commentary. J Neurotrauma 2007;24(Suppl 1):2 p preceding S1.
2. Rutland-Brown W, Langlois JA, Thomas KE, et al. Incidence of traumatic brain injury in the United States, 2003. J Head Trauma Rehabil 2006;21(6):544–8.
3. Langlois JA, Rutland-Brown W, Wald MM. The epidemiology and impact of traumatic brain injury: a brief overview. J Head Trauma Rehabil 2006;21(5):375–8.
4. Selassie AW, Zaloshnja E, Langlois JA, et al. Incidence of long-term disability following traumatic brain injury hospitalization, United States, 2003. J Head Trauma Rehabil 2008;23(2):123–31.
5. Sosin DM, Sniezek JE, Waxweiler RJ. Trends in death associated with traumatic brain injury, 1979 through 1992. Success and failure. JAMA 1995;273(22):1778–80.
6. Adekoya N, Thurman DJ, White DD, et al. Surveillance for traumatic brain injury deaths—United States, 1989-1998. MMWR Surveill Summ 2002;51(10):1–14.
7. Langlois JA, Kegler SR, Butler JA, et al. Traumatic brain injury-related hospital discharges. Results from a 14-state surveillance system, 1997. MMWR Surveill Summ 2003;52(4):1–20.
8. Selassie AW, Pickelsimer EE, Frazier L Jr, et al. The effect of insurance status, race, and gender on ED disposition of persons with traumatic brain injury. Am J Emerg Med 2004;22(6):465–73.
9. Thurman DJ, Alverson C, Dunn KA, et al. Traumatic brain injury in the United States: a public health perspective. J Head Trauma Rehabil 1999;14(6):602–15.
10. Lu J, Marmarou A, Choi S, et al. Mortality from traumatic brain injury. Acta Neurochir Suppl 2005;95:281–5.
11. Carey ME. Analysis of wounds incurred by U.S. Army Seventh Corps personnel treated in Corps hospitals during Operation Desert Storm, February 20 to March 10, 1991. J Trauma 1996;40(Suppl 3):S165–9.
12. Rustemeyer J, Kranz V, Bremerich A. Injuries in combat from 1982-2005 with particular reference to those to the head and neck: a review. Br J Oral Maxillofac Surg 2007;45(7):556–60.
13. Patel TH, Wenner KA, Price SA, et al. A U.S. army forward surgical team's experience in operation Iraqi freedom. J Trauma 2004;57(2):201–7.
14. Holcomb JB, McMullin NR, Pearse L, et al. Causes of death in U.S. Special Operations Forces in the global war on terrorism: 2001-2004. Ann Surg 2007;245(6):986–91.
15. Sariego J. CCATT: a military model for civilian disaster management. Disaster Manag Response 2006;4(4):114–7.

16. Eastridge BJ, Jenkins D, Flaherty S, et al. Trauma system development in a theater of war: experiences from operation Iraqi freedom and operation enduring freedom. J Trauma 2006;61(6):1366–72 [discussion: 1372–3].

17. Stein SC, Chen XH, Sinson GP, et al. Intravascular coagulation: a major secondary insult in nonfatal traumatic brain injury. J Neurosurg 2002;97(6):1373–7.

18. Chesnut RM. Statistical association between surgical intracranial pathology and extracranial traumatic injuries. J Trauma 1993;35(3):492–3.

19. Zwahlen RA, Labler L, Trentz O, et al. Lateral impact in closed head injury: a substantially increased risk for diffuse axonal injury—a preliminary study. J Craniomaxillofac Surg 2007;35(3):142–6.

20. Servadei F, Teasdale G, Merry G. Defining acute mild head injury in adults: a proposal based on prognostic factors, diagnosis, and management. J Neurotrauma 2001;18(7):657–64.

21. Haydel MJ, Preston CA, Mills TJ, et al. Indications for computed tomography in patients with minor head injury. N Engl J Med 2000;343(2):100–5.

22. Ingebrigtsen T, Romner B. Routine early CT-scan is cost saving after minor head injury. Acta Neurol Scand 1996;93(2–3):207–10.

23. Arienta C, Caroli M, Balbi S. Management of head-injured patients in the emergency department: a practical protocol. Surg Neurol 1997;48(3):213–9.

24. Stiell IG, Wells GA, Vandemheen K, et al. The Canadian CT Head Rule for patients with minor head injury. Lancet 2001;357(9266):1391–6.

25. Gittleman AM, Ortiz AO, Keating DP, et al. Indications for CT in patients receiving anticoagulation after head trauma. AJNR Am J Neuroradiol 2005; 26(3):603–6.

26. Wojcik R, Cipolle MD, Seislove E, et al. Preinjury warfarin does not impact outcome in trauma patients. J Trauma 2001;51(6):1147–51 [discussion: 1151–2].

27. Reynolds FD, Dietz PA, Higgins D, et al. Time to deterioration of the elderly, anticoagulated, minor head injury patient who presents without evidence of neurologic abnormality. J Trauma 2003;54(3):492–6.

28. Pieracci FM, Eachempati SR, Shou J, et al. Degree of anticoagulation, but not warfarin use itself, predicts adverse outcomes after traumatic brain injury in elderly trauma patients. J Trauma 2007;63(3):525–30.

29. Mina AA, Knipfer JF, Park DY, et al. Intracranial complications of preinjury anticoagulation in trauma patients with head injury. J Trauma 2002;53(4): 668–72.

30. Ohm C, Mina A, Howells G, et al. Effects of antiplatelet agents on outcomes for elderly patients with traumatic intracranial hemorrhage. J Trauma 2005;58(3):518–22.

31. Ivascu FA, Howells GA, Junn FS, et al. Predictors of mortality in trauma patients with intracranial hemorrhage on preinjury aspirin or clopidogrel. J Trauma 2008;65(4): 785–8.

32. Jones K, Sharp C, Mangram AJ, et al. The effects of preinjury clopidogrel use on older trauma patients with head injuries. Am J Surg 2006;192(6):743–5.

33. Fortuna GR, Mueller EW, James LE, et al. The impact of preinjury antiplatelet and anticoagulant pharmacotherapy on outcomes in elderly patients with hemorrhagic brain injury. Surgery 2008;144(4):598–603 [discussion: 603–5].

34. Spektor S, Agus S, Merkin V, et al. Low-dose aspirin prophylaxis and risk of intracranial hemorrhage in patients older than 60 years of age with mild or moderate head injury: a prospective study. J Neurosurg 2003;99(4):661–5.

35. Davenport ND, Lim KO, Armstrong MT, et al. Diffuse and spatially variable white matter disruptions are associated with blast-related mild traumatic brain injury. Neuroimage 2012;59(3):2017–24.

36. Yallampalli R, Wilde EA, Bigler ED, et al. Acute white matter differences in the fornix following mild traumatic brain injury using diffusion tensor imaging. J Neuroimaging 2010. DOI:10.1111/j.1552-6569.2010.00537.x. [Epub ahead of print].

37. Sharp DJ, Ham TE. Investigating white matter injury after mild traumatic brain injury. Curr Opin Neurol 2011;24(6):558–63.

38. Jager TE, Weiss HB, Coben JH, et al. Traumatic brain injuries evaluated in U.S. emergency departments, 1992-1994. Acad Emerg Med 2000;7(2):134–40.

39. Rockswold GL, Pheley PJ. Patients who talk and deteriorate. Ann Emerg Med 1993;22(6):1004–7.

40. Colohan AR, Oyesiku NM. Moderate head injury: an overview. J Neurotrauma 1992;9(Suppl 1):S259–64.

41. Ling GS, Marshall SA. Management of traumatic brain injury in the intensive care unit. Neurol Clin 2008;26(2):409–26, viii.

42. Medical aspects of the persistent vegetative state (1). The Multi-Society Task Force on PVS. N Engl J Med 1994;330(21):1499–508.

43. Feickert HJ, Drommer S, Heyer R. Severe head injury in children: impact of risk factors on outcome. J Trauma 1999;47(1):33–8.

44. Siegel JH. The effect of associated injuries, blood loss, and oxygen debt on death and disability in blunt traumatic brain injury: the need for early physiologic predictors of severity. J Neurotrauma 1995;12(4):579–90.

45. Agrawal A, Timothy J, Cincu R, et al. Bradycardia in neurosurgery. Clin Neurol Neurosurg 2008;110(4):321–7.

46. Guidelines for the acute medical management of severe traumatic brain injury in infants, children, and adolescents. J Trauma 2003;54(Suppl 6):S235–310.

47. Marion DW, Penrod LE, Kelsey SF, et al. Treatment of traumatic brain injury with moderate hypothermia. N Engl J Med 1997;336(8):540–6.

48. Badjatia N, Carney N, Crocco TJ, et al. Guidelines for prehospital management of traumatic brain injury 2nd edition. Prehosp Emerg Care 2008;12(Suppl 1):S1–52.

49. Wisner DH, Victor NS, Holcroft JW. Priorities in the management of multiple trauma: intracranial versus intra-abdominal injury. J Trauma 1993;35(2):271–6 [discussion: 276–8].

50. Oertel M, Kelly DF, Lee JH, et al. Efficacy of hyperventilation, blood pressure elevation, and metabolic suppression therapy in controlling intracranial pressure after head injury. J Neurosurg 2002;97(5):1045–53.

51. Marion DW. Head and spinal cord injury. Neurol Clin 1998;16(2):485–502.

52. Jia X, Koenig MA, Shin HC, et al. Improving neurological outcomes post-cardiac arrest in a rat model: immediate hypothermia and quantitative EEG monitoring. Resuscitation 2008;76(3):431–42.

53. Wang H, Gao J, Lassiter TF, et al. Levetiracetam is neuroprotective in murine models of closed head injury and subarachnoid hemorrhage. Neurocrit Care 2006;5(1):71–8.

54. Patel HC, Menon DK, Tebbs S, et al. Specialist neurocritical care and outcome from head injury. Intensive Care Med 2002;28(5):547–53.

55. Lazaridis C, Desantis SM, McLawhorn M, et al. Liberation of neurosurgical patients from mechanical ventilation and tracheostomy in neurocritical care. J Crit Care 2011. [Epub ahead of print].

56. Anderson RC, Kan P, Klimo P, et al. Complications of intracranial pressure monitoring in children with head trauma. J Neurosurg 2004;101(Suppl 1):53–8.

57. Stein SC, Georgoff P, Meghan S, et al. Relationship of aggressive monitoring and treatment to improved outcomes in severe traumatic brain injury. J Neurosurg 2010;112(5):1105–12.

58. Liu D, Kahn M. Measurement and relationship of subarachnoid pressure of the optic nerve to intracranial pressures in fresh cadavers. Am J Ophthalmol 1993; 116(5):548–56.

59. Rasulo FA, De Peri E, Lavinio A. Transcranial Doppler ultrasonography in intensive care. Eur J Anaesthesiol Suppl 2008;42:167–73.

60. Fodale V, Schifilliti D, Conti A, et al. Transcranial Doppler and anesthetics. Acta Anaesthesiol Scand 2007;51(7):839–47.

61. Klingelhofer J, Conrad B, Benecke R, et al. Evaluation of intracranial pressure from transcranial Doppler studies in cerebral disease. J Neurol 1988;235(3):159–62.

62. Czosnyka M, Matta BF, Smielewski P, et al. Cerebral perfusion pressure in head-injured patients: a noninvasive assessment using transcranial Doppler ultrasonography. J Neurosurg 1998;88(5):802–8.

63. Soldatos T, Chatzimichail K, Papathanasiou M, et al. Optic nerve sonography: a new window for the non-invasive evaluation of intracranial pressure in brain injury. Emerg Med J 2009;26(9):630–4.

64. Geeraerts T, Duranteau J, Benhamou D. Ocular sonography in patients with raised intracranial pressure: the papilloedema revisited. Crit Care 2008;12(3):150.

65. Geeraerts T, Newcombe VF, Coles JP, et al. Use of T2-weighted magnetic resonance imaging of the optic nerve sheath to detect raised intracranial pressure. Crit Care 2008;12(5):R114.

66. Cruz J. Relationship between early patterns of cerebral extraction of oxygen and outcome from severe acute traumatic brain swelling: cerebral ischemia or cerebral viability? Crit Care Med 1996;24(6):953–6.

67. Figaji AA, Zwane E, Thompson C, et al. Brain tissue oxygen tension monitoring in pediatric severe traumatic brain injury. Part 1: relationship with outcome. Childs Nerv Syst 2009;25(10):1325–33.

68. Koenig MA, Bryan M, Lewin JL 3rd, et al. Reversal of transtentorial herniation with hypertonic saline. Neurology 2008;70(13):1023–9.

69. Ware ML, Nemani VM, Meeker M, et al. Effects of 23.4% sodium chloride solution in reducing intracranial pressure in patients with traumatic brain injury: a preliminary study. Neurosurgery 2005;57(4):727–36 [discussion: 727–36].

70. Barmparas G, Inaba K, Georgiou C, et al. Swan-Ganz catheter use in trauma patients can be reduced without negatively affecting outcomes. World J Surg 2011;35(8):1809–17.

71. Qureshi AI, Suarez JI, Castro A, et al. Use of hypertonic saline/acetate infusion in treatment of cerebral edema in patients with head trauma: experience at a single center. J Trauma 1999;47(4):659–65.

72. Ziai WC, Toung TJ, Bhardwaj A. Hypertonic saline: first-line therapy for cerebral edema? J Neurol Sci 2007;261(1–2):157–66.

73. Schreckinger M, Marion DW. Contemporary management of traumatic intracranial hypertension: is there a role for therapeutic hypothermia? Neurocrit Care 2009;11(3):427–36.

74. Kelly DF, Goodale DB, Williams J, et al. Propofol in the treatment of moderate and severe head injury: a randomized, prospective double-blinded pilot trial. J Neurosurg 1999;90(6):1042–52.

75. Muizelaar JP, Schroder ML. Overview of monitoring of cerebral blood flow and metabolism after severe head injury. Can J Neurol Sci 1994;21(2):S6–11.

76. Bullock MR, Chesnut R, Ghajar J, et al. Surgical management of acute epidural hematomas. Neurosurgery 2006;58(Suppl 3):S7–15 [discussion: Si–iv].

77. Bullock MR, Chesnut R, Ghajar J, et al. Surgical management of acute subdural hematomas. Neurosurgery 2006;58(Suppl 3):S16–24 [discussion: Si–iv].

78. Guerra WK, Gaab MR, Dietz H, et al. Surgical decompression for traumatic brain swelling: indications and results. J Neurosurg 1999;90(2):187–96.
79. Albanese J, Leone M, Alliez JR, et al. Decompressive craniectomy for severe traumatic brain injury: evaluation of the effects at one year. Crit Care Med 2003;31(10):2535–8.
80. Rosenfeld JV, Cooper DJ, Kossmann T, et al. Decompressive craniectomy. J Neurosurg 2007;106(1):195–6 [author reply: 197].
81. Okie S. Traumatic brain injury in the war zone. N Engl J Med 2005;352(20): 2043–7.
82. Schlifka B. Lessons learned from OIF: a neurosurgical perspective. J Trauma 2007;62(Suppl 6):S103–4.
83. Munch E, Horn P, Schurer L, et al. Management of severe traumatic brain injury by decompressive craniectomy. Neurosurgery 2000;47(2):315–22 [discussion: 322–3].
84. Cooper DJ, Rosenfeld JV, Murray L, et al. Decompressive craniectomy in diffuse traumatic brain injury. N Engl J Med 2011;364(16):1493–502.
85. Marion DW. Decompressive craniectomy in diffuse traumatic brain injury. Lancet Neurol 2011;10(6):497–8.
86. Hutchinson PJ, Timofeev I, Kolias AG, et al. Decompressive craniectomy for traumatic brain injury: the jury is still out. Br J Neurosurg 2011;25(3):441–2.
87. Ahmad FU, Bullock R. Decompressive craniectomy for severe head injury. World Neurosurg 2011;75(3–4):451–3.
88. Pompucci A, De Bonis P, Pettorini B, et al. Decompressive craniectomy for traumatic brain injury: patient age and outcome. J Neurotrauma 2007;24(7):1182–8.
89. Jennett B, Bond M. Assessment of outcome after severe brain damage. Lancet 1975;1(7905):480–4.
90. Jennett B, Snoek J, Bond MR, et al. Disability after severe head injury: observations on the use of the Glasgow Outcome Scale. J Neurol Neurosurg Psychiatry 1981;44(4):285–93.
91. Wilson JT, Pettigrew LE, Teasdale GM. Structured interviews for the Glasgow Outcome Scale and the extended Glasgow Outcome Scale: guidelines for their use. J Neurotrauma 1998;15(8):573–85.
92. Pettigrew LE, Wilson JT, Teasdale GM. Assessing disability after head injury: improved use of the Glasgow Outcome Scale. J Neurosurg 1998;89(6):939–43.
93. Teasdale GM, Pettigrew LE, Wilson JT, et al. Analyzing outcome of treatment of severe head injury: a review and update on advancing the use of the Glasgow Outcome Scale. J Neurotrauma 1998;15(8):587–97.
94. Perel P, Arango M, Clayton T, et al. Predicting outcome after traumatic brain injury: practical prognostic models based on large cohort of international patients. BMJ 2008;336(7641):425–9.
95. Hou DJ, Tong KA, Ashwal S, et al. Diffusion-weighted magnetic resonance imaging improves outcome prediction in adult traumatic brain injury. J Neurotrauma 2007;24(10):1558–69.
96. Benson RR, Meda SA, Vasudevan S, et al. Global white matter analysis of diffusion tensor images is predictive of injury severity in traumatic brain injury. J Neurotrauma 2007;24(3):446–59.

Evolving Changes in the Management of Burns and Environmental Injuries

Leopoldo C. Cancio, MD[a], Jonathan B. Lundy, MD[a],
Robert L. Sheridan, MD[b],*

KEYWORDS

- Burns • Inhalation injury • Heat injury • Frostbite • Hypothermia

KEY POINTS

- As in trauma, a formatted initial evaluation of burn patients will minimize missed opportunities for optimal care.
- Fluid resuscitation of burns continues to evolve. Colloid and hourly adjustment play an increasingly important role.
- Critical care of the burn patient has several unique components, particularly pain and anxiety control, environmental control, inhalation injury management, transeschar fluid and electrolyte losses, and nutritional support issues.
- Burn care can be divided into four phases: initial evaluation and resuscitation, initial wound care, definitive wound closure, and rehabilitation and reconstruction.
- Rehabilitation should begin coincident with initial care.
- Injuries due to heat and cold have both systemic and local priorities.
- Freeze-thaw-refreeze should be avoided in frostbite patients. In rare patients with frostbite, there may be a role for thrombolytics.

INTRODUCTION

Burns, soft-tissue wounds, and environmental injuries are common in injured survivors of natural disasters and terrorist incidents. They are also common in those injured

The opinions or assertions contained herein are the private views of the authors and are not to be construed as official or as reflecting the views of the Department of the Army or Department of Defense.

Disclosure: L.C.C. is coinventor of the Burn Resuscitation Decision Support System, a software program that has been licensed by the US Army for commercial production by Arcos, Inc, Galveston, TX.

[a] U.S. Army Institute of Surgical Research, 3698 Chambers Pass, Fort Sam Houston, TX 78234-6315, USA; [b] Department of Surgery, Shriners Hospital for Children, 51 Blossom Street, Boston, MA 02114, USA

* Corresponding author.

E-mail address: rsheridan@partners.org

Surg Clin N Am 92 (2012) 959–986

http://dx.doi.org/10.1016/j.suc.2012.06.002
surgical.theclinics.com

in combat and peacetime deployed military settings. Burns complicate a significant number of explosion injuries.[1] Effective management is facilitated by preestablished protocols, implementation of which require an understanding of the unique contributions of burns to morbidity and mortality. In general, patient management is divided into four phases: initial evaluation and resuscitation, initial wound management, definitive wound closure, and rehabilitation. The focus of this article is on recent advances in the initial hospital care of patients suffering burns and environmental injuries; long-term issues are only briefly acknowledged.

INITIAL EVALUATION
General Approach

The triage and initial evaluation of the burn patient should focus on identification of life-threatening injuries. During the primary survey, the airway takes first priority. Acute airway loss after thermal injury can be a result of direct damage to, and edema of, any portion of the upper airway—from face to glottis. Stridor, hoarseness, and/or respiratory distress identify a patient with inhalation injury who requires urgent intubation. Airway loss may occur during the initial hours postburn, even in the absence of inhalation injury and especially in patients with total body surface area (TBSA) burned equal to or greater than 40%. This is caused by edema of unburned tissue, for which early elective intubation is encouraged. Intubation may also be required for patients who are obtunded due to hypoxia and/or inhalation of toxic products of combustion (carbon monoxide, cyanide).

Children are at high risk of acute airway loss and tolerate hypoxia poorly. When intubating burned children, a cuffed endotracheal tube is preferable. During burn resuscitation, pulmonary compliance decreases, which can result in an uncontrolled air leak around an uncuffed tube. These same patients often develop massive facial edema, making urgent tube exchange treacherous—a situation which is best avoided from the outset.[2]

The inability to oxygenate after such injuries may be a result of airway obstruction, inhalation injury (see later discussion), or concomitant thoracic trauma. In addition, progressive edema of eschar and subjacent tissue of the chest and abdominal wall may lead to loss of thoracic compliance, elevated peak and plateau pressures, and hypoxia—especially if the patient has sustained circumferential, full-thickness torso burns.

Evaluation of adequate circulation and perfusion should include assessment of peripheral pulses, mentation, level of consciousness, and serum markers of hypoperfusion (base deficit, serum bicarbonate, and lactate). In the absence of concomitant mechanical trauma or a long delay in resuscitation, profound hypotension at initial evaluation is uncommon. During initial evaluation, intravenous access should be obtained and a fluid infusion started. In the absence of hypotension or other evidence of profound hypovolemic shock, no bolus should be given. This is in contradistinction to Advanced Trauma Life Support (ATLS) guidelines for mechanical trauma patients.[3]

Neurologic abnormalities during initial evaluation can result from toxin exposure, head or spine injury, or, less frequently, compression of peripheral nerves as a result of eschar or compartment syndrome. The final component of the primary survey concerns the exposure of the patient for identification of other injuries. If mechanical trauma is suspected, cervical spine precautions should be maintained until injury is ruled out. Facial burns place the patient at risk for corneal injury, so examination using a Woods lamp and fluorescein should be performed. Identification of all burns with mapping of the extent using a technique such as the rule of nines or the

Lund-Browder chart will help determine the severity of burn injury as well as predict expected resuscitative needs. Although obviously superficial burns (**Fig. 1**) and markedly deep burns (**Fig. 2**) are easily identified, many severely burned patients have a mix of superficial partial-thickness, deep partial-thickness, and full-thickness burns not readily distinguished acutely after injury. These wounds should be reexamined daily to assist with determination of depth and future surgical planning to achieve wound closure. Also, circumferential burns to extremities or the torso should be identified to alert the clinician to areas that may be at risk for development of eschar syndrome (see later discussion).

A special note should be made on abuse in thermally injured patients. Cases of abuse can occur in all age groups, but most commonly impact the extremes of age. Patterns of intentional thermal injury include cigarette burns (most common type of abuse-related burn, usually not requiring hospital admission), intentional immersion with scald injury to hands, buttocks, and posterior legs and heels, and iron burns of the hand. Abuse-related burns are most commonly seen in children of 2 years old or younger, who typically also demonstrate signs of neglect such as poor hygiene, malnutrition, and delayed psychological development. Suspicion of a burn related to abuse mandates a thorough investigation of the events surrounding the incident and referral to proper personnel to ensure the safety of the patient.

Transfer Criteria

As early as possible during initial evaluation, a determination should be made as to whether the patient merits referral to a burn center. The American Burn Association (ABA) has established criteria for burn center referral[4]:

- Extent ($\geq$10% TBSA)
- Location (face, hands, feet, genitalia, perineum, joints)
- Depth (any full thickness burns)
- Cause (electric, chemical, inhalation injury)
- Complicating factors (patients with special medical or rehabilitation needs).

When patients have mechanical trauma and burns, initial stabilization may be required in a trauma center, followed by burn center transfer. The key to managing the transfer process is early and frequent communication between the referring hospital and the receiving burn center.

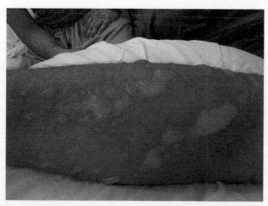

Fig. 1. Superficial thermal injury.

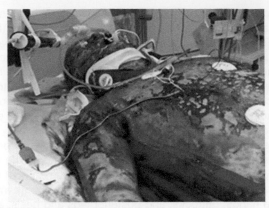

Fig. 2. Full-thickness thermal injury.

FLUID RESUSCITATION
Resuscitation Formulas

Thermal injury leads to progressive loss of intravascular volume, edema in burned and unburned tissue, and a decrease in cardiac output and vital organ perfusion. The amount of fluid lost is roughly a function of TBSA. The two classic and most commonly used burn resuscitation formulas are the modified Brooke formula (2 mL/kg/TBSA administered over 24 hours) and the Parkland formula (4 mL/kg/TBSA).[5,6] However, surveys through the ABA, the International Society for Burn Injuries (ISBI), and the European Burn Association (EBA) demonstrated wide variation in resuscitative techniques. The EBA survey revealed that 72% of burn units responding use either the original Parkland formula or some modification thereof.[7] Similarly, the ABA report showed that almost 70% of burn providers preferred the Parkland formula, followed by the Brooke (7%), Galveston (9%), and Warden hypertonic formulas (6%).[8] The complexity of current resuscitation formulas led Chung and colleagues[8] to develop a simplified technique for the initiation of fluid resuscitation (for adult patients only) termed the Institute of Surgical Research (ISR) rule of tens:

- Estimate TBSA burned to nearest 10%.
- Initial fluid rate (in mL/hr) equals TBSA times 10 (for adult patients with weight between 40 and 80 kg).
- In adults weighing more than 80 kg, increase rate by 100 mL/hr for every 10 kg above 80.

For example, in a 70 kg man with a 50% TBSA burn, the initial fluid resuscitation volume would be 500 mL/hr. Alternatively, in a 100 kg man with a similar 50% TBSA burn, the initial resuscitation volume would be 700 mL/hr. Using a computerized validation tool, these investigators showed that, in 88% of simulated patients, the initial resuscitative fluid rate using the ISR rule of tens fell between initial rates predicted by either the modified Brooke or Parkland formulas.[9]

Multiple studies have documented actual delivered fluid volumes far in excess of target volumes predicted by resuscitation formulas, a phenomenon termed fluid creep.[10] Several hypotheses have been proposed to explain this long-term trend, to include increased use of opioids.[11] It is unclear whether choice of resuscitation formula contributes to fluid creep because there are no randomized controlled trials of the Parkland versus Brooke formulas. However, Chung and colleagues[12] recently reported that, when combat casualties were started on the modified Brooke formula, they actually received 3.8 mL/kg/%TBSA. When started on the Parkland formula, they actually received 5.9 mL/kg/%TBSA. Patients initially begun on the Parkland formula more often surpassed input of 250 mL/kg over 24 hours, a level associated with increased risk of abdominal compartment syndrome (ACS). However, in this study, this overshoot in fluid resuscitation did not result in different outcomes between the groups.

Monitoring

The various formulas only provide a starting point. Fluid input must be titrated hourly based on patient response. Attention to this detail improves outcomes. In combat casualties, Ennis and colleagues[13] showed that compliance with a paper flow sheet for documentation of hourly fluid input and output improved a combined endpoint of mortality and ACS. Urine output remains the indicator most providers use (95%) to titrate resuscitative fluids.[8] In adults, the goal for urine output is 30 to 50 mL/h (alternatively, 0.5–1.0 mL/kg/h); in children it is 1 to 2 mL/kg/h.[5] This is achieved by increasing or decreasing the fluid infusion rate by 20% to 30% every 1 to 2 hours.

The modern era provides an array of techniques for monitoring intravascular volume or organ perfusion. Such technologies were used by 23% of providers in addition to urine output to guide resuscitation in an ABA survey. These included the pulmonary artery catheter (8%), base deficit (7%), lactate (5%), lithium indicator dilution (5%), transpulmonary thermodilution (3%), and hematocrit (1%). Caution should be used in interpreting these results because overenthusiastic attempts to normalize intravascular volume or, worse, achieve a supranormal cardiac output during the first 24 hours postburn place the patient at risk of overresuscitation and compartment syndromes.

Salinas and colleagues[14] recently reported the development of a computerized decision support program that is currently used for resuscitation of all severely burned patients at the US Army Burn Center. The main function of the program is to provide a recommendation each hour for the lactated Ringer's infusion rate based on the trend in the urine output over the past 3 hours, the time postburn, and the patient's burn size. Compared with historical controls, use of this program resulted in a reduction in crystalloid volumes infused during the first 24 and 48 hours, and the urine output was more frequently within the target range. A prospective study is planned.

Fluid of Choice

The most commonly used resuscitative fluid is lactated Ringer's (91% of those surveyed). Almost half of burn providers supplement crystalloid resuscitation with some type of colloid, typically starting 12 to 24 hours postburn.[8] This timing reflects that, during the initial 8 to 12 hours postburn, the microvasculature is incapable of sieving proteins. Use of colloid before hour 8 to 12 hours postburn may be ineffective or, worse, enhance edema formation.

Albumin (5% in normal saline) is the most commonly used colloid. The modified Brooke formula provides the following dose calculation for 5% albumin to be given over 24 hours:

- 0% to 29% TBSA: no albumin is normally given
- 30% to 49% TBSA: 0.3 mL/kg/TBSA
- 50% to 69% TBSA: 0.4 mL/kg/TBSA
- 70% to 100% TBSA: 0.5 mL/kg/TBSA.

The crystalloid infusion rate is then titrated as before, anticipating that it will be possible to decrease it. Fresh frozen plasma has also been used for burn shock. In one study, this practice resulted in fewer instances of elevated intraabdominal pressure.[15]

Adjuncts to Resuscitation

Preclinical data indicate that high-dose intravenous vitamin C reduces lipid peroxidation in the postburn period, ameliorates the increase in postburn vascular permeability, decreases resuscitative volume requirements, and reduces edema associated with thermal injury.[16] Tanaka and colleague's[17] single-center, prospective study in 37 patients admitted with burns greater than 30% TBSA revealed a significant reduction in resuscitative volume, weight gain, wound edema, and pulmonary dysfunction. The dose of vitamin C used in this study was 66 mg/kg/h, begun as rapidly as possible after injury. Although promising, these single-center results need further verification.

Therapeutic plasma exchange (TPE) has resurfaced as an adjunct for patients with refractory burn shock. TPE involves removal of blood from the patient via a large-bore intravenous catheter and separation of components. Plasma is collected and the remaining components are returned to the patient. The efficacy of TPE in inflammatory states is thought to be due to removal of large molecular weight proteins such as cytokines.[18,19]

Decompression

In burn patients, transvascular fluid flux during the first 48 hours postburn causes not only shock but also massive edema formation. Thus, the counterpart to fluid resuscitation in these patients is a decompressive strategy designed to minimize the effects of edema.[20] Circumferential or near-circumferential full-thickness burns involving the torso or extremities can result in a leather-like, noncompliant constrictive band. Progressive edema formation beneath the eschar then compresses underlying structures to include nerves, vessels, muscle, or lungs. This process is termed eschar syndrome. In the chest, it decreases thoracic compliance and may present as increased airway pressure, decreased tidal volume, respiratory acidosis, hypoxia, and, ultimately, cardiac arrest. Thoracic eschar syndrome is treated emergently at the bedside with escharotomy. Bilateral incisions are made through the eschar into underlying viable fat, from the midclavicular line, downwards along the anterior axillary line, and across the midline in the epigastric region (**Fig. 2**). An immediate improvement in compliance should be obvious. An analogous problem occurs in the extremities and is treated with extremity escharotomy (see later discussion).

With massive fluid resuscitation (eg, >250 mL/kg), ACS may develop. ACS requiring decompressive laparotomy is a highly lethal complication in this patient population. Every effort should be taken to anticipate and avoid it. The incidence of ACS in a review at the US Army Burn Center was 1%, with a mortality of 90% (18/20).[21] Latenser and colleagues[22] described a 9-patient pilot study of the use of percutaneous drainage for the treatment of intraabdominal hypertension (bladder pressure >25 mm Hg) in burns. They found that catheter drainage resulted in successful amelioration of the process and prevented progression in five patients. In a recent survey of burn physicians on the subject of ACS, 34% of respondents advocated percutaneous catheter decompression before decompressive laparotomy for ACS.[23]

Vulnerable Organs

Initial care of burn patients is focused, appropriately, on sustaining life. Nevertheless, failure to attend to certain burn-specific vulnerable organs throughout the resuscitation and intensive care course may result in lasting injury. These vulnerable organs include the extremities (the hands especially) and the eyes.

Several factors combine to place burn patients at risk for permanent extremity injury or loss. The most obvious risk is that of the extremity eschar syndrome, which develops during the first 48 hours postburn. In circumferential deep burns of an extremity, edema formation in the soft tissue beneath the inelastic burned skin (eschar) elevates internal pressure within the limb, constricting venous outflow and ultimately arterial inflow. Elevation of the burned extremities reduces the transvascular pressure experienced by the microvasculature during a period of increased permeability, and is essential to decreasing the risk of this syndrome.

Extremity eschar syndrome may be manifested by distal cyanosis (if the fingertips are unburned), numbness, tingling, and other signs and symptoms of vascular compromise. The progressive diminution or loss of distal pulses, which should be monitored hourly by Doppler flowmetry, is the classic indication for escharotomy. In the right clinical setting (ie, circumferential full thickness burns of an extremity) an experienced surgeon may perform escharotomy before a change in peripheral pulses. Escharotomy is commonly performed at the bedside under semisterile conditions using a scalpel and or electrocautery to incise the eschar along the midmedial and midlateral joint lines. Care must be taken to incise all circumferential eschar, to achieve good hemostasis, to incise all the way through the eschar but to stay out of the viable tissue beneath it, and to document pulse restoration (**Fig. 3**).

If the hand is burned, and if limb escharotomies do not restore pulsatile Doppler flow to the palmar arch and digital arteries, then additional hand and finger escharotomies may be required. Dorsal hand escharotomies are performed over the location of the dorsal interossei (between the metacarpals). Finger escharotomies are performed on the radial aspect of the thumb and on the ulnar aspect of the other digits, using care to stay between the extensor mechanism and the neurovascular bundle.

Extremity eschar syndrome must be distinguished from extremity compartment syndrome. The authors use the latter term to refer to the process whereby pressure

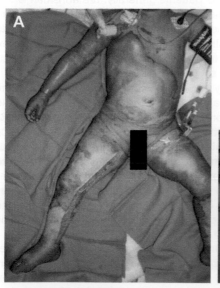
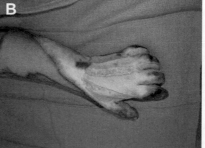

Fig. 3. (*A, B*) Escharotomies.

within the investing fascia of an extremity causes vascular compromise and neuro-muscular damage. Common causes of compartment syndrome include vascular injury and repair, crush injury, or fracture. In a burn patient, compartment syndrome may also result from a delay in escharotomy, leading to ischemia-reperfusion injury; from direct muscle injury (eg, from high-voltage electricity or blast injury); or from massive fluid resuscitation and anasarca. Regardless of the cause, recognize that the treat-ment of eschar syndrome is escharotomy, whereas the treatment of compartment syndrome is fasciotomy. Performing a prophylactic fasciotomy on a patient who requires only an escharotomy exposes uninjured muscle to microbial contamination. Equally, failure to diagnose compartment syndrome in a burn patient places the limb at risk. When diagnosis is delayed, compartment syndrome may present as sepsis with dead, infected muscle anywhere from approximately 12 days to 2 months after injury.

Following successful resuscitation, burned hands remain at high risk until success-ful wound closure and rehabilitation have been achieved. This is a function of depth of injury. Ninety-seven percent of patients with superficial hand burns had normal func-tion at discharge compared with 81% of those who required surgery for deep dermal or full thickness injuries. Furthermore, only 9% of patients with injury to the extensor mechanism, joint capsule, or bone had a normal functional outcome.[24]

The above concepts are well-recognized problems in burn care. Less well docu-mented are postburn peripheral nerve injuries. These may be manifested by weak-ness, numbness, and/or tingling. In a prospective study, symptomatic patients underwent nerve conduction studies, and peripheral neuropathy was diagnosed in 10%. The most commonly involved nerve was the median sensory nerve, followed by the ulnar sensory nerve. All patients but one had sensory and motor involvement of at least two nerves.[25] Risk factors for neuropathy in another study included ICU days, history of alcohol abuse, age, and electric injury. Attention to eschar and compartment syndromes, careful positioning and splinting, avoidance of tight dress-ings, and detailed neurologic examination are keys to prevention and early detection of peripheral neuropathy in burn patients.

It seems likely that burn patients, like ICU patients generally, are at risk for critical illness polyneuropathy (CIP) and critical illness myopathy (CIM). CIP is a distal axonal sensory-motor polyneuropathy affecting the limbs and phrenic nerve. CIM is a primary myopathy not secondary to denervation. CIP and CIM often coexist. Both may present as extremity weakness, difficulty weaning from the ventilator, and months to years of disability.[26] The pathophysiology of these syndromes is not fully understood.

Thermally injured patients are particularly vulnerable to ocular injury throughout their ICU course. In one study, one-quarter of patients with facial burns, TBSA greater than 20%, and/or inhalation injury had ocular complications. Patients receiving mechanical ventilation, with wound infections, and with decreased Glasgow Coma Scale score were at particular risk.[27] Accordingly, all patients with periorbital burns should undergo Wood's lamp examination on admission to rule out corneal abrasions. Posi-tive or doubtful results merit immediate ophthalmologic consultation. Failure to treat corneal abrasion aggressively may lead to corneal ulceration, perforation, and blind-ness. Amniotic membrane transplantation is one technique available to treat signifi-cant corneal injury. For most patients, aggressive treatment with topical antibiotics and daily follow-up by the ophthalmologist is effective.

Like abdominal and extremity compartment syndromes, orbital compartment syndrome (OCS) is increasingly recognized in thermally injured patients who receive large fluid resuscitations. If untreated, OCS can cause blindness. Based on retrospec-tive data, the intraocular pressure (IOP) should be measured daily using a portable tonometer for the first 2 to 3 days postburn, particularly in patients whose 24-hour fluid resuscitation volume exceeds 5.5 mL/kg/% burn. When the IOP is found to be elevated (ie, above 30 mm Hg), orbital release by lateral canthotomy and cantholysis should be considered.[28]

Over time, deeply burned eyelids may scar and contract open, leading to extrinsic ectropion, conjunctivitis, and exposure of the corneas. When this occurs, secondary keratitis again places the corneas at risk. One approach to this problem is tarsorrhaphy. Because this procedure does not correct the underlying scarring process, tarsorrhaphy often fails, damaging the tarsal plates in the process. For this reason, many investigators consider tarsorrhaphy to be contraindicated in this setting.[29] Instead, release of deep eyelid burns should be considered when the patient can no longer protect the corneas. Moisture goggles help protect the corneas until this operation can be performed.

CRITICAL CARE OF THE BURN PATIENT
The Burn ICU

Both the environment of care and a team approach are exceedingly important for successful outcomes in burns. Three characteristics make the burn ICU environment different from other ICUs: infection control, temperature control, and hydrotherapy. Burn centers were the original research institutes for infection control. Individual isolation rooms; rigorous hand washing; personal protective gear such as gowns, gloves, masks, hats, and shoe covers; microbial surveillance; and antibiotic stewardship constituted the infection-control bundle enacted at the US Army Burn Center ICU in 1983, which was associated with eradication of pandemic multiple-drug resistant organisms. Other units have reduced cross-contamination with bacteria-controlled nursing units (BCNUs), which further isolate the patient within a laminar airflow chamber with plastic walls.[30] The importance of housekeeping and the quality of the physical plant in preventing infection cannot be ignored.

Another essential feature of the burn center environment of care is temperature control. Because one of the functions of the skin is to act as a barrier against heat loss, and because injury redirects blood flow to the wound surface, patients with extensive burns are at risk of hypothermia. Even when hypothermia is not overtly recognized as a decrease in body temperature, a normal room temperature increases a burn patient's metabolic rate through the process of nonshivering thermogenesis. This adds to the patient's already hypermetabolic, hypercatabolic state. In the operating room (OR), burn patients are at high risk of hypothermia for several reasons:

- Exposure of multiple wounds
- Significant blood loss and fluid requirements
- Impairment of peripheral vasoconstriction by anesthetic agents.

The main solution to the hypothermia problem is to elevate the room temperature to suit the patient's needs rather than the providers' comfort. This means an ICU room temperature of 85°F and an OR temperature of 90° to 95°F.

A third essential feature is a dedicated tank or shower facility for hydrotherapy. Eighty-three percent of North American burn centers report such a capability. Because hydrotherapy tanks are a potential locus for transmission of nosocomial organisms, they are less common today. Instead, patients can be showered on a special shower cart. Either way, hydrotherapy is widely used to facilitate wound care.[31]

The most important aspect of burn ICU care, however, is not the physical plant but the team approach to care. Just as burns are among the most lethal and disfiguring injuries known to humans, the coordinated efforts of multiple disciplines are required to achieve functional survival. These disciplines include surgery, nursing, rehabilitation, respiratory therapy, nutrition care, psychology, and social work. Multidisciplinary team rounds should be conducted daily. Success is a function not of any one individual, but of an effective burn team. The surgeon's key role is to lead this team by developing and communicating an overall management strategy based on a complete head-to-toe evaluation of the burn patient on admission to the ICU and frequently thereafter.

Pain and Anxiety

Burns and burn treatment is painful. Pain generates anticipatory anxiety that amplifies the experience of pain. Pain makes it difficult for even experienced personnel to perform thorough wound care and rehabilitation. Poorly controlled pain and anxiety may contribute to long-term psychological sequelae. The cornerstone of initial pain management is frequent, small doses of an intravenous narcotic. Opiates, benzodiazepines, and ketamine are useful in procedural sedation but must be carefully monitored. Nonpharmacologic approaches to management of pain and anxiety are an important part of burn care. Available techniques include hypnosis, immersive virtual reality, and music therapy. Anxiety should be specifically managed and benzodiazepines are the pharmacologic tools most frequently used. Dexmedetomidine may play an important role in these procedures in coming years.[32]

Pulmonary

Inhalation injury consists of three processes that can coexist in any single patient: upper airway injury, subglottic injury, and chemical asphyxiant inhalation. Injury to the upper airway—lips, tongue, pharynx, and larynx—causes edema and may cause precipitous airway obstruction during the first 48 hours postburn. Patients presenting with symptomatic inhalation injury should be prophylactically intubated, particularly before interhospital transfer. The same is true of patients with TBSA of approximately 40% or more, even in the absence of inhalation injury, because edema during resuscitation can cause airway obstruction.

Once the patient has been intubated, continuous attention to the security and patency of the endotracheal tube is critical. Adhesive tape does not stick to a burned face and should not be used. Security is ensured by tying the tube using umbilical tape (cotton ties) circumferentially around the head. As the face swells during resuscitation, repositioning of the ties may be needed to ensure that the endotracheal tube remains at the correct distance from the carina. Likewise, the face should be protected from and inspected for lesions that can be caused by the ties. The tube can alternatively be wired to the upper incisors using an arch bar.[29] Patency is achieved by frequent suctioning and by the use of nebulized heparin (5000 units in 5 mL NS every 4 hours, or 10,000 units every 6 hours) to prevent the formation of endoluminal clots and casts in patients with inhalation injury. Early detection of endotracheal tube obstruction is facilitated by end-tidal carbon dioxide monitoring. Fiberoptic bronchoscopy is performed on admission to diagnose inhalation injury and is repeated as needed to perform pulmonary toilet.

Early tracheostomy (within a few days of injury) may facilitate pulmonary toilet in patients with severe inhalation injury and copious cast formation. The larger, shorter, easily replaceable airway provided by the tracheostomy may be lifesaving. In other patients, tracheostomy is often performed after 21 days of endotracheal intubation. It is still unclear, however, whether tracheostomy or prolonged translaryngeal intubation is preferable in burn patients.[33] In one retrospective study, translaryngeal endotracheal intubation was safe and effective in thermally injured children for up to 3 months.[34] Increasingly, chronic pathologic conditions following prolonged intubation or tracheostomy in burn patients have been documented. These problems include dysphagia; dysphonia; granulation tissue; vocal cord paresis, fixation, or fusion; arytenoid dislocation; and bronchial, tracheal, or subglottic stenosis.[35]

The second form of inhalation injury is injury to the subglottic airways and pulmonary parenchyma, mediated by toxic gases and particulate matter. Distinct from other causes of acute lung injury, smoke inhalation injury attacks the small airways more so than the alveolar-capillary membrane.[36] Major mechanisms active in inhalation injury include oxidative[37] and nitrosative stress[38]; activation of coagulation and inhibition of fibrinolysis[39,40]; increased bronchial blood flow[41]; hypersecretion of mucus[42]; bronchiolar obstruction[43]; and ventilation-perfusion mismatch. Therapies directed at maintaining small airway patency are, therefore, key to the treatment of patients with this injury. Examples include inhaled heparin (see previous discussion) and high-frequency percussive ventilation (Volumetric Diffusive Respiration [VDR], Percussionaire, Sandpoint, Idaho, USA). A randomized controlled trial of VDR versus low-tidal-volume ventilation according to the ARDSnet algorithm—in burn patients with or without inhalation injury—demonstrated a higher rescue need (ie, transition to another mode due to failure to meet ventilation and oxygenation goals) for the ARDSnet group.[44] Inhaled beta agonists, such as albuterol, are routinely given to patients with inhalation injury to prevent bronchoconstriction. A recent preclinical study demonstrated that inhaled epinephrine improves pulmonary function after inhalation injury by reducing airway blood flow (and, in turn, airway edema, mucus secretion, inflammation, and ventilation-perfusion mismatch).[45]

The third form of inhalation injury is systemic toxicity caused by the absorption into the blood of the chemical asphyxiants present in smoke. Carbon monoxide (CO) binds to hemoglobin more avidly than does oxygen, forming carboxyhemoglobin (COHb). This has two deleterious consequences for oxygen delivery: the hemoglobin binding sites occupied by CO are not available to carry oxygen, causing a relative anemia; and CO binding alters the hemoglobin such that the oxygen dissociation curve is shifted toward the left. CO also binds to the terminal cytochrome oxidase on the mitochondrial electron transport chain.[46] This causes impaired cellular respiration and oxidative stress. Oxidative stress and inflammation also result from several other pathways.[47] Symptoms of CO toxicity range from mild (eg, headache, nausea) to severe (eg, coma, myocardial infarction, death). Treatment of CO poisoning consists of 100% oxygen until the COHb is less than 5%.[48] Because 100% oxygen decreases the half life of COHb from approximately4 hours to approximately1 hour, use of hyperbaric oxygen (HBO) to further accelerate CO elimination–particularly in unstable burn patients–may be impractical. However, a randomized controlled trial demonstrated that HBO (within 24 hrs of end of exposure) prevented delayed neurologic sequelae of CO,[49] likely by mechanisms other than hemoglobin binding.

Cyanide (CN) also binds to the terminal cytochrome oxidase, albeit at a different site than CO. By interfering with the cell's ability to use oxygen, CN produces rapid cardiovascular collapse and unconsciousness.[50] The prevalence of CN poisoning in patients with smoke inhalation injury is debated; the diagnosis is made difficult by the lack of a rapid assay, but it can be suspected in patients with lactic acidosis on initial presentation out of proportion to the burn size. Several antidotes are available for CN poisoning. Amyl and sodium nitrite convert hemoglobin to methemoglobin, which chelates CN. This treatment is risky, however, because methemoglobin is incapable of carrying oxygen and causes vasodilatation. Recently, high-dose hydroxocobalamin (Cyanokit) has become available for the treatment of CN poisoning; it also chelates

CN without the side effects of the nitrites.[50] Finally, sodium thiosulfate serves as a sulfur donor for hepatic rhodanase, which converts CN to thiocyanate. It has a slower onset of action than the other drugs.

Renal, Fluid, and Electrolyte Issues After Resuscitation

Successful resuscitation of a patient with burn shock is signaled by a sustained decrease in the fluid infusion rate required to maintain a urine output in the target range to maintenance levels, and usually occurs by 48 hours postburn. Other indicators of successful resuscitation include hemodynamic stability, resolution of lactic acidosis, and normalization of the base deficit. Patients can then be expected to offload the large amounts of resuscitation fluids during the ensuing 10 days or so. Assessment of volume status and of the adequacy of end-organ perfusion can be challenging in these patients, whose burn-induced hypermetabolic state and systemic inflammatory response syndrome drives an elevated heart rate, increased cardiac output, and decreased systemic vascular resistance even in the absence of any infection or other complications. When volume status is in doubt, measurement of the base deficit, lactate, central venous pressure, central venous saturation of oxygen, stroke-volume variability and, most important, of the response to a therapeutic intervention, such as a bolus of fluid, are diagnostically useful.

Frequent (eg, twice daily) measurement of serum electrolytes, including calcium, magnesium, and phosphate, is important during the management of critically ill burn patients. The most striking feature of fluid and electrolyte balance in these patients after resuscitation is evaporative water loss, which will result in hypernatremia if untreated. Such water loss is proportional to the open wound size. Water losses during a 24-hour period can be estimated as 1 mL/kg/(open burn size,%). This provides an estimate of water requirements. Water intake can be provided enterally (as a component of tube feedings or as additional water flushes), and/or intravenously (as 5% dextrose in water [D5W] or D5W in half-normal saline). Water intake is then adjusted based on daily or twice daily measurements of the serum sodium level. With wound healing, the open wound size gradually decreases and with it the daily water requirement. Burn patients are also at risk for hyponatremia, particularly if allowed to drink freely. Hypophosphatemia requiring intravenous replacement is common in patients with major thermal injury, particularly during days 3 to 5 postburn. Potassium and magnesium levels should be checked daily and replaced as needed.

Acute kidney injury (AKI) classified according to Acute Kidney Injury Network (AKIN) or Risk, Injury, Failure, Loss, End-Stage (RIFLE) criteria, is fairly common in burn patients. Using the RIFLE criteria, AKI occurred in 27% of 304 patients with burns equal to or greater than 10% TBSA.[51] Risk factors for AKI in this study included inhalation injury and sepsis. Failure (RIFLE, F) was an independent predictor of mortality. To address this problem, Chung and colleagues[52] implemented a continuous renal replacement therapy program for adult burn patients at the US Army Burn Center. This program is managed by intensivists and operated by specially trained ICU nurses. Patients undergo continuous venovenous hemofiltration (CVVH) if they meet AKIN 2 (with shock) or AKIN 3 criteria. Compared with historical controls, CVVH decreased mortality and pressor requirements. A multicenter study of CVVH for this patient population is underway.

Gastrointestinal

Abdominal complications occurred in 7% of patients admitted to one burn center and are more likely with increasing burn size.[21] ACS is a feared intraabdominal catastrophe, the avoidance of which is a principal goal during the initial fluid resuscitation of burn patients; however, it can also occur at other times during the ICU course, for example following massive perioperative resuscitation.[21]

Another cause of intraabdominal catastrophe in thermally injured patients is nonocclusive mesenteric ischemia (NOMI). This highly lethal complication (mortality approximately 70%) presents as necrosis of variable portions of the small and/or large bowel.[21] The onset of NOMI is usually later in the course than ACS, although some ACS patients also have NOMI at laparotomy. The cause of NOMI in burn patients is unknown. Retrospective efforts to relate it to pressor use, massive burn wound excision, and/or hyperosmolar enteral feeding have been inconclusive. Diagnosis is often made by CT scan, but diagnostic peritoneal lavage can be used in the unstable patient.

Whereas stress gastroduodenal ulceration in burn patients (Curling's ulcer) is now uncommon, it is important to recall that thermal injury causes a dose-related ulcer diathesis with evidence of mucosal injury (in untreated patients) within 12 hours of injury. In the era before antacids, H_2 blockers, and proton-pump inhibitors, this led to laparotomy for control of hemorrhage or perforation in a significant number of patients, highlighting the importance of prevention in this patient population.

Impaired bowel function is both a marker of critical illness and a frequent consequence of narcotic administration in burn patients. Critically ill burn patients are also at risk of pancreatitis. Forty percent of patients with burns greater than 20% TBSA had hyperamylasemia and or hyperlipasemia in one review, of whom 82% had symptoms of pancreatitis.[53] The burn patient with elevated cholestatic enzymes and evidence of infection merits evaluation for acute cholecystitis, which may be successfully treated with percutaneous cholecystostomy in many cases.

Nutrition and Metabolism

No population has greater nutritional requirements than thermally injured patients, whose metabolic rate may increase to over twice normal. As a rule of thumb, patients cannot meet their nutritional requirements orally if their total burn size is equal to or greater than 30%, and enteral tube feeding should be initiated as soon as hemodynamic stability is achieved. In a review of critically ill burn patients enrolled in the Inflammation and the Host Response to Injury (Glue Grant) study, enteral feeding was begun within 24 hours of burn in 80% of patients, with no increase in complications and a shorter ICU stay.[54] Whenever possible, the enteral route is preferred, but some centers cautiously use partial parenteral nutrition to make up the difference in patients unable to tolerate full enteral nutrition.[55] Malnutrition is a real risk: 61% of children, with burn size equal to or greater than 20% and chronically open wounds transferred to a burn center between 3 and 24 weeks postburn, were classified as malnourished.[56]

A variety of formulas are in use to estimate the caloric requirements of burn patients. These requirements are proportional to the burn size and decrease over time as healing occurs. Because of differences in healing rate, infections, or other factors, this formula becomes inaccurate at a month postburn, and we perform metabolic cart studies (indirect calorimetry) to measure the resting energy expenditure (REE). Even at discharge and despite successful wound closure, the measured energy expenditure remains elevated in patients with large burns.[57] This phenomenon persists for up to 3 years postburn and is accompanied by elevations in cortisol, catecholamines, cytokines, and acute phase proteins.[58]

Nitrogen requirements are likewise elevated. Skeletal muscle breakdown in patients with large burns provides a pool of amino acids that the rest of the body uses for wound healing, acute phase protein synthesis, and gluconeogenesis.[59] It stands to reason, therefore, that enteral protein intake should be augmented in these patients. A high-protein enteral feeding formula was shown to improve outcomes in thermally injured children, including decreased bacteremia and increased survival. Therefore, high-protein nutrition is routinely provided to burn patients (ie, 1.5–2.0 g/kg/d for adults and 2.5–3.0 g/kg/d for children). Also, a lower nonprotein calorie-to-nitrogen formula should be used (ie, 100 kcal/g or lower). Visceral protein levels including prealbumin, retinol-binding protein, and transferrin correlate weakly with nitrogen balance. We measure urine urea nitrogen levels and estimate nitrogen balance weekly. Even when a positive nitrogen balance is maintained, proteolysis continues throughout the hospital stay. With wound closure, proteolysis decreases.[59] However, total protein turnover is increased compared with normal children even at discharge, reflecting the persistent hypermetabolic state.[60]

Glutamine, a conditionally essential amino acid, is greatly decreased in burn patients. This may contribute to immune failure and intestinal mucosal atrophy. Intravenous glutamine supplementation has been associated with decreased bacteremia, improved measures of nutrition, and decreased measures of inflammation. Pending larger studies, we provide glutamine supplementation to critically ill burn patients.

Trace elements such as copper, selenium, and zinc are depleted in burn patients.[61] This may impair wound healing and, because selenium is a component of glutathione peroxidase, may degrade the intracellular antioxidant system.[62] We routinely replace these elements in critically ill patients and await outcome results of this treatment strategy.

Stress-induced hyperglycemia is common in thermally injured patients. A tight glucose-control strategy improved outcomes in burned children.[63] There are multiple therapeutic effects of insulin beyond glucose control, including a reduction in inflammation,[64] an improvement in wound healing,[65] and maintenance of lean body mass (see later discussion). The ideal glucose target in critically ill patients is controversial.[66] We currently use intravenous insulin to achieve a target glucose level of 100 to 150 mg/dL and have found a computerized decision support system useful in dosing continuous insulin infusions.[67]

Patients with major thermal injury are catabolic for the duration of their hospital stay and beyond, resulting in significant loss of lean body mass despite adequate replacement of calories, nitrogen, and other nutrients. This phenomenon has been addressed in various ways. Unfortunately, feeding more calories than 1.2 times REE leads to fat deposition instead of than lean body mass accretion.[68] An anabolic steroid, oxandrolone, maintained net protein balance and lean body mass in severely burned children, with increased gene expression for functional muscle proteins.[69] Oral propranolol (targeted to achieve a 20% decrease in the heart rate) decreased REE while increasing net muscle protein balance in burned children.[70] Intraarterial insulin infusion resulting in extremity hyperinsulinemia caused an increase in muscle protein synthesis but did not affect proteolysis.[71] Based on these data, we routinely administer oxandrolone and propranolol to our patients with severe thermal injury, but studies of propranolol efficacy in adult burn patients are still needed. The desire to achieve the anabolic effects seen with higher doses of insulin without the risk of hypoglycemia has pointed researchers to metformin, fenofibrate, and related agents.[72,73]

BURN-SPECIFIC MANAGEMENT
Wound Care: Topical Antimicrobials

Initial wound care should be performed as soon as the patient is hemodynamically stable. Most burn centers have dedicated wound care rooms for this purpose. The

OR is also appropriate. Use of analgesics and anesthetics must be carefully managed because patients with total burn size equal to or greater than 20% are likely to be hypovolemic during this period. The principles of wound care include total exposure of the patient, aggressive debridement of all nonviable tissue, and thorough cleansing with a surgical skin antiseptic. The solution of choice for this is chlorhexidine gluconate (except for infants and on the face).

The method of topical care developed at the US Army Burn Center is twice-daily cleansing with chlorhexidine gluconate (including removal of all previously applied creams), followed by application of an opaque layer of mafenide acetate (Sulfamylon) cream in the morning, and of silver sulfadiazine in the evening. This method maximizes the advantages and minimizes the disadvantages of either drug used alone. 0.5% silver nitrate solution (aqueous) may be used instead of burn creams. Patients are dressed in 8-ply gauze dressings and the solution is applied to the dressings once every 2 hours.[74]

Several dressings now exist that provide alternatives to the original antimicrobial agents. Careful patient selection and understanding of the products are essential for effective use. Biobrane (Mylan, Canonsburg, PA, USA) is a bilaminar artificial material composed of an inner collagen-impregnated polyethylene mesh (dermal equivalent) and a perforated silicone layer (epidermal equivalent). We use it in patients with new (≤48 hours), clean, superficial partial thickness burns such as scalds. After the Biobrane is applied, it is kept covered with gauze for 24 hours and then inspected. Accumulation of pus under the material indicates need for immediate removal and conversion to topical antimicrobials. Otherwise, it is left in place until the wound is healed. In the right patients, this material reduces hospital days, healing times, and pain. It should be noted that Biobrane contains no antimicrobial agent. Instead, any method of wound closure, if successful, acts per se to decrease bacterial burden on a wound surface.

The other major class of new dressings provides silver in a variety of slow-release formats (eg, Silverlon [Argentum Medical, Geneva, IL, USA] and Acticoat [Smith & nephew, St Petersburg, FL, USA]). An advantage of such dressings is that they can be left in place for up to 7 days with sustained release of silver cations onto the wound surface. However, safe use for such a period of time without wound inspection presumes a low risk of an adverse outcome from an infection, should one occur. Thus, we prefer to use silver dressings mainly in patients with deeper burns (who thus are not candidates for Biobrane), but whose wounds are clean and of limited size. Newer silver dressings have been engineered to enhance the local wound healing environment. One such dressing is Mepilex Ag (Molnlycke Health Care, Norcross, GA, USA), a soft silicone foam dressing that is changed every 3 to 5 days initially and then every 5 to 7 days. Compared with silver sulfadiazine, this product was associated with less pain, fewer dressing changes, and no difference in healing.[75] A Cochrane review identified a paucity of data on the treatment of burns with silver preparations, indicating the need for more well-designed studies.[76]

Wound Care: Surgery

Rapid and lasting wound closure is the main effort in the care of burn patients. The time to closure of full-thickness burns was an independent predictor of survival in a 1983 study in which standardized mortality rates differed by a factor of two among burn centers.[77] In children with burn size equal to or greater than 40%, delays in excision and grafting of the burn wound were associated with longer length of stay, delayed wound closure, and increased rates of invasive wound infection and sepsis.[78] In the authors' experience, patients with larger burns are at greater risk of failure to take skin grafts and to heal (so-called wound failure). The explanation for this is no doubt multifactorial.

In view of this, the authors' goal for patients with major thermal injuries is to excise all areas of full thickness burn (and those areas of deep partial thickness burn judged too deep to heal within 21 days of injury) as soon as hemodynamic stability can be achieved, normally within 2 to 3 days of injury. For patients with TBSA less than 50%, donor sites are available such that the excised burns can be closed with the patient's own skin (autograft). For patients with larger burns, cadaver allograft is used to make up the difference until the donor sites have healed and can be reharvested. Allograft can be used to cover excised wound beds, or it can be applied over widely meshed (eg, 3:1 or 4:1) autograft in a sandwich technique. Close postoperative attention to the graft sites by an experienced surgeon is essential to gauge the success of surgery and to preemptively address areas of wound infection.

Given the importance of wound closure, several technologies have emerged to provide more skin for the patient with massive wounds. None of these is a panacea and they should only be used in burn centers with a multidisciplinary commitment to their safe use. Cultured autologous epithelium consists of keratinocytes grown in tissue culture from small skin biopsies. We perform such cultures for patients with massive burns (≥80% TBSA) and thus limited donor sites. We typically achieve closure of a limited (5%–10%) portion of the body, anticipating that many patients will experience delayed loss of the cells even if initial engraftment is achieved.

Integra (Integra LifeSciences, Plainsboro, NJ, USA) is a bilaminar dermal regeneration matrix. The dermal layer is made of a matrix of cross-linked collagen and glycosaminoglycan. The temporary epidermal layer is made of silicone. About 14 to 21 days after application to the wound, the dermal layer engrafts, the patient is taken back to the OR, the outer layer is peeled off, and a thin autograft (0.04–0.08 in) is grafted onto the dermal layer. Ryan and colleagues[79] documented a decreased length of stay in high-risk burn patients, possibly related to more rapid wound closure. As of yet, a mortality benefit for Integra has not been demonstrated. In a postapproval multicenter study, the infection rate was 16% (13% superficial and 3% invasive)[80]; this risk should be considered when using Integra.

StrataGraft (Stratatech Corporation, Madison, WI, USA) was developed as a substitute for cadaver allograft. It consists of an epidermal layer of keratinocytes from a single human donor, grown on a collagen matrix embedded with fibroblasts from a second human donor. ReCell (Avita Medical, Northridge, CA, USA) is a technology whereby a 2 cm by 2 cm autograft is processed in the OR to yield a suspension of noncultured autologous epithelial cells. This cell suspension is then immediately sprayed onto the wound.[81] Clinical trials of these products are underway.

Infection

Immune failure, open wounds, and invasive devices place burn patients at high risk of infection. Infections are a leading cause of death in burn patients, but the location of these infections and the causative organisms have gradually shifted. In a recent autopsy series, cause of death included infection in 61%. Common organisms involved were true fungi, Pseudomonas aeruginosa, and Klebsiella pneumoniae. Of lesser importance were gram-positive organisms, to include methicillin-resistant Staphylococcus aureus, and the multiple-drug resistant but relatively indolent Acinetobacter baumanni complex. The location of these infections was predominantly wound and lung.[82] Even when infection has been eliminated, systemic inflammation—induced by tissue injury and multiple infectious episodes—may cause death by multisystem organ failure.

Before the discovery of effective topical antimicrobial agents, patients commonly died of invasive gram-negative burn wound infection.[83] Currently, invasive infection by true fungi (eg, Aspergillus, Fusarium, and Mucor) is more common than bacterial invasion. Diagnosis of invasive burn wound infection is made by inspection of the wound and by histopathology. In a patient with clinical evidence of sepsis, changes in the color of the wound (tinctorial changes) may suggest infection and merit biopsy. Patients with smaller burns are at risk of burn wound cellulitis, which is manifested by erythema spreading more than a centimeter from the wound margin. *Streptococcus* is the most common causative organism but, because some of these patients are infected with methicillin-resistant *S aureus*, we often initiate treatment with intravenous vancomycin.

Intubated burn patients are at high risk for pneumonia. The presence of inhalation injury and the severity thereof increase the risk of pneumonia. Bundles to prevent ventilator-associated pneumonia are appropriate for these patients.[33] Animal studies confirmed that smoke inhalation injury predisposes to pneumonia by several synergistic mechanisms. Small airway damage and obstruction lead to distal atelectasis, colonization, and infection. Damage to the mucociliary apparatus and deleterious effects on immune function interfere with host response. Thus, it is unclear whether pneumonia in intubated patients with inhalation injury should be termed ventilator-associated pneumonia or inhalation-injury-associated pneumonia. High-frequency percussive VDR was associated with a decrease in pneumonia in patients with inhalation injury. One likely mechanism for this benefit is enhanced clearance of material from the distal airways. No therapy, however, is superior to weaning and extubation, which requires a multidisciplinary approach to daily sedation breaks, spontaneous breathing trials, and physical therapy of intubated patients.

Because burns in excess of about 20% TBSA induce a systemic inflammatory response syndrome—manifested by fever, tachycardia, increased cardiac output, elevated white blood cell count, decreased peripheral vascular resistance—the diagnosis of infection in these patients may be particularly difficult.[84,85] A high index of suspicion and attention to nontraditional indicators of sepsis is required. A consensus conference sponsored by the ABA proposed that the following indicators be used as triggers for a search for infection[86]:

- Temperature (>39° or <36.5°C)
- Progressive tachycardia
- Progressive tachypnea
- Thrombocytopenia
- Hyperglycemia (or insulin resistance)
- Enteral feeding intolerance (distension, high residuals, or diarrhea).

Prospective validation of these indicators is needed.[85] In the presence of clinical evidence of sepsis, we usually initiate broad-spectrum antibiotics while aggressively searching for a source. On the other hand, because burn patients have protracted ICU lengths of stay (1–2 days per percent burn, on average) and multiple bouts of infection, indiscriminant use of antibiotics only exerts pressure for the development of multiple-drug resistant organisms, without improving outcome: making judicious use of antibiotics imperative.

Rehabilitation

Although rehabilitation has been an integral part of the care of burn patients for decades, the scientific understanding of its impact on pathophysiology and on outcomes is in its infancy. The magnitude of the burn rehabilitation problem is indicated by a meta-analysis that showed a return-to-work rate of only 72% in previously employed burn patients with a mean burn size of 18%.[87] Similarly, 67% of surviving combat casualties returned to duty, whereas the remaining 33% were medically discharged.[88] Rehabilitation is increasingly recognized not as a phase of care that transpires after wound healing has been completed but as an integral part of all phases of care—from resuscitation, through ICU care, to reintegration. The priorities and the time investment by the therapy team change during these phases, but the hospital course of a burn patient is simply too long to postpone rehabilitation. Furthermore, the authors propose not only that rehabilitation be integrated into ICU care, but also that it be re-envisioned as a way to change ICU outcomes such as ventilator days.

Burn patients should be evaluated by a burn therapist within 24 hours of admission.[89] Early priorities in rehabilitation are to preserve fine motor function and gross motor strength, to facilitate wound healing, and to counteract scar contracture formation. During resuscitation, the therapist evaluates the patient for functional deficits and elevates the upper extremities to decrease edema formation. While in the ICU, the therapist works with the other team members to combat the deleterious effects of prolonged bed rest, CIP-CIM, and mechanical ventilation. The feasibility of physical therapy despite endotracheal intubation to include sitting, standing, and ambulation, has recently been demonstrated in a prospective trial in medical ICUs.[90] In burn patients unable to transition rapidly to standing, devices such as the tilt table and the Moveo exercise platform (Chattanooga, Inc, Vista, CA, USA) are commonly used.

As healing progresses, contracture formation threatens the patient's mobility, particularly across the joints. Range-of-motion exercises, splinting, and positioning are used to counteract this process. Following excision and grafting of the burn wound, splinting is performed to maximize graft take, followed by gradual mobilization beginning about 5 days postburn. As the patient transitions from the ICU to the ward, he or she becomes able to participate in physical and occupational therapy in a clinic setting and relearns the activities of daily living.

OUTCOMES

A systematic approach to burn care by multidisciplinary teams has resulted in significant improvements in survival and functional recovery from burn injuries. Overall mortality relates to the age of the patient, the size of burn, and the number of underlying comorbidities. The National Burn Repository (2007) indicates a 4.35% mortality rate for women and a 4.72% mortality rate for men.[91] In multiple studies, rural locales that refer patients to a burn center,[92] urban areas with significant burn resources,[93] and international burn care centers[94] all demonstrate significant improvements in burn outcomes over time. As survival increases, emphasis has been appropriately placed on measures of functional outcome.[95]

INJURIES DUE TO HEAT AND COLD

Injuries due to heat and cold can be primary presenting problems or can complicate the management of patients suffering blunt or penetrating injuries. The later is particularly common in patients injured in disaster scenarios or combat operations where prompt access to medical care is commonly impossible. Local and systemic manifestations of heat and cold exposure can occur together or separately. The systemic manifestations can be quite subtle and dangerous and should be considered in all casualties in whom a delay in initial care has occurred.

Heat Injury

The local effect of heat is thermal injury (see previous discussion). The systemic effects constitute a spectrum of conditions called heat illness. Heat illness is a graded elevation of core body temperature due to a failure of normal thermoregulation.[96] It is different from fever, which is a centrally regulated response. Body temperature is tightly controlled in mammals because so many metabolic reactions are susceptible to variations in temperature. Mammals have two major categories of cooling mechanisms: autonomic and behavioral. Humans evolved in a hot environment and are hairless to improve heat dissipation. Core temperature is controlled by the anterior hypothalamus via the autonomic nervous system. Major autonomic cooling mechanisms are conductive (cutaneous vasodilation) and evaporative (sweating). Conductive cooling becomes less effective as ambient temperature rises. Evaporative cooling becomes less effective as ambient humidity rises. Behavioral cooling strategies include seeking shade, reducing activity, and removing clothing.

Causes and consequences of hyperthermia

There are three primary causes of systemic hyperthermia: exertional, nonexertional, and iatrogenic. Exertional heat illness occurs in soldiers and other athletes whose activity-related heat generation exceeds their autonomic cooling capabilities. Behavioral cooling methods are often suppressed to accomplish a task. The consequences can be severe, and use of the Heat Stress Index and planning for heat management is an important component of mission success.[97] Nonexertional hyperthermia results from conditions that impair normal autonomic or behavioral thermoregulation. Principal causes are psychiatric or neurologic problems, obesity, hyperthyroidism, or behavioral limits seen in those at the extremes of age. Iatrogenic causes of systemic hyperthermia include neuroleptic malignant syndrome, malignant hyperthermia, and the use of anticholinergic drugs. For management of nonenvironmental hyperthermia, the reader is referred to many available references.[98]

Hyperthermia is deleterious for several reasons. Initially, O_2 consumption and CO_2 production are increased with greater demand placed on ventilation. Above 42°C (108°F), oxidative phosphorylation is impaired in mitochondria, interfering with cellular oxygen use. At higher temperatures, many enzyme systems cease to function; cell membranes become incompetent, and multiorgan failure develops, eventually leading to death.

Clinical presentation of hyperthermia

Heat illness occurs when behaviors, generally exercise in hot environments, exceeds autonomic cooling mechanisms and behavioral cooling mechanisms are voluntarily suppressed. Initial symptoms are mild and constitutional but can progress to cardiovascular failure, multiple organ failure, and death if not addressed.[99,100]

The initial symptoms of heat illness are called heat cramps. The symptoms consist of sweating, fatigue, and cramping of major torso and/or extremity muscle groups. With continued exercise or systemic heating, symptoms progress to heat exhaustion that is characterized by heavy sweating, pallor, muscle cramps, weakness, headache, vomiting, and often fainting. Core temperature is by definition less than 40.5°C (105°F). With continued exercise or systemic heating, symptoms progress to heat stroke. In addition to the findings of heat exhaustion, symptoms of heat stroke include confusion, coma, seizures, respiratory failure, and cardiovascular collapse. Core temperature is, by definition, greater than 40.5°C (105°F).

Physical and laboratory findings also present a spectrum. Early heat illness has little in the way of hard physical abnormalities. As the disease progresses through heat exhaustion, heavy sweating, and high temperature (under 105°F or 40.5°C) are noted. This is followed by cutaneous vasodilation, tachypnea, tachycardia, and an altered sensorium. Heat stoke is signaled by temperatures in excess of 105°F (40.5°C) and cessation of sweating. Neurologic dysfunction ranges from confusion through seizures and coma. Rhabdomyolysis occurs. Noncardiogenic pulmonary edema and hypotension lead to cardiovascular collapse. Disseminated intravascular coagulation and renal and hepatic failure follow with corresponding laboratory findings.

Management of hyperthermia

The spectrum of response is guided by the severity of the individual's condition. Heat cramps and exhaustion are managed with hydration, rest, and external cooling via clothing removal, shower, sponge bath, and enhanced evaporative cooling by fanning.[101] Heat stroke, in contrast, is a medical emergency with a mortality of up to 20% even with prompt treatment. Management principles include standard airway management, if needed, and restoration of circulating volume.[102] A rapid but controlled core temperature reduction to an initial target of 39°C (102.2°F) is appropriate. A combination of evaporative and conductive cooling is used by unclothing the patient and spraying him or her with tepid water adjacent to a fan. Core temperature should be monitored via rectal or esophageal probe. In general, tepid water is preferable to ice water because the latter may cause cutaneous vasoconstriction and thus reduce the rate of heat dissipation. Intravascular volume is usually low and should be promptly replenished.

In the critically ill patient with hyperthermia, sedation and/or anticonvulsants may be needed.[103] Hypoglycemia may occur and should be promptly corrected. One-third of these patients may develop rhabdomyolysis. In the presence of urine pigment from rhabdomyolysis, urine output of 2 to 3 mL/kg/h should be targeted. There may be a limited role for alkalinization of the urine and/or mannitol. Electrolyte abnormalities may occur, including hyperkalemia, hypocalcemia, and hyperphosphatemia. Coagulopathy may develop and, in rare cases, patients may require blood product transfusion. Noncardiogenic pulmonary edema should be managed with positive pressure support. Renal failure may occur and should be managed as in nonhyperthermia patients. Cerebral and intracompartmental edema may develop in severe cases and should also be managed as in the nonhyperthermia patient. It is important to exclude these complications in critically ill hyperthermia patients.

Cold Injury

Cold injury has both local and systemic manifestations that are seen in similar circumstances, including wilderness experience and military deployment. Both have similar exacerbating factors, including tobacco, alcohol, drugs, diabetes, and neuropathies. Prevention strategies include training and situational awareness.[104] Both local and systemic cold injury are described by a confusing archaic nomenclature and are described here as stages 1 to 3 (**Table 1**).

Hypothermia

Systemic cold injury, or hypothermia, presents with a range of symptoms from violent shivering and piloerection through confusion to paradoxic behaviors, arrhythmias, organ failures, and death. It is generally useful to describe this spectrum in stages associated with specific temperatures but, in reality, one stage blends gradually into another. Paradoxic behaviors are seen in later stages of hypothermia and are thought to originate with cold-induced hypothalamic dysfunction resulting in a sensation of extreme heat. This leads to the classic paradoxic behaviors of undressing and burrowing into snow that are seen in about half of those who die of hypothermia.

Hypothermia is best prevented through training, use of proper equipment, and situational awareness. Treatment requires prompt systemic rewarming using external or internal means.[105] External rewarming involves the use of blankets, hot-air covers,

Table 1 Stages of local and systemic cold injury			
Cold Injury Type	Stage One	Stage Two	Stage Three
Hypothermia (Systemic Cold Injury)	35–37°C (95–98.6°F) Strong shivering and piloerection Poor fine-motor coordination, hands become numb Shallow breathing, fatigue, nausea, visual disturbance	33–35°C (91–94.9°F) Violent shivering that then stops, pallor, distal cyanosis Poor gross motor coordination, stumbling Confusion, alertness maintained	Below 32°C (89.6°F) Shivering stops, reduced level of consciousness progressing to stupor Paradoxic behaviors, terminal burrowing and undressing Bradyarrhythmias and tachyarrhythmias, reduced respiration Cold diuresis, organ failures, death
Frostbite (Local Cold Injury)	Burning and numbness Pallor warms to erythema	Insensate Pallor warms to blistering Perfusion after warming	Insensate Frozen warms to hemorrhagic blisters Variable perfusion or necrosis after warming

and/or warm-water immersion. Internal methods primarily involve administration of warm intravenous fluids and warm humidified air. More invasive techniques include nasogastric, peritoneal, or pleural warm-water lavage. Venovenous perfusion and cardiopulmonary bypass have been reported as effective but are rarely used in clinical practice. Providers should be aware that dehydration is extremely common in hypothermic patients because of the situations in which the injury occurs as well as the profound tubular dysfunction and diuresis that follows renal cooling. Patients in later stages of hypothermia are prone to arrhythmias; care should be taken when moving and repositioning patients and with placement of upper body central venous catheters. Finally, profoundly hypothermic patients can seem clinically dead, so resuscitation should be continued until they have been rewarmed.

Frostbite
Local cold injury, or frostbite, also presents with a range of symptoms from burning and numbness, through loss of sensation and hemorrhagic blistering, to small vessel thrombosis and necrosis after rewarming (see **Table 1**). Treatment requires prompt local rewarming using passive and/or active means. Passive rewarming involves external covers and the use of the patient's body heat (eg, placing a hand in an axilla) or the body heat of another person. Friction should not be used because this aggravates local tissue injury. Active rewarming generally involves application of, or immersion in, warm (40°C/104°F) water. Care must be taken not to burn the insensate part. Refreezing of frozen parts must be avoided because this has been shown to exacerbate tissue loss. Rewarming of frozen parts should be carefully considered in the field and only done when it is clear that refreezing will not occur during evacuation.

There are a large number of anecdotally reported and poorly supported adjuncts, including nonsteroidal antiinflammatory drugs, hyperbaric oxygen, dextran, Coumadin, heparin, vasodilators, calcium-channel blockers, alpha-blockers, pentoxifylline, aspirin, vitamin C, and surgical sympathectomy. None of these are established as standard of care. Imaging with Tc-99 or PET scanning has been reported but has not been shown to improve outcome. Fasciotomy is generally not helpful because

Table 2
Thrombolytic screening checklist: patients are potential candidates if all queries are answered "yes"

Query	"Yes" or "No" Answer
Does the patient demonstrate stable gas exchange and hemodynamics?	
Is flow absent flow after rewarming (No capillary refill, no Doppler signals)?	
Is the cold ischemia (frozen) time <24 h?	
Is the warm ischemia time <12–24 h?	

the tissue necrosis is caused by small vessel thrombosis instead of intracompartmental edema.

In rare patients, acute thrombolytic therapy may be useful. In stage 3 frostbite, in which involved parts are frozen, small vessel thrombosis may follow rewarming and can lead to nonperfusion and necrosis. The pathophysiology is related to endothelial cell disruption from freezing with secondary thrombosis of smaller vessels. The experience has been mixed, with patients treated who show no perfusion immediately after rewarming being potential candidates. Ideal patients have little warm ischemia time. A thrombolytic treatment screening tool has been reported (**Table 2**).[106] Patients should demonstrate stable gas exchange and hemodynamics, have no detectable perfusion after rewarming, have a cold ischemia time fewer than 24 hours, and a warm ischemia time fewer than 24 hours. Potential candidates are taken to

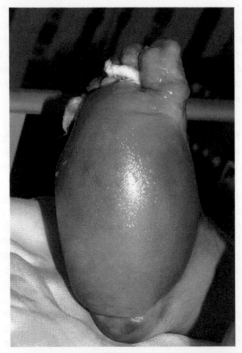

Fig. 4. Frostbite. After rewarming, initial wound care is generally conservative, with minimal debridement unless infection occurs. Blisters are allowed to collapse when possible.

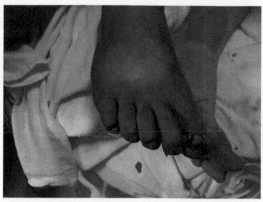

Fig. 5. Frostbite. When necrosis is clearly demarcated, excision and closure is performed.

angiography for a diagnostic study with intraarterial vasodilators. If there is no flow in the affected part, intraarterial tissue plasminogen activator (tPA) is given. Angiography is repeated in 24 hours; tPA is stopped for restoration of flow, bleeding complications, or absence of flow at 72 hours. Empiric prophylactic anticoagulation is given for 1 month.

After rewarming, initial wound care is generally conservative, with minimal debridement unless infection occurs (**Fig. 4**). When necrosis is clearly demarcated, excision and closure is performed.[107] This may require a creative combination of grafts and flaps depending on the individual wound (**Fig. 5**). Long-term challenges are generally related to the wounds, but some patients will develop neuropathic pain and sensory and motor dysfunction depending on ischemia time. Many of these symptoms will improve with time.

SUMMARY

Burns, soft-tissue, and environmental injuries are common in survivors of natural disasters, terrorist incidents, and combat. Many other patients will suffer from such exposures in addition to their primary injury as a consequence of delays inherent in dangerous and chaotic environments. Effective and organized initial care will enhance survival and optimize long-term outcome.

REFERENCES

1. Kauvar DS, Wolf SE, Wade CE, et al. Burns sustained in combat explosions in Operations Iraqi and Enduring Freedom (OIF/OEF explosion burns). Burns 2006;32:853–7.
2. Sheridan RL. Uncuffed endotracheal tubes should not be used in seriously burned children. Pediatr Crit Care Med 2006;7:258–9.
3. Advanced Trauma Life Support. Available at: http://www.facs.org/trauma/atls/index.html. Accessed June 28, 2012.
4. American Burn Association. Burn center referral criteria. 2006. Available at: www.ameriburn.org. Accessed June 28, 2012.
5. Pham TN, Cancio LC, Gibran NS. American Burn Association practice guidelines: burn shock resuscitation. J Burn Care Res 2008;29:257–66.
6. Alvarado R, Chung KK, Cancio LC, et al. Burn resuscitation. Burns 2009;35: 4–14.

7. Boldt J, Papsdorf M. Fluid management in burn patients: results from a European survey—more questions than answers. Burns 2008;34:328–38.
8. Greenhalgh DG. Burn resuscitation: the results of the ISBI/ABA survey. Burns 2010;36:176–82.
9. Chung KK, Salinas J, Renz EM, et al. Simple derivation of the initial fluid rate for the resuscitation of severely burned adult combat casualties: in silico validation of the rule of 10. J Trauma 2010;69(Suppl 1):S49–54.
10. Saffle JR. The phenomenon of "fluid creep" in acute burn resuscitation. J Burn Care Res 2007;28:382–95.
11. Wibbenmeyer L, Sevier A, Liao J, et al. The impact of opioid administration on resuscitation volumes in thermally injured patients. J Burn Care Res 2010;31: 48–56.
12. Chung KK, Wolf SE, Cancio LC, et al. Resuscitation of severely burned military casualties: fluid begets more fluid. J Trauma 2009;67:231–7 [discussion: 7].
13. Ennis JL, Chung KK, Renz EM, et al. Joint Theater Trauma System implementation of burn resuscitation guidelines improves outcomes in severely burned military casualties. J Trauma 2008;64:S146–51 [discussion: S51–2].
14. Salinas J, Chung KK, Mann EA, et al. Computerized decision support system improves fluid resuscitation following severe burns: an original study. Crit Care Med 2011;39:2031–8.
15. O'Mara MS, Slater H, Goldfarb IW, et al. A prospective, randomized evaluation of intra-abdominal pressures with crystalloid and colloid resuscitation in burn patients. J Trauma 2005;58:1011–8.
16. Dubick MA, Williams C, Elgjo GI, et al. High-dose vitamin C infusion reduces fluid requirements in the resuscitation of burn-injured sheep. Shock 2005;24: 139–44.
17. Tanaka H, Matsuda T, Miyagantani Y, et al. Reduction of resuscitation fluid volumes in severely burned patients using ascorbic acid administration: a randomized, prospective study. Arch Surg 2000;135:326–31.
18. Klein MB, Edwards JA, Kramer CB, et al. The beneficial effects of plasma exchange after severe burn injury. J Burn Care Res 2009;30:243–8.
19. Neff LP, Allman JM, Holmes JH. The use of therapeutic plasma exchange (TPE) in the setting of refractory burn shock. Burns 2010;36:372–8.
20. Orgill DP, Piccolo N. Escharotomy and decompressive therapies in burns. J Burn Care Res 2009;30:759–68.
21. Markell KW, Renz EM, White CE, et al. Abdominal complications after severe burns. J Am Coll Surg 2009;208:940–7 [discussion: 7–9].
22. Latenser BA, Kowal-Vern A, Kimball D, et al. A pilot study comparing percutaneous decompression with decompressive laparotomy for acute abdominal compartment syndrome in thermal injury. J Burn Care Rehabil 2002;23:190–5.
23. Burke BA, Latenser BA. Defining intra-abdominal hypertension and abdominal compartment syndrome in acute thermal injury: a multicenter survey. J Burn Care Res 2008;29:580–4.
24. Sheridan RL, Hurley J, Smith MA, et al. The acutely burned hand: management and outcome based on a ten-year experience with 1047 acute hand burns. J Trauma 1995;38:406–11.
25. Gabriel V, Kowalske KJ, Holavanahalli RK. Assessment of recovery from burn-related neuropathy by electrodiagnostic testing. J Burn Care Res 2009;30: 668–74.
26. Latronico N, Bolton CF. Critical illness polyneuropathy and myopathy: a major cause of muscle weakness and paralysis. Lancet Neurol 2011;10:931–41.

27. Smith SB, Coffee T, Yowler C, et al. Risk factors for ophthalmic complications in patients with burns. J Burn Care Res 2010;31:911–7.
28. Singh CN, Klein MB, Sullivan SR, et al. Orbital compartment syndrome in burn patients. Ophthal Plast Reconstr Surg 2008;24:102–6.
29. Friedstat JS, Klein MB. Acute management of facial burns. Clin Plast Surg 2009; 36:653–60.
30. Weber JM, Sheridan RL, Schulz JT, et al. Effectiveness of bacteria-controlled nursing units in preventing cross-colonization with resistant bacteria in severely burned children. Infect Control Hosp Epidemiol 2002;23:549–51.
31. Davison PG, Loiselle FB, Nickerson D. Survey on current hydrotherapy use among North American burn centers. J Burn Care Res 2010;31:393–9.
32. Stoddard FJ Jr, Sorrentino EA, Ceranoglu TA, et al. Preliminary evidence for the effects of morphine on posttraumatic stress disorder symptoms in one- to four-year-olds with burns. J Burn Care Res 2009;30:836–43.
33. Mosier MJ, Pham TN. American Burn Association Practice guidelines for prevention, diagnosis, and treatment of ventilator-associated pneumonia (VAP) in burn patients. J Burn Care Res 2009;30:910–28.
34. Kadilak PR, Vanasse S, Sheridan RL. Favorable short- and long-term outcomes of prolonged translaryngeal intubation in critically ill children. J Burn Care Rehabil 2004;25:262–5.
35. Cancio LC. Airway management and smoke inhalation injury in the burn patient. Clin Plast Surg 2009;36:555–67.
36. Cancio LC, Batchinsky AI, Dubick MA, et al. Inhalation injury: pathophysiology and clinical care proceedings of a symposium conducted at the Trauma Institute of San Antonio, San Antonio, TX, USA on 28 March 2006. Burns 2007;33: 681–92.
37. Park MS, Cancio LC, Jordan BS, et al. Assessment of oxidative stress in lungs from sheep after inhalation of wood smoke. Toxicology 2004;195:97–112.
38. Enkhbaatar P, Wang J, Saunders F, et al. Mechanistic aspects of inducible nitric oxide synthase-induced lung injury in burn trauma. Burns 2011;37: 638–45.
39. Hofstra JJ, Vlaar AP, Knape P, et al. Pulmonary activation of coagulation and inhibition of fibrinolysis after burn injuries and inhalation trauma. J Trauma 2011;70:1389–97.
40. Midde KK, Batchinsky AI, Cancio LC, et al. Wood bark smoke induces lung and pleural plasminogen activator inhibitor 1 and stabilizes its mRNA in porcine lung cells. Shock 2011;36:128–37.
41. Morita N, Enkhbaatar P, Maybauer DM, et al. Impact of bronchial circulation on bronchial exudates following combined burn and smoke inhalation injury in sheep. Burns 2011;37:465–73.
42. Bhattacharyya SN, Dubick MA, Yantis LD, et al. In vivo effect of wood smoke on the expression of two mucin genes in rat airways. Inflammation 2004;28: 67–76.
43. Cox RA, Burke AS, Soejima K, et al. Airway obstruction in sheep with burn and smoke inhalation injuries. Am J Respir Cell Mol Biol 2003;29:295–302.
44. Chung KK, Wolf SE, Renz EM, et al. High-frequency percussive ventilation and low tidal volume ventilation in burns: a randomized controlled trial. Crit Care Med 2010;38:1970–7.
45. Lange M, Hamahata A, Traber DL, et al. Preclinical evaluation of epinephrine nebulization to reduce airway hyperemia and improve oxygenation after smoke inhalation injury. Crit Care Med 2011;39:718–24.

46. Lee HM, Hallberg LM, Greeley GH Jr, et al. Differential inhibition of mitochondrial respiratory complexes by inhalation of combustion smoke and carbon monoxide, in vivo, in the rat brain. Inhal Toxicol 2010;22:770–7.
47. Kao LW, Nanagas KA. Toxicity associated with carbon monoxide. Clin Lab Med 2006;26:99–125.
48. Weaver LK. Clinical practice. Carbon monoxide poisoning. N Engl J Med 2009; 360:1217–25.
49. Weaver LK, Hopkins RO, Chan KJ, et al. Hyperbaric oxygen for acute carbon monoxide poisoning. N Engl J Med 2002;347:1057–67.
50. Fortin JL, Desmettre T, Manzon C, et al. Cyanide poisoning and cardiac disorders: 161 cases. J Emerg Med 2010;38:467–76.
51. Coca SG, Bauling P, Schifftner T, et al. Contribution of acute kidney injury toward morbidity and mortality in burns: a contemporary analysis. Am J Kidney Dis 2007;49:517–23.
52. Chung KK, Lundy JB, Matson JR, et al. Continuous venovenous hemofiltration in severely burned patients with acute kidney injury: a cohort study. Crit Care 2009;13:R62.
53. Ryan CM, Sheridan RL, Schoenfeld DA, et al. Postburn pancreatitis. Ann Surg 1995;222:163–70.
54. Mosier MJ, Pham TN, Klein MB, et al. Early enteral nutrition in burns: compliance with guidelines and associated outcomes in a multicenter study. J Burn Care Res 2011;32:104–9.
55. Prelack K, Dylewski M, Sheridan RL. Practical guidelines for nutritional management of burn injury and recovery. Burns 2007;33:14–24.
56. Dylewski ML, Prelack K, Weber JM, et al. Malnutrition among pediatric burn patients: a consequence of delayed admissions. Burns 2010;36:1185–9.
57. Milner EA, Cioffi WG, Mason AD, et al. A longitudinal study of resting energy expenditure in thermally injured patients. J Trauma 1994;37:167–70.
58. Jeschke MG, Gauglitz GG, Kulp GA, et al. Long-term persistence of the pathophysiologic response to severe burn injury. PLoS One 2011;6:e21245.
59. Prelack K, Yu YM, Dylewski M, et al. The contribution of muscle to whole-body protein turnover throughout the course of burn injury in children. J Burn Care Res 2010;31:942–8.
60. Borsheim E, Chinkes DL, McEntire SJ, et al. Whole body protein kinetics measured with a non-invasive method in severely burned children. Burns 2010;36:1006–12.
61. Berger MM, Baines M, Raffoul W, et al. Trace element supplementation after major burns modulates antioxidant status and clinical course by way of increased tissue trace element concentrations. Am J Clin Nutr 2007;85: 1293–300.
62. Dylewski ML, Bender JC, Smith AM, et al. The selenium status of pediatric patients with burn injuries. J Trauma 2010;69:584–8 [discussion: 8].
63. Jeschke MG, Kulp GA, Kraft R, et al. Intensive insulin therapy in severely burned pediatric patients: a prospective randomized trial. Am J Respir Crit Care Med 2010;182:351–9.
64. Jeschke MG, Kraft R, Song J, et al. Insulin protects against hepatic damage postburn. Mol Med 2011;17:516–22.
65. Tuvdendorj D, Zhang XJ, Chinkes DL, et al. Intensive insulin treatment increases donor site wound protein synthesis in burn patients. Surgery 2011;149:512–8.
66. Preiser JC, Devos P. Clinical experience with tight glucose control by intensive insulin therapy. Crit Care Med 2007;35:S503–7.

67. Mann EA, Jones JA, Wolf SE, et al. Computer decision support software safely improves glycemic control in the burn intensive care unit: a randomized controlled clinical study. J Burn Care Res 2011;32:246–55.
68. Hart DW, Wolf SE, Herndon DN, et al. Energy expenditure and caloric balance after burn: increased feeding leads to fat rather than lean mass accretion. Ann Surg 2002;235:152–61.
69. Wolf SE, Thomas SJ, Dasu MR, et al. Improved net protein balance, lean mass, and gene expression changes with oxandrolone treatment in the severely burned. Ann Surg 2003;237:801–10 [discussion: 10–1].
70. Herndon DN, Hart DW, Wolf SE, et al. Reversal of catabolism by beta-blockade after severe burns. N Engl J Med 2001;345:1223–9.
71. Gore DC, Wolf SE, Sanford AP, et al. Extremity hyperinsulinemia stimulates muscle protein synthesis in severely injured patients. Am J Physiol Endocrinol Metab 2004;286:E529–34.
72. Gauglitz GG, Williams FN, Herndon DN, et al. Burns: where are we standing with propranolol, oxandrolone, recombinant human growth hormone, and the new incretin analogs? Curr Opin Clin Nutr Metab Care 2011;14:176–81.
73. Williams FN, Branski LK, Jeschke MG, et al. What, how, and how much should patients with burns be fed? Surg Clin North Am 2011;91:609–29.
74. D'Avignon LC, Chung KK, Saffle JR, et al. Prevention of infections associated with combat-related burn injuries. J Trauma 2011;71:S282–9.
75. Silverstein P, Heimbach D, Meites H, et al. An open, parallel, randomized, comparative, multicenter study to evaluate the cost-effectiveness, performance, tolerance, and safety of a silver-containing soft silicone foam dressing (intervention) vs. silver sulfadiazine cream. J Burn Care Res 2011;32:617–26.
76. Storm-Versloot MN, Vos CG, Ubbink DT, et al. Topical silver for preventing wound infection. Cochrane Database Syst Rev 2010;(3):CD006478.
77. Wolfe RA, Roi LD, Flora JD, et al. Mortality differences and speed of wound closure among specialized burn care facilities. JAMA 1983;250:763–6.
78. Xiao-Wu W, Herndon DN, Spies M, et al. Effects of delayed wound excision and grafting in severely burned children. Arch Surg 2002;137:1049–54.
79. Ryan CM, Schoenfeld DA, Malloy M, et al. Use of Integra artificial skin is associated with decreased length of stay for severely injured adult burn survivors. J Burn Care Rehabil 2002;23:311–7.
80. Heimbach DM, Warden GD, Luterman A, et al. Multicenter postapproval clinical trial of Integra dermal regeneration template for burn treatment. J Burn Care Rehabil 2003;24:42–8.
81. Wood FM, Giles N, Stevenson A, et al. Characterisation of the cell suspension harvested from the dermal epidermal junction using a ReCell kit. Burns 2012;38:44–51.
82. Gomez R, Murray CK, Hospenthal DR, et al. Causes of mortality by autopsy findings of combat casualties and civilian patients admitted to a burn unit. J Am Coll Surg 2009;208:348–54.
83. Brown TP, Cancio LC, McManus AT, et al. Survival benefit conferred by topical antimicrobial preparations in burn patients: a historical perspective. J Trauma 2004;56:863–6.
84. Murray CK, Hoffmaster RM, Schmit DR, et al. Evaluation of white blood cell count, neutrophil percentage, and elevated temperature as predictors of bloodstream infection in burn patients. Arch Surg 2007;142:639–42.
85. Mann EA, Baun MM, Meininger JC, et al. Comparison of mortality associated with sepsis in the burn, trauma, and general intensive care unit patient: a systematic review of the literature. Shock 2012;37:4–16.

86. Greenhalgh DG, Saffle JR, Holmes JH, et al. American Burn Association consensus conference to define sepsis and infection in burns. J Burn Care Res 2007;28:776–90.
87. Mason ST, Esselman P, Fraser R, et al. Return to work after burn injury: a systematic review. J Burn Care Res 2012;33:101–9.
88. Chapman TT, Richard RL, Hedman TL, et al. Military return to duty and civilian return to work factors following burns with focus on the hand and literature review. J Burn Care Res 2008;29:756–62.
89. Holavanahalli RK, Helm PA, Parry IS, et al. Select practices in management and rehabilitation of burns: a survey report. J Burn Care Res 2011;32:210–23.
90. Pohlman MC, Schweickert WD, Pohlman AS, et al. Feasibility of physical and occupational therapy beginning from initiation of mechanical ventilation. Crit Care Med 2010;38:2089–94.
91. Miller SF, Bessey P, Lentz CW, et al. National burn repository 2007 report: a synopsis of the 2007 call for data. J Burn Care Res 2008;29(6):862–70.
92. Blaisdell LL, Chace R, Hallagan LD, et al. A half-century of burn epidemiology and burn care in a rural state. J Burn Care Res 2012;33(3):347–53.
93. Gomez M, Cartotto R, Knighton J, et al. Improved survival following thermal injury in adult patients treated at a regional burn center. J Burn Care Res 2008;29(1):130–7.
94. Brusselaers N, Monstrey S, Vogelaers D, et al. Severe burn injury in Europe: a systematic review of the incidence, etiology, morbidity, and mortality. Crit Care 2010;14(5):R188.
95. Pereira C, Murphy K, Herndon D. Outcome measures in burn care. Is mortality dead? Burns 2004;30(8):761–71.
96. Becker JA, Stewart LK. Heat-related illness. Am Fam Physician 2011;83:1325–30.
97. Wexler R. Preventing heat illness in athletes. South Med J 2006;99:334.
98. Gurunluoglu R, Swanson JA, Haeck PC, et al. Evidence-based patient safety advisory: malignant hyperthermia. Plast Reconstr Surg 2009;124(Suppl 4):68S–81S.
99. Nelson NG, Collins CL, Comstock RD, et al. Exertional heat-related injuries treated in emergency departments in the U.S., 1997–2006. Am J Prev Med 2011;40:54–60.
100. Rav-Acha M, Hadad E, Epstein Y, et al. Fatal exertional heat stroke: a case series. Am J Med Sci 2004;328:84–7.
101. Hadad E, Rav-Acha M, Heled Y, et al. Heat stroke: a review of cooling methods. Sports Med 2004;34:501–11.
102. American College of Sports Medicine, Armstrong LE, Casa DJ, et al. American College of Sports Medicine position stand. Exertional heat illness during training and competition. Med Sci Sports Exerc 2007;39:556–72.
103. Bouchama A, Dehbi M, Chaves-Carballo E. Cooling and hemodynamic management in heatstroke: practical recommendations. Crit Care 2007;11:R54.
104. Armed Forces Health Surveillance Center (AFHSC). Update: cold weather injuries, U.S. Armed Forces, July 2006–June 2011. MSMR 2011;18:14–8.
105. van der Ploeg GJ, Goslings JC, Walpoth BH, et al. Accidental hypothermia: rewarming treatments, complications and outcomes from one university medical centre. Resuscitation 2010;81:1550–5.
106. Sheridan RL, Goldstein MA, Stoddard FJ Jr, et al. Case records of the Massachusetts General Hospital. Case 41-2009. A 16-year-old boy with hypothermia and frostbite. N Engl J Med 2009;361:2654–62.
107. Petrone P, Kuncir EJ, Asensio JA. Surgical management and strategies in the treatment of hypothermia and cold injury. Emerg Med Clin North Am 2003;21:1165–78.

Management of Complex Extremity Injuries

Tourniquets, Compartment Syndrome Detection, Fasciotomy, and Amputation Care

Robert M. Rush Jr, MD[a],*, Edward D. Arrington, MD[b],
Joseph R. Hsu, MD[c]

KEYWORDS

- Extremity injury • Mangled extremity • Amputation • Compartment syndrome
- Fasciotomy • Prosthesis

KEY POINTS

- Save the patient first.
- Tourniquets save lives and limbs.
- Most patients with mangled limbs require resuscitation with blood products and operative intervention.
- Damage control options for extremity trauma include tourniquets, shunts, splints, external fixators, amputation, adequate initial débridement, and fasciotomy (both therapeutic and prophylactic). For mangled extremities, the initial procedure is rarely the last.
- Save the injured limb if possible—and reasonable—at first. If there is a question on whether or not limb salvage or amputation should be undertaken, get another surgeon's opinion.
- A reasonable conversation with the patient after limb salvage could include the following: "We saved your extremity for now, but it may or may not be as functional as a prosthetic limb. Time will tell. You (and your family) will be included in the decision to either continue with limb salvage or to opt for amputation."
- Regardless of your initial decision to amputate or salvage, a patient's preinjury socioeconomic status and personality greatly influence the patient's rehabilitation potential and ultimate functional result.
- Orthotic devices for dysfunctional, salvaged limbs are improving.

The opinions or assertions contained herein are the private views of the authors and are not to be construed as official or as reflecting the views of the Department of the Army or the Department of Defense.

The authors have nothing to disclose.

[a] Department of Surgery, Madigan Army Medical Center, Tacoma, WA 98431, USA; [b] Department of Orthopedic Surgery, Madigan Army Medical Center, Tacoma, WA 98431, USA; [c] Department of Orthopedic Surgery and Rehabilitation, San Antonio Military Medical Center, Fort Sam Houston, TX 78234, USA

* Corresponding author.

E-mail address: robert.rush1@us.army.mil

INTRODUCTION

When it comes to traumatic injuries, the extremities are the most exposed and most frequently affected body part. The arms and legs are exposed to a wide range of wounding mechanisms from falls to high-speed vehicular crashes and industrial accidents. Similarly, combat injures to the extremities result from blasts, multiple fragment munitions, and high-velocity weapons. The heavy toll of these injuries is especially apparent when caring for patients sustaining multiple proximal amputations or mangled limbs from the impact of an improvised explosive device. As the devastation of modern weaponry has increased over the past decade of war, so have the remarkable advances in the management of complex extremity trauma.

Complex extremity injuries, or mangled extremities, are those that have sustained a combination of bony, vascular, skin, and soft tissue and/or nerve injury in which amputation may be necessary. When embarking on salvaging a severely injured limb, not only does a patient's acute injury and hemodynamic status need to be taken into account but also the ability to provide a functional outcome needs to be considered.

Herein is a discussion of some of the highlights of recent advances in the treatment of complex extremity trauma (illustrated in **Fig. 1**).

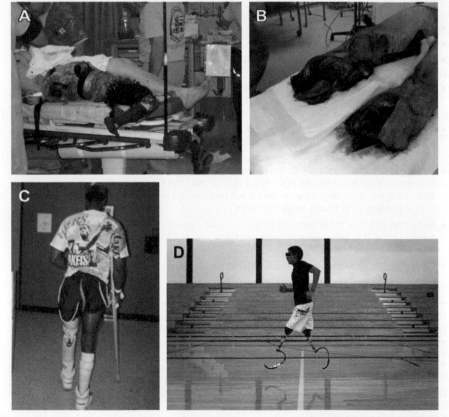

Fig. 1. Complex extremity trauma and amputation care have advanced greatly over the past decade. The progression from (*A*) initial presentation to (*B*) initial débridement to (*C*) early rehabilitation and through (*From* Hermes LM. Military lower extremity amputee rehabilitation. Phys Med Rehabil Clin N Am 2002;13:45–66; with permission.) (*D*) the process of recovery back to full function. (*Courtesy of* Reuters/Jason Reed; with permission.)

PREHOSPITAL CARE

Recent advances in the prehospital management of trauma patients are discussed in detail in the article by Kerby and colleagues elsewhere in this issue. For patients sustaining extremity trauma, the emphasis is on saving life over limb; priorities include

- Compressing sites of external bleeding
- Protecting patient airway via the simplest means possible
- Decompressing suspected tension pneumothraces
- Immobilizing fractures and potential spinal injuries
- Preventing hypothermia.

Patients are expeditiously transferred to an emergency department or first surgical capability as soon as possible.

Care at the point of injury as well as care en route and in emergency rooms includes the following and differs slightly depending on the environment and the number injured. First and foremost, ensure the safety of medical personnel—either by moving the patients to a safe location or by nullifying the danger—such as returning fire to suppress immediate enemy threats in a military setting. Once provider safety is established, direct pressure at the site of bleeding followed by a compressive dressing are the first and second maneuvers in the treatment of any bleeding wound. Given that the leading cause of preventable death from trauma is hemorrhage, if a patient has obvious external bleeding from the extremities that a simple tourniquet or hemostatic dressing could stop, then these maneuvers may be as important as establishing an airway. For traumatic amputations, a tourniquet should be applied to an intact portion of the extremity proximal to the injury.

Tourniquet Placement

Although any type of strap that can be wrapped around an extremity and held in place can work, tourniquets with a windlass are effective in stopping arterial bleeding when placed appropriately (**Fig. 2**). The most important factor in successfully placing a windlass tourniquet is to ensure that the strap/belt portion is fitted as tightly as possible around a casualty's injured extremity before tightening the windlass. With most windlass tourniquets, the amount of tightening, once appropriately strapped onto a limb, is 3 cm of linear length (not radial distance). Some investigators advocate field

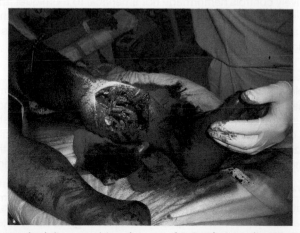

Fig. 2. Lower extremity injury requiring the use of 2 Combat Application Tourniquets.

pneumatic tourniquets (similar to a large blood pressure cuff) that are reported to apply more effective pressure over a wider area, although field-testing in combat has not been reported.[1] The Israeli Defense Forces use a simple elastic band as a tourniquet (described in the article by Soffer elsewhere in this issue). Regardless of the tourniquet type, reassessment is essential, especially as patients are resuscitated—as intravascular volume is restored and blood pressure increases, the more likely an initial tourniquet is to fail if not retightened. All large military series have shown a survival benefit from the early use of tourniquets for complex extremity injuries and there have been no permanent adverse effects of tourniquet application in several large series reported from the battlefield, including no tourniquet-caused amputations.[2–6]

Pitfalls

The application and maintenance of a tourniquet is not always easy. Recognizing when to apply a tourniquet requires training. During the course of patient transport or resuscitation, reapplication or the placement of additional tourniquets proximally may be required. The time and circumstances of tourniquet application must be communicated to the transport team and to the receiving facility. Tourniquets must be placed as distally as possible to stop the bleeding but limit ischemic tissue and nerve compression. Frequent re-evaluation to ensure there is no pooling of blood under sheets, equipment bags, or drapes is mandatory. Limb cooling may have an added protective effect if the tourniquet time is prolonged greater than 4 to 6 hours, although this technique is best performed with other systemic warming measures in place because hypothermia kills patients more quickly than a prolonged tourniquet.[7] Recent preclinical evidence suggests that the duration of ischemia should be limited as much as possible, especially in the setting of shock.[8,9] Practically speaking, tourniquets should be removed as soon as surgical control of the hemorrhage can be obtained.

Hemostatic Dressings

One of the most controversial developments over the past decade of war is the multitude of hemostatic dressings available to augment hemorrhage control. The US Army now fields Combat Gauze (Z-Medica Corporation, Wallingford, CT, USA), a kaolin-impregnated gauze that activates the natural clotting cascade by activating factor XII and initiates platelet adhesion. Some studies have found this hemostatic dressing effectively controls hemorrhage not amenable to tourniquet application.[10–12] Most common sites for use are in the groin and axilla, though any of these dressings can be used to augment hemorrhage control provided by tourniquets as well as potentially decreasing tourniquet time.[13]

Splints

Temporary skeletal fixation is important to minimize further bleeding; minimize further injury to exposed and unexposed nerves, soft tissue, and vessels; and reduce pain. Splints can be applied over tourniquets as long as both the tourniquet and bleeding portions of the open wound remain accessible and visible. The principles of splinting are to immobilize the joints above and below the fracture/injury site. If the extremity is mangled and thus fractured in many places, extend the splint to fit the entire extremity.

Other Considerations at Point of Injury

Gather amputated parts and transport with patients because this tissue can sometimes be used as spare parts for reimplantation or bone graft. Administer an antibiotic and/or tetanus if transport time to an emergency room or first surgical capability is delayed. Make sure all this is communicated in the handoff. Field débridement of wounds is not advocated except in extreme circumstances (eg, patient extraction can only be accomplished by amputating the limb).

SCORING SYSTEMS: AMPUTATE OR SALVAGE?

Although many have been proposed, no scoring system is definitive in making the decision for limb salvage versus amputation in managing patients with complex extremity trauma. All the studies done in this area rely on applying well thought-out descriptions of extremity system derangements but are applied to a cohort retrospectively or in a prospective observational method—none are by prospective randomization of patients to amputation versus salvage groups.[14–20] Each does provide perspective and a framework in which to address these complex management problems. None of the scoring systems, however, reliably guides management when evaluated on other retrospective cohorts.[21–23]

Bosse and colleagues[24] published a large prospective study of severely injured lower extremities, the Lower Extremity Assessment Project (LEAP). This study of 601 patients was conducted at 8 level 1 trauma centers and eventually included 556 limbs in 539 patients with severe extremity injuries. The objective of this study was to prospectively evaluate 5 limb salvage scoring systems. Gustilo classification was recorded as well as treatment (salvage, immediate amputation, or delayed amputation). The treating surgeon was also asked to record the critical components of the Mangled Extremity Severity Score (MESS); the Limb Salvage Index; the Predictive Salvage Index; the Nerve Injury, Ischemia, Soft-Tissue Injury, Skeletal Injury, Shock, and Age of Patient score; and the Hannover Fracture Scale-97 during the study period. All these scoring systems were compared with treatment for sensitivities and specificities of predicting the need for amputation. The investigators determined that a low score was predictive of limb salvage whereas a high score did not necessarily predict the need for amputation. The investigators cautioned against the use of these scoring systems in clinical decision making when considering primary amputation.[14] The same group published an article that concluded that 2-year functional outcomes were in between limb salvage patients and amputation patients for lower extremity injuries and questioned the usefulness of heroic limb salvage efforts.[24]

Most validating studies for these scoring systems took place at level 1 trauma centers with specialists, resources, and multidisciplinary teams. Thus, the applicability of these data to smaller centers and military and rural settings, where misguided limb salvage could have fatal consequences, should be considered. The decision to amputate a severely injured extremity remains a difficult one that no single scoring system performed at the bedside or in the operating room is likely to simplify. It makes intuitive sense that a surgeon is not likely to calculate a complex score during an operation. By being aware of these systems and what predicts salvage, however, these scoring systems have given surgeons a thought process to aid in this difficult decision. These reports have also provided a common language with which new results may be reported and compared.

In another study performed by the Lower Extremity Assessment Project (LEAP) Study Group, looking at factors that led to decisions to amputate or salvage,[25] the most important factors considered were (1) muscle injury (as this relates to ultimate function), (2) absence of sensation (although this is controversial), and (3) injury to deep veins and arteries (especially the popliteal artery). This is how expert orthopedic and trauma surgeons thought through their decisions as prospectively recorded, thus outlining their priorities and their results. As medicine and techniques advance, surgeons still have to rely on good judgment and on allocation of resources at the facility to abide by the old dictum, life over limb—not only limb but also an expedient recovery to a functional limb.

Decision to Amputate

Complex extremity trauma, also referred to as a mangled extremity, applies to those severely injured arms or legs where primary amputation may be considered a treatment option. There are no studies that have prospectively evaluated the factors that are involved in a decision to amputate or salvage a mangled limb. Ultimately, the decision for limb salvage or primary amputation must be made by the treating surgeon although input from additional colleagues or specialists is encouraged.

Base the decision on the known information. An adequate evaluation of the injury needs to be done depending on patient condition. If a patient is unstable, the evaluation needs to be done in the operating room where vascular control can be obtained and other life-threatening hemorrhage or injuries can be simultaneously addressed so that there is a live patient. If stable, a more thorough vascular and neurologic assessment can be completed after initial skeletal alignment in an emergency department.[26] The questions to ask are

1. Is limb salvage feasible (considering the damaged extremity systems)?
2. Is limb salvage advisable (given patients hemodynamic status)?
3. If embarking on salvage, what are the management priorities?
4. When should secondary amputation be considered?

If possible, include the patient and patient's family in the decision early (sometimes not possible). Scalea and colleagues and the Western Trauma Association[26] have provided an excellent and up-to-date algorithm to help with the management of immediate postinjury mangled extremities that are sustained in civilian trauma settings (**Box 1**). In military populations where high-energy ballistic injuries are prevalent, civilian scoring systems do not necessarily apply. Brown and colleagues[27] found that the ischemia and generally poor condition of the patients sustaining high-energy combat wounds led to a greater need for primary amputation. Conversely, a MESS score greater than or equal to 7 did not mandate amputation. The LEAP study goes a bit further and is helpful in that the degree of soft tissue injury as it relates to best-guess functional outcome is important, ensuring that factors, such as a patient's means (ie, economic and social) to perform rehabilitation and multiple limb reconstructive procedures, is present.

Sometimes secondary amputation is desired and should not be considered a failure. This has become evident as results from the military LEAP study are released, where it was found that most soldiers undergoing amputation attained a better level of postinjury function more quickly than those undergoing complex extremity salvage (James Ficke, COL, personal communication, 2012).

INITIAL EVALUATION AND MANAGEMENT

Most patients sustaining complex extremity trauma require resuscitation with blood products and operative intervention. Patients with a mangled extremity are at some risk for both early and late death from one of several mechanisms:

- Unrecognized or ongoing hemorrhage from the limb
- Hemorrhage from other injuries
- Wound sepsis from inadequate débridement or necrotizing soft tissue infections

---

Box 1
Predictors of amputation in complex extremity trauma

Systemic factors

Age >50 y

High-energy transfer

Persistent hypotension (<90 mm Hg)

Bony skeletal factors

Gustilo type III A with significant tissue loss or nerve injury, associated with fibular fracture and displacement of >50% and comminuted segmental fracture or high probability of need for bone graft

Gustilo type III B and type III C tibial fractures

Gustilo type III open fractures of the pilon

Gustilo type III B open fractures of the ankle

Severe open injury to the hindfoot or midfoot

Soft tissue factors

Large, circumferential tissue loss

Extensive closed soft tissue loss or necrosis

Compartment syndrome with myonecrosis

Neurologic factors

Confirmed nerve disruption, in particular, the tibial nerve

Vascular factors

Prolonged warm ischemia time, >6 h

Degree of vascular segment loss

Proximal vascular injury (femoral greater risk than popliteal or more distal)

Absence of viable distal anastomotic target

Data from Scalea TM, Dubose J, Moore EE, et al. Western Trauma Association critical decisions in trauma: management of the mangled extremity. J Trauma 2012;72(1):86–93.

- Unrecognized massive ischemia leading to renal and multiorgan failure
- Thromboembolic events.

Patients with traumatic amputations die from the same causes.

Priorities

As with prehospital care, the management priorities in these patients emphasize saving life over limb. These priorities include

1. A live patient—what needs to be done immediately to ensure this:
   a. Stop the bleeding.
   b. Establish/maintain an airway.
   c. Ensure respiration/breathing.
   d. Damage control resuscitation—the order of these steps depends on a patient's stability and individual injury pattern but ideally should be addressed in a multiteam or simultaneous approach.

2. Do no more harm to the live patient:
   a. Limit further disability (head and spine trauma).
   b. Control contamination/infection (tetanus and initial antibiotics).
   c. Prevent hypothermia.
3. Operative management (highly dependent on local resources):
   a. Damage control principals—do as much or as little as possible at each operative intervention or point of care to ensure that the patient stays alive.
   b. Ensure hemostatic resuscitation continues (blood/platelets/plasma).
   c. Replace field tourniquets with pneumatic tourniquets while assessing injuries.
   d. Give tetanus prophylaxis and appropriate antibiotics depending on the degree of contamination of the wounds. Do not forget to redose if necessary.
   e. Decide on an order between skeletal fixation and revascualization procedures knowing that shunting of vascular injuries and external fixation are excellent damage control techniques that should not require a lot of time to perform. Shunts have been used successfully to keep an extremity perfused over prolonged periods of time as well as over great evacuation distances and have proved a key advancement over the past 10 years of war.[28–32] Although nothing is better than autologous vein graft from an unaffected limb, there may not be time to perform bypass grafting in many settings involving complex extremity trauma because most of these patients have sustained polytrauma. If the major artery and vein of an extremity are both damaged, attempt to shunt or repair both as long as the patient can tolerate the length of the procedure. Otherwise, at least establish inflow if limb salvage is to be undertaken.
   f. Ensure adequate débridement of all devitalized soft tissue (no irrigation under high pressure because this may extend contamination into clean tissue plains).
   g. Consider primary and/or prophylactic fasciotomy of damaged and distal compartments
   h. Maintain as much nerve length as possible and mark nerve ends if patient hemodynamic status permits. These nerves can be used to restore some muscle innervation, which may prevent atrophy and improve limb or prosthetic function.
   i. Use wound vacuum-assisted closure (VAC) devices liberally once the wound bed is clean. For massively contaminated, high-energy open wounds, a vacuum dressing may need to be deferred for one or several operations.
4. Multiteam approach:
   a. Triage and timing of care is critical in the management plan. The trauma surgeon coordinating a patient's care is the team leader and negotiates with consultants as to the timing and complexity of procedures, simultaneous procedures, and length of anesthesia as well as allowable blood loss.
   b. For cases of single limb injuries and in multitrauma patients, several teams are necessary—one for each major body cavity and limb. Each limb may have multiple teams involved in the injury management (eg, vascular, orthopedics, and plastics).
   c. Team priorities must be made by the trauma surgeon in charge regardless of that surgeon's primary surgical discipline.

COMPARTMENT SYNDROME AND FASCIOTOMY

In at-risk extremities, compartment syndrome must be anticipated, investigated, and treated. Fascial compartments swell and become tight when they are ischemic for a prolonged period of time (usually >4–6 hours) and then reperfused or when the extremity is directly injured by impact or energy transfer. In a mangled extremity, both mechanisms are at play. After such an insult, tissue within the fixed fascial envelopes of the extremity begins to swell, and, as this process continues, intracompartmental pressure rises until venous obstruction occurs.

Once the low intramuscular arteriolar pressure is exceeded, blood is shunted away from end muscular capillary beds. This reduced flow generally occurs at compartment pressures of 3 mm Hg to 40 mm Hg or greater for longer than 8 to12 hours. Arterial inflow continues at first, increasing tissue edema, leading to what Mubarak and Owen[33] define as compartment syndrome, an elevation of the interstitial pressure in a closed osseofascial compartment that results in microvascular compromise. Arterial inflow can continue despite the presence of compartment syndrome and the loss of a distal pulse is thus a late finding.

Nerve tissue is affected first by the subsequent end-tissue hypoxia causing pain on passive motion seen early in the development of compartment syndrome, sparing distal pulses until late in the course. Damage to muscle can occur even with normal flow into a compartment when pressures reach 30 mm Hg to 40 mm Hg for 8 hours. Studies have shown that pressures of 40 mm Hg sustained for 14 hours did not cause nerve dysfunction. Higher compartment pressure, however, take less time to cause permanent functional loss of nerve and muscle function.[34] Reperfusion of the extremity after vascular repair can cause massive swelling of some of the compartments, resulting in a secondary compartment syndrome, even after short-term disruption of blood flow (2–6 h). This can place a potentially viable limb at risk for amputation if compartment syndrome is missed.[35,36]

Detection

The diagnosis of compartment syndrome can be challenging. Missing this injury is usually devastating and can result in a Volkmann contracture or ischemic contracture of the compartment musculature, compounding the severity of the original injury and further compromising limb salvage and eventual function. Compartments with noncompliant surrounding structures or tissue are generally more at risk, especially the anterior and deep compartments of the lower leg and the volar compartment of the forearm. Anatomy of the compartments of the lower leg and forearm is shown in **Fig. 3**. Other compartments that are susceptible to increased pressures are in the hands and feet, thigh, and gluteal fascial envelopes.

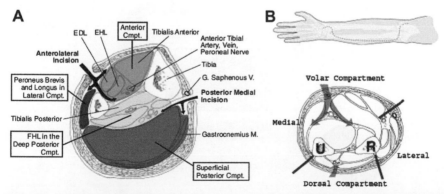

Fig. 3. (*A*) Lower extremity cross-section at the midcalf depicting locations of 4 compartments requiring fasciotomy for the treatment or prevention of compartment syndrome. (*B*) Forearm cross-section showing compartments requiring fasciotomy for upper extremity compartment syndrome. Also shown is the required incision for fasciotomy of the forearm needed for release of volar compartments (*B*). Cmpt, compartment; EDL, extensor digitorum longus; EHL, extensor hallucis longus; FHL, flexor hallucis longus; G, greater; M, muscle; R, radius; U, ulna; V, vein.

Injuries to the extremities, such as fractures, massive soft tissue trauma (by blunt and penetrating high energy mechanisms), intracompartmental bleeding, arterial or venous injury, limb compression, and burns (especially circumferential and electrical), warrant a heightened index of suspicion.[37] In awake patients, a tight compartment associated with the appropriate mechanism of injury may lead to suspicion of the diagnosis. Pain out of proportion to the injury at that level on passive motion—as the compromised muscle slides through the affected compartment—is the most common early finding. Paresthesias and numbness can be early signs. The loss of 2-point discrimination is a sensitive sign in differentiating compartment syndrome from raised intracompartmental pressure alone.[38] In dealing with the mangled extremity, however, most patients have sustained multisystem trauma (especially those sustaining concomitant head injuries) that may preclude a reliable examination, are frequently taken back to the operating room for damage control and subsequent procedures, and remain sedated. In these patients, intracompartmental pressures should be measured.

There are several methods for measuring intracompartmental pressures. Most involve needles and/or catheters. Using the Stryker compartment measuring device is an easy way to do this (**Fig. 4**).[39] McQueen and Court-Brown[40] used a pressure differential of less than 20 mm Hg between the compartment measurement and diastolic pressure (or <30–40 mm Hg from mean arterial pressure) to determine the need for fasciotomy. At a pressure differential equal to or greater than 20 mm Hg, as opposed to absolute compartment pressures, no compartment syndromes were missed and no unnecessary fasciotomies were performed in tibial diaphyseal fracture patients in this study.

Recently, near-infrared spectroscopy, a continuous but noninvasive method for detecting compartment syndrome, has been shown to have a higher positive predictive value of detecting truly increased compartment pressures than measuring compartment pressures via needles or catheters.[41,42] Near-infrared spectroscopy transmits light that passes through skin and subcutaneous tissue but is reflected or absorbed by hemoglobin, depending on the oxygenation-reduction state of the molecule. This can be related to the ischemic state of muscle as in compartment syndrome. The measurements seem to be accurate even in states of circulatory shock.[43]

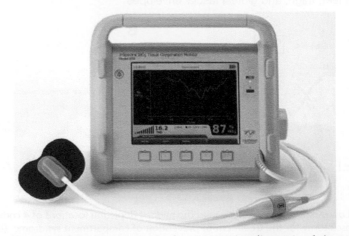

Fig. 4. Portable near-infrared spectrometer for noninvasive diagnosis of decreased tissue blood flow. (*From* Vorwerk C, Coats TJ. The prognostic value of tissue oxygen saturation in emergency department patients with severe sepsis or septic shock. Emerg Med J 2011 Sep 21. [Epub ahead of print]; with permission.)

Regardless of the initial state of the compartment, a prophylactic fasciotomy is sometimes warranted. This is especially applicable to military settings, in cases of delayed transports in rural settings, and in managing mass casualties from disasters. In such circumstances, if a patient is currently at risk for a compartment syndrome or could develop a compartment syndrome, prophylactic fasciotomy should be strongly considered. Long-term complications of an inappropriate fasciotomy can lead to severe venous congestion, infections, scarring, and decreased range of motion of the joints above and below the fasciotomy in some cases. These risks must be weighed when contemplating the use of prophylactic fasciotomy.

Treatment

The treatment of compartment syndrome consists of fasciotomy, completion fasciotomy, and sometimes the judicial use of prophylactic or preventive fasciotomy. Ensure that previously applied casts, splints, and dressings are removed first. For the lower leg, 2 longitudinal incisions must be made, an anterolateral incision to decompress the anterior and lateral compartments and a posteromedial incision aimed at the posterior superficial and deep compartments (**Fig. 5**). Pitfalls include incomplete fasciotomy, where incisions in the fascia are not extended to the compartment limits both distally and proximally, thus not completely relieving the swelling and tightness along the length of the compartment. It is important to ensure that the length of the

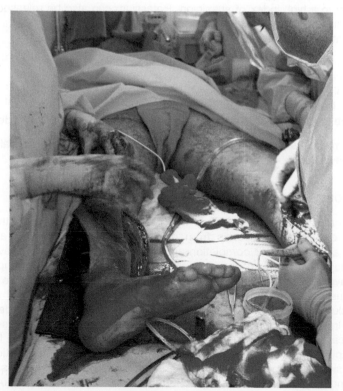

Fig. 5. Double incision (medial and lateral) through which a complete 4-compartment fasciotomy of lower leg has been performed.

incision is long enough because there are reports in which the skin continued to cause compression after fasciotomy performed through short incisions.[44] A caveat to this is that compartment syndrome can still exist in open wounds and fractures and may require fasciotomies despite being open. Peripheral motor and sensory nerves must be avoided in the fascial incisions, especially the deep posterior compartment of the lower leg, where the posterior tibial neurovascular bundle runs just deep to the investing fascia.[45]

Fasciotomy Wound Management

Skin tension should be applied when there is skin available to minimize the need for skin grafts. Sterile dressings should be applied and changed frequently or a wound VAC device applied. On the resolution of underlying compartmental muscle swelling, the fascia and skin can be reapproximated in many cases. Finally, splint the extremity in the position of function after compartment releases. When closing the fasciotomy sites, close the medial wound first at expense of the lateral wound.

Crush/Ischemia/Reperfusion Injury and Rhabdomyolysis

Extremity trauma resulting from crush injures and ischemia-reperfusion injuries may result in rhabdomyolysis, hyperkalemia, or both. In these cases, myoglobin from the damaged tissue can be released with the potential of causing renal failure. For the detection of rhabomyolysis, marked elevation of tissue creatinine kinase of greater than 10,000 IU/L is suggestive. If there is no laboratory, "crankcase" or dark urine should lead to a high index of suspicion. Potassium can also be released, causing hyperkalemia and the potential of cardiac arrhythmias.

Treatment of rhabdomyolysis and of hyperkalemia is similar:

- Check for tourniquets and remove if possible.
- Restore intravascular volume.
- Alkalinize urine with sodium bicarbonate infusion.
- Infuse insulin, glucose, furosemide, and calcium.
- Ensure fasciotomies are complete and that any dead tissue is fully débrided.

If these measures prove unsuccessful, patients may require urgent dialysis if this therapy is available.

AMPUTATIONS

One of the most difficult decisions is when to amputate a mangled extremity. If a patient is delivered in extremis from multiple injuries that include a mangled extremity, an emergent or completion amputation can be life saving, even if limb salvage may have been an option in a more stable patient. When amputation is decided, avoid guillotine (straight perpendicular cut across the axis of the extremity) amputations because viable soft tissue may be lost—better to save all viable soft tissue, including skin, muscle, fascia, and nerves. This requires débridement and irrigation. Irrigation should be copious but not under pressure because this has shown to cause microscopic debris and bacteria to lodge in good tissue. If performing an amputation in a damage control setting or if there is contamination, do not close the skin. Also ensure that the bone is left as long as possible (as long as it is viable and has periosteal covering) so that it can act as a tension-producing splint for the soft tissue envelope. The bone can be cut back at the time of a more definitive repair.

When an amputation is decided on for the treatment of a severely injured extremity, there are several universal principles that should be considered:

1. Ensure that the level of the amputation is as low as possible while débriding all devitalized tissue. Avoid guillotine amputations because these remove elements of the soft tissue envelope surrounding the cut bone.
2. Salvage any viable flaps possible because the soft tissue is more important than the bone in the amputation. The posterior flap is the most important part of the soft tissue coverage of the bone for a below-the-knee amputation.
3. The definitive amputation procedure and stump closure do not have to be done at the time of the primary or at the time of secondary amputation procedure or washout.
4. In a contaminated wound, serial débridements may be required before final stump closure. Use wound VAC devices for open stumps and other open wounds usually after second débridement, because the time between first and second operations is usually between 12 and 24 hours, which sometimes nullifies the effectiveness of this form of dressing.
5. Keep tension on the remaining skin flaps directed distally.
6. Ask patients if they have seen or know the extent of damage to their extremity and include them and their families in on the decision-making process, if feasible. They should always be informed that amputation could be considered at any time during the course of reconstruction and rehabilitation.

The specific technique in performing an amputation is as follows[46]:

- Surgically prepare the entire limb, because planes of injury may be higher than they appear on the surface.
- Place a pneumatic tourniquet, if available; otherwise, use a prehospital tourniquet and prep it into the surgical field.
- Excise nonviable tissue: (1) debride necrotic skin and subcutaneous tissue, (2) remove devascularized, noncontracting muscle, (3) sharply debride tendons back to the level of viable muscle, and (4) excise grossly contaminated bone devoid of soft tissue that cannot be covered.
- Identify and ligate major vascular structures, including veins.
- Identify and gently pull nerves distally while cutting or ligating proximally to allow them to retract to a covered area for definitive amputations of the lower extremity. Upper extremity and proximal lower extremity nerves should be preserved in length, because these nerves can be used for innervation in reconstructive procedures using muscle flaps and advanced prosthetics. Large nerves should always be ligated.
- Place preserved muscle and skin flaps on gentle tension to avoid retraction, thus preserving maximal stump length.
- Do not initially close grossly contaminated stumps completely (**Fig. 6**).

Level of Amputation

The different levels of amputation are as many as the number of limbs needing to be amputated. A common misconception is that amputating through joints is not indicated when, in actuality, a knee disarticulation, for example, is much more functional than an above-the-knee amputation. Leaving the distal femur allows patients better balance when sitting and prosthetics for through-knee amputations are improving. If any of the tibia or surrounding tissue can be spared in a damage control setting,

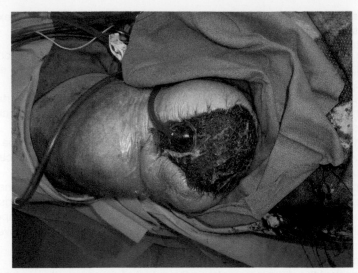

Fig. 6. Aftermath of second débridement of a grossly contaminated stump wound on an amputated lower extremity with a wound VAC device applied.

however, save it because this allows for better skin and muscle tension for definitive repair. For ray amputations of the foot, removing the big toe in most cases is worse than a transmetatarsal amputation due to lack of balance in gait with the absence of the main digit. In the upper extremity, retention of limb length is more important than for lower extremity amputations, due to the difficulty in moving several prosthetic joints simultaneously (elbow and wrist). Moving two joints simultaneously is not possible and must be done sequentially leading to cumbersome and awkward movements, especially in transhumeral amputees. Furthermore, forearm amputations should attempt to retain at least half the radius for maximal function. Another important point for the mangled upper extremity is that even a very dysfunctional limb is better than an amputation as long as infection is avoided in the initial wound.

Complications

Complications exist in patients with amputated extremities and are a major reason the amputation group was found to have an almost equal degree of functional problems postinjury in the LEAP study as compared to the limb salvage group. Stump skin ulcers or blisters affect most patients occasionally, sometimes leading to wound breakdown with or without cellulitis. Chronic osteomyolitis can develop from the start or develop over time if a stump is not cared for properly. Psychologically, patients must go through a period of psychosocial adaptation and part of this process is mourning the loss of the extremity. Those with better support systems are able to shorten this process significantly and are more likely to return to better function than those without—similar to the functional outcomes in salvaged extremities. Although every patient has a sensation that the limb is still present, phantom limb pain, characterized by searing, burning, and throbbing pain in the "amputated" limb, occurs infrequently. Nerve blocks and other chronic pain medications usually control these symptoms. Mirror therapy has also been described as a useful therapeutic tool.[47] Revisional surgery is sometimes required for deep infections and bony protrusions of the skin. Dermatologic complications develop and mild forms of rashes are treated with lanolin or hydrocortisone cream. Low-grade skin infections and carbuncles can be treated with oral tetracycline.

Verrucous hyperplasia, or chronic venous congestion of the distal limb, occurs from lack of total contact with the prosthesis and requires refitting.

Heterotopic ossification (HO), the aberrant formation of mature, lamellar bone in nonosseous tissue, has emerged as a common complication of both amputated and salvaged mangled extremities over the past decade of war.[48–50] The increased prevalence of high-energy blast injuries is thought to be a major cause due to the marked activation or presence of osteogenic connective tissue progenitor cells found in these wounds.[51] In civilian trauma, complex lower extremity injuries in conjunction with traumatic brain injury and an elevated injury severity score are most commonly associated with later development of HO. Although operative excision remains the treatment of choice for symptomatic HO, preventive measures for high-risk limbs are being developed so that prophylactic treatment can begin closer to the time of injury. Radiation therapy given within 48 hours postoperatively or the administration of nonsteroidal anti-inflammatory drugs is shown to minimize the development of HO. Neither has been a viable option in the combat setting to this point but further risk stratification and diagnostic techniques may be able to identify patients most likely to develop HO after high-energy, combat-related wounds to further direct prophylactic treatment.[52]

PROSTHETICS AND REHABILITATION

Postinjury rehabilitation is vital for patients suffering severe extremity trauma whether the limb was salvaged or required amputation. Depending on the complexity of the extremity injury, rehabilitation of a salvaged mangled extremity can be more difficult than rehabilitation after a primary or secondary amputation. Rehabilitation often is accompanied by further reconstructive work, such as

- Limb-lengthening procedures, sometimes using the Ilizarov external external skeletal fixation device, as well as new frontiers in regenerative medicine (cortical bone scaffolding, muscle stem cell replantation, and nerve cell growth)
- Rotational skin flaps
- Myocutaneous transposition flaps (keep original vascular pedicle intact)
- Microvascular free flaps (complete autotransplantation of muscle or myocutaneous tissue group)
- Flaps or grafts from "spare parts"—using portions of a patient's own amputated limbs in reconstructing other injured extremities.

Lower limb and upper limb orthotics and prosthetics have undergone revolutionary improvements over the past decade mainly due to the United States' emphasis on helping military amputees return to and lead a productive life. There are many designs available for upper extremity and lower extremity prostheses, but, for the most part, the more proximal the amputation the more complex the prosthesis needs to be—because there are more joints to be mimicked and the more degrees of freedom needed.

New developments in lower extremity orthotics have been found to allow better functioning of salvaged extremities. Reasons for this are multifactorial and include the access to and development of supporting programs available to train with the new devices. Design of lower extremity orthotics must include the ability to maintain stability, relieve neurogenic pain, and allow for strength across a fused joint.[53] Several orthotics are available, including the Intrepid Dynamic Exokseletal Orthosis (IDEO) (**Fig. 7**). When using this energy-storing ankle-foot orthosis device for soldiers with salvaged lower extremities from combat injuries, the Center for the Intrepid in San Antonio, Texas, was able to return all the patients back to some form of athletic

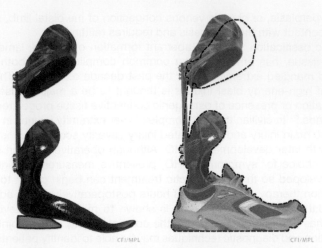

Fig. 7. The IDEO. (*From* Owens JG, Blair JA, Patzkowski JC, et al. Return to running and sports participation after limb salvage. J Trauma 2011;71(Suppl 1):S120–4; with permission.)

training and 8 patients to full running.[53] The orthosis alone was not the key component but the entire sequential rehabilitative sequence, including gait and exercise training, was essential for success. This is a major point brought out by the studies done by the LEAP group—that patients' pre-existing socioeconomic status and postinjury access to programs/equipment are key for them to becoming productive members of society after complex limb trauma.

Secondary or late amputation is a viable alternative for patients due to the rapid development of functional lower limb prosthetics as well as the rehabilitation resources dedicated to teaching patients, especially military amputees, how to use the new appendage. The recent Military Extremity Trauma Amputation/Limb Salvage (METALS) analysis of injured American warriors who sustained complex extremity trauma, including amputations, shows that both unilateral and bilateral lower extremity amputees scored better on the Short Musculoskeletal Functional Assessment index than did those who underwent limb salvage and the multiple, numbers of reoperations and courses of rehabilitation. Although there was no significant difference in return to work/active duty, depression, and chronic pain between amputation and limb salvage, amputees reported as engaging in more vigorous sports were less likely to have post-traumatic stress.[54] Another important note in this study is that 20% of the amputees underwent secondary amputation more than 1 month from original injury. The Center for the Intrepid at both the Walter Reed National Military Medical Center and at Brooke Army Medical Center focuses on this care and provide all returning amputees a near ideal environment for treatment and rehabilitation.

The arm is more complicated in duplicating than any type of lower extremity segment. Because of this, upper extremity limb salvage attempts should be more rigorous than lower extremity limb salvage. A dysfunctional upper limb can allow for stabilization of gait and apposition. Arm prosthetics have evolved from cosmetic or 1-D functional devices to myointegrated advanced limbs that look like and have nearly as many degrees of freedom as a real limb (eg, the DEKA [or Luke] arm designed by Kamen [**Fig. 8**]). Control of this arm can be done with a footplate device in the shoe and/or by connected residual nerves to pectoral muscles that can interface with electrodes on a breastplate. Although the human arm has 22° of freedom, the DEKA arm has 18°. As with orthotics for salvaged limbs, the rehabilitation and continued training

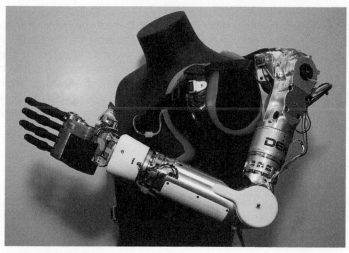

Fig. 8. DEKA arm with straps.

needed for these and other amputations to attain optimal postinjury function is essential and requires a systematic and multidisciplinary approach, including surgeon, physiatrist, physical therapist, psychologist, prosthetist, and patient's family.[55] Additionally, the Defense Advanced Research Projects Agency has funded research in cortical neural control prosthetics whereby electrode sensors/transducers are implanted on the surface of the cortex of the brain, and, through rigorous training, patients are able to control the prosthetic by actual thinking instead of having to perform some physical motion or muscle stimulation (such as the pectoralis implantation). Work by Ling and associates is on the forefront of limb replacement options.[56,57]

Although upper extremity replantation and transplantation is extremely technical, research in arm transplantation is evolving. There are case reports of several successful hand and arm transplants that have resulted in partial function. Common complications are rejection and lack of complete function.[58–61] Arm and hand replantation requires a clean-cut injury and is inappropriate for blast, crush, and high-energy mechanism injuries.

Lower limb prosthetics are somewhat simpler because there are fewer degrees of freedom to replace. The same technology is available for nerve implantation to control prosthetic ankle joints and knee joints. As with energy-transferring orthotics, lower extremity amputees can attain good function with energy transfer prosthesis. In general, the higher the amputation, the more energy that is required by patient to ambulate with a prosthesis. One of the key factors in prosthetics of the lower extremity is the socket fit of the stump—because this is where the most energy transfer occurs and where the new weight-bearing surface is located. Typically, regardless of the prosthetic, patients undergo multiple adjustments of their prosthetic in the socket area over a lifetime and may require stump revision as well.[62]

SUMMARY

Extremity injuries are common and can present a significant injury burden for patients, especially if an extremity is mangled. Those injuries requiring the need for a surgeon to decide on amputation versus limb salvage are less common except in the deployed military population, where this is a daily occurrence. For a bleeding, mangled limb, or traumatic amputation, a correctly applied tourniquet saves lives and limbs.

Following the treatment algorithms developed in civilian and military arenas over the past decade reduces morbidity and mortality in patients sustaining these injuries regardless of amputation or limb salvage. The decision to amputate or salvage a mangled limb can be difficult but if patients' hemodynamic status at presentation and what function they are likely to attain are taken into account, it can be easier. Secondary or delayed amputation is becoming a more viable option as prosthetics continue to improve at remarkable rates. Nonetheless, it is preferable to involve the patient, the patient's family, and other specialists on the treatment team in this complex decision, if possible.

REFERENCES

1. Taylor DM, Vater GM, Parker PJ. An evaluation of two tourniquet systems for the control of prehospital lower limb hemorrhage. J Trauma 2011;71(3):591–5.
2. Beekley AC, Sebesta JA, Blackbourne LH, et al. Prehospital tourniquet use in Operation Iraqi Freedom: effect on hemorrhage control and outcomes. J Trauma 2008; 64(Suppl 2):S28–37.
3. Kragh JF Jr, Walters TJ, Baer DG, et al. Practical use of emergency tourniquets to stop bleeding in major limb trauma. J Trauma 2008;64(Suppl 2):S38–49.
4. Kragh JF Jr, Walters TJ, Baer DG, et al. Survival with emergency tourniquet use to stop bleeding in major limb trauma. Ann Surg 2009;249(1):1–7.
5. Kragh JF Jr, O'Neill ML, Walters TJ, et al. Minor morbidity with emergency tourniquet use to stop bleeding in severe limb trauma: research, history, and reconciling advocates and abolitionists. Mil Med 2011;176(7):817–23.
6. Lakstein D, Blumenfeld A, Sokolov T, et al. Tourniquets for hemorrhage control on the battlefield: a 4-year accumulated experience. J Trauma 2003;54(Suppl 5): S221–5.
7. Kragh JF Jr, Baer DG, Walters TJ. Extended (16-hour) tourniquet application after combat wounds: a case report and review of the current literature. J Orthop Trauma 2007;21(4):274–8.
8. Burkhardt GE, Gifford SM, Propper B, et al. The impact of ischemic intervals on neuromuscular recovery in a porcine (Sus scrofa) survival model of extremity vascular injury. J Vasc Surg 2011;53(1):165–73.
9. Hancock HM, Stannard A, Burkhardt GE, et al. Hemorrhagic shock worsens neuromuscular recovery in a porcine model of hind limb vascular injury and ischemia-reperfusion. J Vasc Surg 2011;53(4):1052–62.
10. Kheirabadi B. Evaluation of topical hemostatic agents for combat wound treatment. US Army Med Dep J 2011;25–37.
11. Gordy SD, Rhee P, Schreiber MA. Military applications of novel hemostatic devices. Expert Rev Med Devices 2011;8(1):41–7.
12. Ran Y, Hadad E, Daher S, et al. Quik Clot Combat Gauze use for hemorrhage control in military trauma: January 2009 Israel Defense Force experience in the Gaza Strip—a preliminary report of 14 cases. Prehosp Disaster Med 2010;25(6):584–8.
13. MacIntyre AD, Quick JA, Barnes SL. Hemostatic dressings reduce tourniquet time while maintaining hemorrhage control. Am Surg 2011;77(2):162–5.
14. Bosse MJ, MacKenzie EJ, Kellam JF, et al. A prospective evaluation of the clinical utility of the lower-extremity injury-severity scores. J Bone Joint Surg Am 2001; 83A(1):3–14.
15. Gregory RT, Gould RJ, Peclet M, et al. The mangled extremity syndrome (M.E.S.): a severity grading system for multisystem injury of the extremity. J Trauma 1985; 25(12):1147–50.

16. Howe HR Jr, Poole GV Jr, Hansen KJ, et al. Salvage of lower extremities following combined orthopedic and vascular trauma. A predictive salvage index. Am Surg 1987;53(4):205–8.
17. Johansen K, Daines M, Howey T, et al. Objective criteria accurately predict amputation following lower extremity trauma. J Trauma 1990;30(5):568–72.
18. McNamara MG, Heckman JD, Corley FG. Severe open fractures of the lower extremity: a retrospective evaluation of the Mangled Extremity Severity Score (MESS). J Orthop Trauma 1994;8(2):81–7.
19. Seekamp A, Regel G, Ruffert S, et al. Amputation or reconstruction of IIIB and IIIC open tibial fracture. Decision criteria in the acute phase and late functional outcome. Unfallchirurg 1998;101(5):360–9 [in German].
20. Sudkamp N, Haas N, Flory PJ, et al. Criteria for amputation, reconstruction and replantation of extremities in multiple trauma patients. Chirurg 1989;60(11): 774–81 [in German].
21. Bonanni F, Rhodes M, Lucke JF. The futility of predictive scoring of mangled lower extremities. J Trauma 1993;34(1):99–104.
22. Durham RM, Mistry BM, Mazuski JE, et al. Outcome and utility of scoring systems in the management of the mangled extremity. Am J Surg 1996;172(5):569–73.
23. Hoogendoorn JM, van der Werken CC. The mangled leg. Eur J Trauma 2002; 28:1–10.
24. Bosse MJ, MacKenzie EJ, Kellam JF, et al. An analysis of outcomes of reconstruction or amputation after leg-threatening injuries. N Engl J Med 2002;347(24): 1924–31.
25. MacKenzie EJ, Bosse MJ, Kellam JF, et al. Factors influencing the decision to amputate or reconstruct after high-energy lower extremity trauma. J Trauma 2002;52(4):641–9.
26. Scalea TM, Dubose J, Moore EE, et al. Western Trauma Association Critical Decisions in Trauma: management of the mangled extremity. J Trauma 2012; 72(1):86–93.
27. Brown KV, Ramasamy A, McLeod J, et al. Predicting the need for early amputation in ballistic mangled extremity injuries. J Trauma 2009;66(Suppl 4):S93–7.
28. Borut LT, Acosta CJ, Tadlock LC, et al. The use of temporary vascular shunts in military extremity wounds: a preliminary outcome analysis with 2-year follow-up. J Trauma 2010;69(1):174–8.
29. Brounts LR, Wickel D, Arrington ED, et al. The use of a temporary intraluminal shunt to restore lower limb perfusion over a 4,000 mile air evacuation in a special operations military setting: a case report. Clinical Medicine Insights: Trauma and Intensive Medicine 2012;1(1):5–9. Available at: http://www.la-press.com/the-use-of-a-temporary-intraluminal-shunt-to-restore-lower-limb-perfus-article-a1007. Accessed March 1, 2012.
30. Taller J, Kamdar JP, Greene JA, et al. Temporary vascular shunts as initial treatment of proximal extremity vascular injuries during combat operations: the new standard of care at Echelon II facilities? J Trauma 2008;65(3):595–603.
31. Chambers LW, Green DJ, Sample K, et al. Tactical surgical intervention with temporary shunting of peripheral vascular trauma sustained during Operation Iraqi Freedom: one unit's experience. J Trauma 2006;61(4):824–30.
32. Rasmussen TE, Clouse WD, Jenkins DH, et al. The use of temporary vascular shunts as a damage control adjunct in the management of wartime vascular injury. J Trauma 2006;61(1):8–12.
33. Mubarak SJ, Owen CA. Double-incision fasciotomy of the leg for decompression in compartment syndromes. J Bone Joint Surg Am 1977;59(2):184–7.

34. Rorabeck CH, Clarke KM. The pathophysiology of the anterior tibial compartment syndrome: an experimental investigation. J Trauma 1978;18(5):299–304.
35. Place RJ, Rush RM Jr, Arrington ED. Forward surgical team (FST) workload in a special operations environment: the 250th FST in Operation ENDURING FREEDOM. Curr Surg 2003;60(4):418–22.
36. Rush RM Jr, Stockmaster NR, Stinger HK, et al. Supporting the Global War on Terror: a tale of two campaigns featuring the 250th Forward Surgical Team (Airborne). Am J Surg 2005;189(5):564–70.
37. Azar F. Traumatic disorders. In: Canale S, Beaty J, editors. Campbell's operative orthopedics. 11th edition. Philadelphia: Mosby Elsevier; 2007. p. 2737–46.
38. Gelberman RH, Garfin SR, Hergenroeder PT, et al. Compartment syndromes of the forearm: diagnosis and treatment. Clin Orthop Relat Res 1981;161:252–61.
39. Tiwari A, Haq AI, Myint F, et al. Acute compartment syndromes. Br J Surg 2002; 89(4):397–412.
40. McQueen MM, Court-Brown CM. Compartment monitoring in tibial fractures. The pressure threshold for decompression. J Bone Joint Surg Br 1996;78(1):99–104.
41. Gentilello LM, Sanzone A, Wang L, et al. Near-infrared spectroscopy versus compartment pressure for the diagnosis of lower extremity compartmental syndrome using electromyography-determined measurements of neuromuscular function. J Trauma 2001;51(1):1–8.
42. Giannotti G, Cohn SM, Brown M, et al. Utility of near-infrared spectroscopy in the diagnosis of lower extremity compartment syndrome. J Trauma 2000;48(3): 396–9.
43. Arbabi S, Brundage SI, Gentilello LM. Near-infrared spectroscopy: a potential method for continuous, transcutaneous monitoring for compartmental syndrome in critically injured patients. J Trauma 1999;47(5):829–33.
44. Cohen MS, Garfin SR, Hargens AR, et al. Acute compartment syndrome. Effect of dermotomy on fascial decompression in the leg. J Bone Joint Surg Br 1991;73(2): 287–90.
45. Pearse MF, Harry L, Nanchahal J. Acute compartment syndrome of the leg. BMJ 2002;325(7364):557–8.
46. Emergency war surgery, 3rd United States Revision. Washington, DC: Borden Institute; 2004.
47. Chan BL, Witt R, Charrow AP, et al. Mirror therapy for phantom limb pain. N Engl J Med 2007;357(21):2206–7.
48. Forsberg JA, Pepek JM, Wagner S, et al. Heterotopic ossification in high-energy wartime extremity injuries: prevalence and risk factors. J Bone Joint Surg Am 2009;91(5):1084–91.
49. Forsberg JA, Potter BK. Heterotopic ossification in wartime wounds. J Surg Orthop Adv 2010;19(1):54–61.
50. Potter BK, Burns TC, Lacap AP, et al. Heterotopic ossification following traumatic and combat-related amputations. Prevalence, risk factors, and preliminary results of excision. J Bone Joint Surg Am 2007;89(3):476–86.
51. Davis TA, O'Brien FP, Anam K, et al. Heterotopic ossification in complex ortho-paedic combat wounds: quantification and characterization of osteogenic precursor cell activity in traumatized muscle. J Bone Joint Surg Am 2011; 93(12):1122–31.
52. Potter BK, Forsberg JA, Davis TA, et al. Heterotopic ossification following combat-related trauma. J Bone Joint Surg Am 2010;2(Suppl 92):74–89.
53. Owens JG, Blair JA, Patzkowski JC, et al. Return to running and sports participation after limb salvage. J Trauma 2011;71(Suppl 1):S120–4.

54. Doukas WC, Hayda RA, Frisch HA, et al. Lower limb amputees fare better than limb-salvage patients in military population. AAOS 2012;4(12). Available at: http://www.aaos.org/news/aaosnow/dec10/clinical12.asp. Accessed April 15, 2012.
55. Resnik L, Meucci MR, Lieberman-Klinger S, et al. Advanced upper limb prosthetic devices: implications for upper limb prosthetic rehabilitation. Arch Phys Med Rehabil 2012;93(4):710–7.
56. Thakor NV, Moore DF, Miranda RA, et al. Special issue of DARPA NEST proceedings. IEEE Trans Neural Syst Rehabil Eng 2012;20(2):113–6.
57. Moore DF, Miranda R, Ling GS. DARPA Nest. IEEE Pulse 2012;3(1):14.
58. Jablecki J, Kaczmarzyk L, Kaczmarzyk J, et al. Unilateral arm transplant 28 years after amputation: fourteen-month result. Transplant Proc 2011;43(9):3563–5.
59. Cavadas PC, Landin L, Thione A, et al. The Spanish experience with hand, forearm, and arm transplantation. Hand Clin 2011;27(4):443–53.
60. Cavadas PC, Ibanez J, Thione A, et al. Bilateral trans-humeral arm transplantation: result at 2 years. Am J Transplant 2011;11(5):1085–90.
61. Landin L, Cavadas PC, Nthumba P, et al. Preliminary results of bilateral arm transplantation. Transplantation 2009;88(5):749–51.
62. Fergason J, Keeling JJ, Bluman EM. Recent advances in lower extremity amputations and prosthetics for the combat injured patient. Foot Ankle Clin 2010;15(1):151–74.

Verification and Regionalization of Trauma Systems

The Impact of These Efforts on Trauma Care in the United States

Jeffrey Bailey, MD[a,*], Scott Trexler, MD[b], Alan Murdock, MD[c], David Hoyt, MD[d]

KEYWORDS

- Trauma systems • Verification • Regionalization

KEY POINTS

- A trauma system is a coordinated and organized approach to the delivery of care to injured patients within a community implemented to enhance community health and to ensure the effective use of resources.
- Efforts to develop trauma systems in the United States have resulted in the implementation of a system of care for the seriously injured in most states and within the US military, particularly in relation to recent major conflicts in the Middle East and Southwest Asia.
- The methodology intended to verify trauma systems is focused on performance based on patient-centered outcomes.
- Trauma systems are effectively regionalized to the extent that the most seriously injured patients in a community are cared for at designated tertiary care trauma centers.
- Outcome measures, beyond hospital-based mortality, such as risk-adjusted rates of preventable morbidity and quality-of-life indicators, may serve as a future means to verify trauma systems.

DoD disclaimer: The opinions or assertions contained herein are the private views of the authors and are not to be construed as official or as reflecting the views of the US Air Force, the Army Medical Command, the US Department of the Army, or the US Department of Defense.

Grant support/financial disclosure: None.

Conflict of interest statement: The authors have no conflicts to report.

[a] US Army Institute of Surgical Research, Joint Trauma System, 3611 Chambers Pass, Building 3611, Fort Sam Houston, TX 78234, USA; [b] Department of Surgery, San Antonio Military Medical Center, Fort Sam Houston, TX, USA; [c] US Air Force Medical Service and University of Pittsburgh, Pittsburgh, PA, USA; [d] Department of Surgery, American College of Surgeons, Chicago, IL, USA

* Corresponding author.

E-mail address: Jeffrey.a.bailey3@amedd.army.mil

Surg Clin N Am 92 (2012) 1009–1024

doi:10.1016/j.suc.2012.04.008

0039-6109/12/$ – see front matter Published by Elsevier Inc.

surgical.theclinics.com

INTRODUCTION AND BACKGROUND

A trauma system is an organized approach to the delivery of care to injured patients within a community. Trauma systems operate within defined geographic boundaries and serve to provide multidisciplinary care to injured patients. Through statewide coordination, trauma systems serve to not only enhance community health but to also ensure efficient use of medical resources.

In 1966, the National Academy of Sciences published their landmark article, "Accidental Death and Disability: The Neglected Disease of Modern Society,"[1] bringing to light the need for an organized approach to the treatment of injured patients. With the publication of the American College of Surgeons Committee on Trauma guideline "Optimal Hospital Resources for the Care of the Seriously Injured"[2] a decade later, the framework for what would become the modern trauma system was established.

In 2007, Hoyt and Coimbra[3] published a comprehensive article detailing the history, organization, and future directions of trauma systems within the United States. This article serves to provide an update of the developments that have occurred in trauma systems in the areas of system verification and regionalization in the intervening years since the original publication.

STATES WITH TRAUMA SYSTEMS

As indicated, trauma systems, as opposed to trauma centers, represent a coordinated and organized approach to the care of the injured in a region versus a medical treatment facility. It is important to recognize that regions of trauma care may cross state and even international boundaries (as is the case of the US Military Joint Trauma System). Although the term region is geography-centric and defined by boundaries, the term system is patient-centric and defined by a coordinated and organized approach to trauma care. At the time of publication of the original article, approximately 50% of states had statewide trauma systems,[3] which increased to 90% as of October 2011.[4]

US MILITARY TRAUMA SYSTEMS

The development of the civilian trauma system has been closely tied to lessons learned by America's military during armed conflict through the last 2 centuries. Although it contributed early to the formation of the civilian trauma system, in the absence of armed conflict, the United States military trauma system stagnated in the 1980s and found itself unprepared for the delivery of trauma care in the deployed environment during Operations Desert Shield and Desert Storm.[5] In response to the terrorist attacks of September 11, 2001, Operation Enduring Freedom (OEF) and Operation Iraqi Freedom (OIF) were initiated. An effort to develop a military trauma system modeled after the civilian system while accounting for the unique situations encountered in the battlefield environment was initiated in May 2004. In November 2004, the Joint Theater Trauma System (JTTS) was implemented as a result of these efforts. **Table 1** differentiates some of the conventional and symmetric definitions of the agents, ways, means, and ends of violence and its intended or unintended consequence in a region or population. Terrorist activity may exploit conventional definitions and understandings of the agents, ways, means, and ends of violence in a population; as such, its domain is asymmetrical and overlaps the military and civilian community.

To allow for ongoing performance improvement and research, the Joint Theater Trauma Registry (JTTR) was developed. This comprehensive database includes injury

Table 1 Conventional definitions of the agents, ways, means, and ends of violence on the battlefield and civilian community		
	Battlefield	**Civilian Community**
Agents	Military combatants	Criminals, constabulary responders
Ways	Military operations	Criminal activity and law enforcement
Means	High-energy weapons and explosives	Low-energy weapons, motor vehicle crashes, falls, natural disasters
Ends	Military objectives	Illegal purposes, maintenance of civil order

and outcome data entered into a central database from a concise form (**Fig. 1**). In 2 recent reviews by Eastridge and colleagues,[6,7] the positive impact that the JTTS has had on the care delivered to the injured soldier, airman, sailor, and marine is evident. In a review of 3 of the 27 evidence-based clinical practice guidelines (CPGs) implemented after the formation of the JTTS,[6] clinically and statistically significant improvements were seen in the following areas:

- Burn resuscitation-associated abdominal compartment syndrome mortality
- Hypothermia on presentation
- Massive transfusion mortality (damage control resuscitation).

To further highlight the effectiveness of the JTTS, this article demonstrates a 5.2% mortality rate after battlefield hospital admission, which is comparable to an age-matched cohort case fatality rate of 4.3% from the National Trauma Data Bank. In their more recent review of the JTTS, Eastridge and colleagues[7] show the significant impact that this trauma system has had in the care of the wounded service member, demonstrating a 54% decrease in aggregate postinjury complications after the development and implementation of the aforementioned 27 evidence-based CPGs. The implemented CPGs are available at http://www.usaisr.amedd.army.mil/cpgs.html.

In 2010, the joint trauma system (JTS) concept was introduced in the Department of Defense (DoD). The newly described JTS organization would serve as a consulting agency to each of the regional or theater US military combatant commands as a resource for deploying a JTTS if conflict- or disaster-related contingencies required an organized oversight of trauma care.[8] This organization has been formally recognized and funded in the DoD for the next 5 years, and a tactical plan to operationalize its funding resources is in development.

Funding that continues beyond the duration of the current conflict in the US Central Command Area of Responsibility supports the primary goal of the JTS: to serve as an enduring resource for DoD trauma care and trauma systems, regardless of region, command, or contingency. To maintain that capability and relevance in trauma care and systems, the JTS is positioned to be sustained as a surgeon lead joint military service entity that remains agile and current with advances in injury care.

To ensure its perpetual relevance and excellence in DoD trauma care, the JTS has strengthened its relationship with the American College of Surgeons Committee on Trauma (ACS COT) and aligned its activities with COT trauma systems by seeking appointment of its trauma surgeon leadership to COT military region leadership positions and development of a US military manual entitled: *Joint Trauma System: Development, Conceptual Framework, and Optimal Elements*. This document is

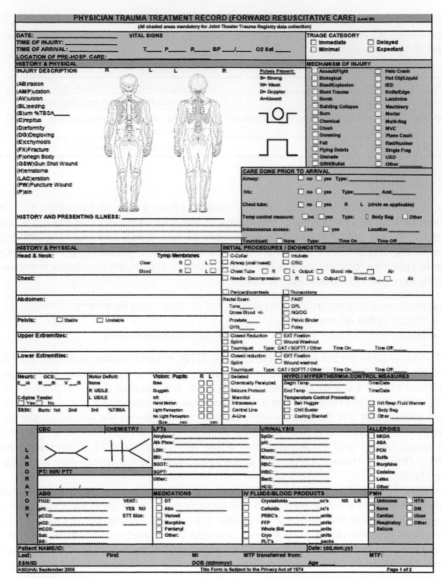

Fig. 1. JTTR record.

intended to serve as the ACS COT regional trauma systems manual. It is to be a perpetual and regularly updated resource for US military trauma systems definition. These efforts mirror the important relationship that has developed between US military and civilian trauma care providers and systems in the decade preceding and since the September 11th attacks.[8]

In addition to the publication of a trauma systems manual, the development of a *theater* operations manual to describe the structure, function, and tactical deployment of a trauma system to future contingencies, regions, and commands has been recently recommended to the Defense Health Board. This recommendation is now under review for implementation at JTS. This manual is intended to capture all currently available stand-up and operational procedures for all elements of the theater trauma system and accelerate the speed and efficacy of future JTTS.[9]

LEGISLATIVE ACTIVITY AND AUTHORIZATION
Funding

To plan, implement, and evaluate statewide or regional trauma systems, sufficient funding is required. All components of the trauma system require funding, including the following[10]:

- Prehospital care
- Acute-care medical facilities
- Rehabilitation centers
- Prevention programs.

Of the 45 states with statewide trauma systems, only 60% of them are funded.[4]

In his comprehensive review of trauma system funding, Geehan[11] discusses many of the changes in the medical landscape of today that have affected the funding of trauma centers. It is difficult to accurately assess the cost of a functioning trauma center, although recent estimates have ranged between $2.7 million and $4.5 million yearly.

Given the unpredictable nature of injured-patient arrivals, trauma centers must have their facilities and staff at the ready at all times. At present, there is no effective method to bill for this readiness. The Current Procedural Terminology coding system does make an allowance for physician standby time, but there is a 30-minute time limit. Additionally, the code is assigned a low relative value unit of 1.2 and is not routinely reimbursed by Medicare or Medicaid.[11] A revenue code (68x) was approved by the American Hospital Association to charge for trauma activation. To bill for this code, patients must arrive at the trauma center by trained prehospital care providers, meaning that those patients that are brought in by privately owned vehicles or who bring themselves to the trauma center are not eligible for use of this code. Despite being available for use since 2002, a recent survey conducted to determine the usage rate of this code found that payers only variably accept it.[12]

Because of the difficulty in billing for readiness, a stream of sustainable funding is desirable for any trauma system. **Box 1** lists various funding methods states have used to support trauma systems.[4,10]

Given the frequently encountered difficulties in securing and maintaining adequate funding, it behooves the trauma center (and the trauma system) to limit costs. Methods that have been proposed to achieve this end include varying staffing throughout the day based on peak patient-volume times and minimizing staff turnover to prevent excess expenditure on recruitment and training of new personnel.

Box 1
Funding mechanisms for state-supported trauma systems
Moving traffic violation fees
Driver's license renewal fees
Gambling revenue compacts
Cigarette taxes
Crime victim funds
911 call surcharge

VERIFICATION OF US TRAUMA SYSTEMS AND THE IMPACT ON TRAUMA CARE
Valuation of US Trauma Systems

Public valuation and expectations of trauma systems have been consistently demonstrated.[13,14] This perception has almost certainly buoyed the acceptance and subsequent development of trauma systems in the United States.[4] Nonetheless, the same level of commitment has not applied to the willingness of electorates and government to consistently underwrite the cost of trauma systems. This factor is likely the primary factor that has generated the mismatch between public perception and expectation and the realities of the current state of US systems.[13–15] Three years before the 2007 Hoyt/Coimbra SCNA review[3] of US trauma systems, the National Foundation for Trauma Care (now known as The Trauma Center Association of America) described a crisis in trauma care because of the loss of trauma centers across the United States.[16] Unfortunately, the crisis has been exacerbated by recent unfavorable trends in reimbursements set against the backdrop of an evolving global financial crisis.[11,17] In this environment of austerity, the impact of effort that verifies the benefit and potentially the requirement of trauma systems as an imperative for public health would be difficult to understate. So, given the continued erosion and the real potential for outright collapse of US trauma systems, a body of work that seeks to evaluate the positive impact of US trauma systems on patient care continues to be accumulated and refined. Whether this can win appropriated fiscal support to sustain the US trauma system remains to be seen.

Verification of Trauma Systems as Opposed to Trauma Centers

The elements that constitute a trauma center are quantifiable in component or elemental form, but their organized application is the process that produces the favorable results that are attributed to the care of the injured in designated hospitals. Verification that a hospital has demonstrated the capability and ongoing potential to operate as a trauma center involves the evaluation of the following areas:

- Institutional commitment
- Injury volume and acuity
- Facility layout, dedicated material, and human resources
- Operation of the clinical trauma program
- Trauma performance improvement program.

Although most centers look to verification by the lead external agency for care of the injured, the ACS, some centers have opted out of that process to rely on an internal validation process. Factors that ultimately result in trauma center *designation*, a governmental action, may include review and consideration of an internal or external verification process. The relationship between formal trauma *center* verification and improved outcomes has been empirically reported and has been demonstrated across a spectrum of quality indicators that include in-hospital mortality, lengths of stay, lethal injury complex outcomes, and resource use.[18–21] These results are particularly compelling in that trauma centers care for a more seriously injured patient population with a paradoxically higher burden of predicted morbidity and mortality.[18–20]

Reasons that underlie this paradox are presumably based largely on the commitment of facility resources to trauma care. However, beyond the use of facility material resources, resultant improvements in patient outcome have also been attributed to the synergy that results from the commitment of facility leadership and staff. It is this commitment that is presumed to drive a shift in organizational culture that energizes and sustains a constant state of readiness focused on the care of the seriously injured and in effect transforms a hospital into a trauma center.[11],[19] That culture of commitment and readiness may encompass the continuum of injury care from out of the hospital to hospital and through rehabilitative phases when the continuum is organized as a trauma *system*. Although individual components may be functioning optimally, it does not necessarily follow that when integrated across the continuum of care, they perform at the same high level as a system.[22],[23] As reported by Hoyt and Coimbra in 2007, the 2006 publication, "Model Trauma System Planning and Evaluation," by the US Department of Health and Human Services, Health Resources and Services Administration outlined a public health model for the evaluation of trauma systems defined by system assessment, policy development, and assurance (**Fig. 2**).[23] In this era of fiscal austerity, the continued development, evaluation, and sustainment of trauma systems within this model hinges on evidence that verifies trauma systems provide a measureable and positive impact on patient outcomes while containing costs.

System Evaluation and Verification Efforts and Performance Measures

The evaluation of trauma center performance has relied on the assessment of quality indicators that exist in 4 principle domains as summarized in **Table 2**. Although a large

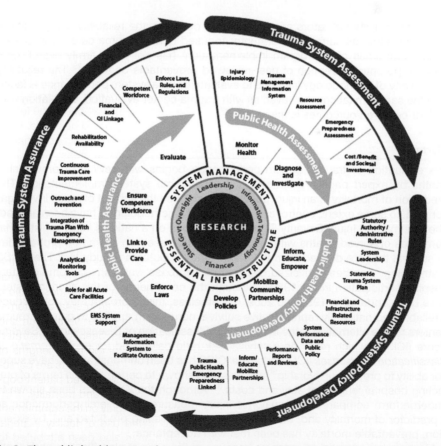

Fig. 2. The public health approach to trauma system development. (*Data from* United States Department of Health and Human Services Health Resources and Services Administration. Model trauma system planning and evaluation August 2006.)

Table 2 Quality indicators for trauma center performance	
Phases of care	Prehospital Hospital Posthospital Secondary prevention
Structure	Field triage Advanced imaging availability Rehabilitation referral practices Alcohol screening
Process	EMS response time ED dwell time Rehabilitation facility wait time Alcohol recidivism
Outcome	Death Admission to long-term care Recurrent injury

Abbreviations: ED, emergency department; EMS, emergency medical services.

number of quality indicators arise from these domains, the reliability and validity of these indicators as surrogates for center-focused quality trauma care (ie, improved patient outcomes after program implementation) has not been firmly established, with the potential exception of peer-reviewed preventable death.[24,25] The reliability and validity of methodology intended to evaluate trauma system performance is faced with the same limitations; however, as with trauma center evaluation, correlation with patient-centered outcomes is the goal.[26,27]

Mortality

The evaluation of trauma system performance begins with review of preventable deaths by expert panels, pretrauma and posttrauma system implementation. The prediction of mortality in an injury population has been the subject of much investigation and, to some extent, controversy. Two primary methodologies have been applied. The Trauma and Injury Severity Score (TRISS) relies on a national injury registry that compares observed deaths with predicted deaths based on estimated probabilities of survival that are derived from the Major Trauma Outcome Study.[13,28] The TRISS methodology has been criticized because its database was derived from voluntary hospital participation in the 1980s, although the coefficients for this scoring system have been updated in 1995 and 2009. Nonetheless, this approach may not produce a reliable and nationally representative survival norm when applied to current trauma centers.[29] The alternative is the International Classification of Diseases Injury Severity Score (ICISS), which relies on a survival risk ratio calculated for each *International Classification of Diseases (ICD)* code. The ICISS has been demonstrated to have superior ability to predict survivorship[30] and was also shown to perform well in terms of predicting hospital lengths of stay and costs.[31] Although the ICISS has been shown to underperform compared with anatomic injury measures, its overall performance as a predictor of mortality and, thus, as a tool for establishing predicted and, by extension, preventable mortality has been met with acceptance.

Mortality is an appealing outcome because of the ease of classification and identification within a data set. A meta-analysis of 14 studies between 1992 and 2003 reported a 15% mortality reduction when trauma care was provided in trauma centers in an established trauma system based on an odds ratio assessment.[29] Since this publication, several studies have demonstrated reductions in mortality, up to 25%, either by comparing outcomes based on facility (trauma center vs nontrauma center) or chronology (pretrauma and posttrauma system implementation).[15,27,30,31] The implementation of a trauma system in the OIF/OEF theaters of combat operations was demonstrated to be associated with lower mortality from burns and abdominal compartment syndrome from 36% to 18% and with massive transfusion from 32% to 20%. This finding has been attributed to the adoption of evidence-based theater clinical practice guidelines that were deployed across the system.[5,6] It should be noted that these results were primarily associated with the care of the combat injured in OIF where the United States played a much larger role in implementation and assurance of the JTTS versus OEF (Afghanistan) where the trauma system has a much larger component of international participants, primarily from the European continent and the United Kingdom. A case-matched comparison of trauma outcomes in these two very different systems has yet to be accomplished, but it is likely that results pertaining to mortality outcomes are comparable. This assumption is based on the observation that the implementation of trauma systems outside of North America has realized comparable improvements in injury-related mortality.[32]

The overall effectiveness of relying on the mortality advantage to establish the value of a trauma system has its limitations because of the low proportion of deaths within a trauma population. This point is particularly relevant in a system with a realistic potential of providing quality care and, thus, influencing favorable outcomes in the population where it is most likely to matter: the one between the populations who are likely to recover and those for whom effective care is not a reasonable possibility.[33] The limitation of mortality as a facile indicator is exacerbated in systems whereby patient volumes and visibility are low but relative risk of adverse outcome is high, such as the rural setting where, although small in absolute magnitude, the relative opportunity to impact care, lower risk, and improve outcomes is high.[34] In addition, longitudinal evaluations are unlikely to demonstrate continued dramatic reductions in mortality once the system matures.[31,33] So, once system maturity has been achieved, a stabilized reduction in mortality may serve to reset the bar of public expectation; early gains made in mortality rates may be lost to public memory. Although the inclusive trauma system has won preference to the exclusive system, a halo effect in the mature trauma system has also been described, which may also lead to public misperceptions because of the misattribution of trauma-center care outcomes to non-trauma hospitals.[27,30,35]

Beyond In-Hospital Mortality

Although mortality has been described as low-hanging fruit in the verification of trauma systems, several other indicators have been evaluated in the effort to verify the impact of trauma systems on trauma care in the United States. This body of work has primarily focused on the in-hospital phase of care. Efforts to verify the impact of trauma systems on out-of-hospital care have largely focused on the value of system-based out-of-hospital decision making by evaluating outcomes, again largely as a function of mortality, although the effect of appropriate triage has also been reported in terms of cost savings.[36–38] Following implementation of a rural trauma system in Iowa, investigators reported a significant reduction in the risk of death associated with traumatic brain injury.[39] Although the ideal approach and algorithm to guide out-of-hospital decision making remains in question, the value of an organized approach in this phase of care is not in dispute,[40,41] and continued efforts to verify the value of system-based trauma care in addition to efficacy of triage include emergency medical services response time and prehospital deaths. However, the enduring hospital-centric, surgical audit-based system for data collection for the evaluation of the system complicates the process of effective capture and evaluation of prehospital data.[24] Although not yet linked to a direct outcome measure, the implementation of the US Military Joint Trauma System Clinical Practice guideline (JTS web site: http://usaisr.amedd.army.mil/joint_trauma_system.html) for the prevention of hypothermia, primarily addressed to the out-of-hospital phase of care, resulted in a 7-fold reduction in the percent of patients demonstrating hypothermia on presentation.[6] The overarching implication of this body of work suggests that the acceptance and practice of trauma care in accordance with theater clinical practice guidelines resulted in a reduction in variance across the system (primarily in the out-of-hospital setting in this case) that was realized in improved hypothermia rates. The validation of this implication requires an assessment of out-of-hospital patient care practice. Effective capture of prehospital data in a combat theater of operations has been a difficult challenge; but early efforts have demonstrated improvement in that capability, although, to date, no means other than case-by-case expert evaluation of out of standards missions (based on response times) is the sole means of evaluating impacts on patient outcomes. As efficacy of system-based registration of out of hospital phases of care improves, system based evaluation of out of hospital care and related patient outcomes will likely continue to improve.[8]

The evaluation of system impact on the posthospital phase of trauma care is in its early stages but may be linked to more profound indicators of quality outcomes that relate to a potential reduction in the burden of long-term disability and years of productive life lost.[27] Inclusion of long-term psychological and emotional sequelae, such as injury-associated posttrauma stress disorder, although not a consistent measure of injury-related functional recovery, may be included in a more far-reaching evaluation of structural and process trauma systems outcomes.[42] The practical application of such investigation will rely on effective means of identifying and evaluating injury-related disability in populations. Adapting a combination of existing generic disability assessment tools may facilitate work in this area.[43,44]

The economic burden of trauma and its related disability is large. In a pay-for-performance culture, the practical value of demonstrating the ability of trauma systems to contain costs has been another avenue of outcomes-related investigation. In response to failure of a state trauma system to win legislative funding, Durham and colleagues[15] produced a report designed to address the effectiveness of trauma systems, which was questioned by the governor in vetoing the legislation. The governor stated: "Trauma centers save lives, but so do hospitals that are not designated trauma centers. What is the difference derived from adherence to our (trauma system) regulations? If state government is to initiate trauma center unique payments, we must first know we are paying for performance."[15] The investigation generated in response to this statement and its related mandate was designed to answer 3 key questions: (1) Does treatment at a trauma center versus a nontrauma center improve survival? (2) Is the system cost effective? (3) Is access to the system equitable?

The investigation showed a mortality reduction of 18% in trauma patients cared for in designated trauma centers, which is comparable with the survival advantage that has been attributed to trauma systems. Although the absolute cost for care at a trauma center was higher than a nontrauma center by $21,875 in charges, the marginal cost per life saved ranged from $32,514 to $122,750, which translated to $746 to $2815 per life-year saved; a savings that is in parity with other major public health programs. Access was found to be superior to the national average but could be improved by the addition of trauma centers in underserved areas. The investigators also reported an oversaturation of one region of the state with level II trauma centers, limiting volumes (from 202 to 368 patients), which the investigators attributed to political reasons, indicating that 1 of the 8 key criteria for trauma system development (authority to designate, certify, identify, or categorize trauma centers) was beyond the reach of the system in that region during the period in study.[10,15]

The cost-effectiveness of trauma-center care was demonstrated in a subsequent study that assessed the value of trauma-center care based on a national outcomes registry representing 14 US states. This investigation showed that the value was most favorable in patients with an injury of higher severity and that these costs were effective in comparison with other life-saving inventions for care of cardiac arrest, severe sepsis, acute respiratory failure, and other general critical care interventions. Moreover, the investigators attributed the cost-effective performance of the individual centers to *regionalization* of trauma care within the 14 states they assessed.[21]

REGIONALIZATION OF US TRAUMA SYSTEMS AND THE IMPACT ON TRAUMA CARE

Trauma systems are effectively *regionalized* to the extent that the most seriously injured patients (injury severity score >15) in a region are cared for at designated tertiary care trauma centers. This concept is reflective of the notion that an effectively regionalized trauma system is shaped to meet the right patient, right injury, right care, right time paradigm. These centers may be designated by either a regional or state trauma system authority or by the ACS verification process.

In addition, regionalized trauma systems place a limit on the number of tertiary care centers to avoid ineffective redundancy of effort and to sustain trauma care experience within the system based on the concern that lower-volume centers will have insufficient experience to provide optimal trauma care. The ACS COT currently recommends that a level I trauma center admit a minimum of 1200 trauma patients per year and that at least 240 of these patients fall into the seriously injured category, although this threshold has been challenged.[45]

Regionalization of trauma systems may be further impacted by the extent to which the systems are exclusive (ie, all trauma patients go to a limited number of centers for care) or inclusive (ie, all acute care hospitals in a region participate in the care of the injured) based on their capability. Inclusive systems have generally been favored over exclusive systems in that they enable the full capacity of the system to care for the injured while at the same time regulate the most seriously injured to the centers with the greatest capability to care for them. Another potential advantage of the inclusive system is the distribution of regional injury care resources, which would be more favorable in the event of a natural or man-made disaster or act of war or terrorism as discussed by Sofer and Klausner elsewhere in this issue.[21,35,45,46] A potential weakness of the inclusive system is excessive dilution of each center's volume of seriously injured patients thereby creating a suboptimal practice experience for some centers. So, one may assess the effectiveness of an inclusive trauma system by evaluating the distribution of patients within the system based on the severity of the injury bearing in mind that the experience imperative will be served by concentrating the most seriously injured in the higher-volume centers.[45] This methodology has been advanced because it is more effective in providing a functional (high-acuity patients to high-volume centers) as opposed to elemental (high-acuity patients to designated trauma centers) assessment of the system. It also offers an assurance tool in that trauma systems may redesignate centers based on this functional evaluation.[35,45]

In an evaluation of the US trauma system, Diggs and colleagues[45] reported that approximately 7% of US hospitals meet the high threshold volume but that, on average, based on actual distribution of the seriously injured, the empirically derived threshold that separates a high-volume from low-volume center was 915 patient admissions per year. All categories of seriously injured patients were included in these findings, with the exception of the elderly, most of whom were not admitted to high-volume higher-acuity centers. The study has important implications on 2 major accounts: First, the empiric threshold for a high-volume center was 915, which suggests that the ACS threshold of 1200 may need to be reassessed. Second, elderly patients were not regulated to the high-volume high-acuity centers, indicating that trauma systems exercise a different standard for regionalization of trauma care of the elderly, which is a topic for further study.[45]

Triage Implications in a Regionalized Trauma System

Another important indicator of effective regionalization is the efficacy of primary response or early appropriate transfer of the seriously injured to designated trauma centers within a region. In evaluating investigations designed to provide such an assessment, it is important to consider that this may be difficult to measure on a large regional or national level if the investigation was based on the evaluation of a large-volume admission or discharge patient databases. Although a conventional methodology, these investigations may miss the emergency-department-to-emergency-department transfer, which may represent inappropriate initial triage of patients from the scene of the injury.[47]

Although undertriage is an important indicator of ineffective regionalization, secondary overtriage (transfer of patients with minor or no injuries to tertiary care trauma centers) has also been demonstrated as a suboptimal performance consequence in an immature trauma system. This situation leads to overburdened transport and tertiary care resources (not to mention geographic displacement of patients with injuries well within their community's trauma care capabilities).[47] An evolving consequence of patient transfer, certainly amplified by secondary overtriage in immature trauma systems, is the growing problem of repeat imaging because of ineffective regionalization, use, and application of advanced imaging technology. Although the issue appeals to a technical solution, a more effective systems-based approach will include the application of good clinical practice guidelines in image-ordering decision schemes.[48]

In an evaluation of triage and mortality, Utter and colleagues[35] found that the most seriously injured patients were more likely to survive in states with the most inclusive trauma systems (ie, largest proportion of designated trauma centers) but that this did not seem to result from differences in triage patterns. They speculate the reasons that underlie this finding include better early care of severely injured patients by transferring hospitals presumably because of an improved state of readiness and capability to care for the injured that is more distinctive of inclusive trauma systems.[35] In addition, there is evidence that in mature trauma systems, a rigid leveling hierarchy may be less relevant in the regionalization of the severely injured; patient outcomes may be comparable in level I and level II centers.[49] It is important to keep in mind that these results have been demonstrated in retrospect and that in the prospective development of trauma systems such findings are not necessarily generalizable across all centers or systems.[50] They do, however, provide a best-evidence opportunity for shaping the regionalization of a maturing system based on past and potential future performance. Finally, optimal regionalization calls for development of an inclusive regional trauma system that operates based on established and effective primary and secondary triage guidelines and transfer agreements.[45]

A FUTURE DIRECTION IN EVALUATING THE IMPACT OF VERIFICATION AND REGIONALIZATION ON TRAUMA CARE: RISK-ADJUSTED OUTCOME MEASURES AND COMPARISONS AS AN INDICATOR OF SYSTEM AS OPPOSED TO CENTER PERFORMANCE

In recognition of the demonstrated positive impact of the National Surgical Quality Improvement Program on patient outcomes, the ACS has developed a Trauma Quality Improvement Program (TQIP), which is modeled to provide a validated, risk-adjusted, outcomes-based program to evaluate and improve the quality of trauma care. A system of confidential report cards has been implemented in order for participating trauma centers to compare their performance within a peer group according to risk-adjusted mortality benchmarks. This measure represents the first systematic measure and reporting of trauma care quality.[24,51] Future outcome measures, beyond hospital-based mortality, such as rates of preventable morbidity, and quality-of-life indicators, such as measures of functional recovery, may serve to benchmark additional risk-adjusted outcomes. This prospect offers the promise of a robust, validated, and facile assessment and assurance tool to assist with the development and refinement of trauma systems.[24] It has been proposed that the review of trauma center risk-adjusted outcomes may be included in determining trauma center status.[52] Such an assessment would most likely be focused on a review of trauma center performance-improvement applications initiated in response to risk-adjusted trauma center indicators. Although not yet designed, aggregation of validated, risk-adjusted outcome measures within a region may similarly serve as a powerful verification tool in the evaluation of effective regionalization of a trauma system.

The application of performance improvement to trauma system disaster response has been demonstrated to improve regionalization of the severely injured to system trauma centers. Cryer and colleagues[53] report a measureable improvement in the distribution of severely injured patients associated with 2 mass casualty incidents. This report is an excellent example of the application of trauma systems as a public health resource in mass casualty and disaster response. However, it stands in relative isolation as a formally reported *and measured* indicator of the maturation of US or regional trauma systems in mass casualty and disaster response since the 2007 Hoyt and Coimbra *Surgical Clinics of North America* review of US trauma systems.

SUMMARY

Trauma systems allow for improvement of community health in the populations they serve by promoting the effective and efficient use of medical resources. Statewide trauma systems have become more prevalent since the time of initial publication of Hoyt and Coimbra's article,[3] with 90% of US states now having statewide systems.

Trauma systems are regionalized to attempt to meet the right patient, right injury, right care, right time paradigm and to limit tertiary trauma center redundancy. Inclusive systems (ie, those systems whereby all participating hospitals care for injured patients based on their capabilities) have traditionally been favored over the exclusive system, and Utter and colleagues[35] retrospectively demonstrated that this may lead to improved outcome. However, the inclusive system is not without flaws, and the patient volume needed to be designated a high-volume center as well as effective regulation of triage across all patient populations need to be further examined.[45]

With the significant cost of maintaining trauma systems, poor reimbursement, and the evolving global financial crisis, a sustainable source of funding remains a substantial hurdle to be overcome in the ongoing fight to prevent the collapse of US trauma systems. The positive impact that robust trauma systems can have on the outcome of injured patients has recently been demonstrated in review articles reporting on the experience of the US military's implementation of the JTTS in OEF and OIF.[5-7] Funding for sustainment of the JTS beyond the recent conflict in Iraq and current conflict in Afghanistan has been programmed. The most effective use of those resources requires the JTS and future JTTS are surgeon lead, agile, and current with advancements in trauma care.

Several studies in the civilian literature have demonstrated a mortality benefit associated with care of the injured in a trauma system.[15,29-31] However, these studies assessed mortality benefit, a benefit that matures along with the trauma system and may not indicate actual success in smaller communities given lower patient numbers. Ongoing publication into the measureable and positive impact that trauma systems have on their communities beyond a mortality benefit is essential to ensure continued funding. Work continues on assessment of prehospital and posthospital care and long-term outcomes. In an environment of sustained fiscal austerity with trauma systems competing for limited financial resources, TQIP performance-based outcome measures may more effectively demonstrate trauma system value and garner improved financial support.

REFERENCES

1. Accidental death and disability: the neglected disease of modern society. Washington, DC: National Academy of Sciences; 1966.
2. Committee on Trauma, American College of Surgeons. Optimal hospital resources for care of the seriously injured. Bull Am Coll Surg 1976;61:15–22.
3. Hoyt DB, Coimbra R. Trauma systems. Surg Clin North Am 2007;87:21–35.
4. Summary of trauma systems and funding mechanisms by state. Available at: http://www.facs.org/trauma/tsepc/pdfs/traumasystemsfundingbystate.pdf. Accessed November 15, 2011.
5. Eastridge BJ, Jenkins D, Flaherty S, et al. Trauma system development in a theatre of war: experiences from operation Iraqi Freedom and Operation Enduring Freedom. J Trauma 2006;61(6):1–8.
6. Eastridge BJ, Costanzo G, Jenkins D, et al. Impact of joint theater trauma system initiatives on battlefield injury outcomes. Am J Surg 2009;198:852–7.
7. Eastridge BJ, Wade CE, Spott MA, et al. Utilizing a trauma systems approach to benchmark and improve combat casualty care. J Trauma 2010;69(Suppl 1): S5–9.
8. Joint Theater Trauma System/Joint Theater Trauma Registry. Annual report for federal fiscal year 2010. Fort Sam Houston (TX): US Army Institute of Surgical Research; 2011.
9. Presentation of Michael Rotondo MD, Chairman American College of Surgeons Committee on Trauma to Defense Health Board. In: Theater system review. Washington, DC, November 14, 2011.
10. Regional trauma systems: optimal elements, integration, and assessment systems consultation guide. Committee on Trauma, American College of Surgeons. Chicago (IL): Trauma System Evaluation and Planning Committee; 2008.
11. Geehan D. The big hurt: trauma system funding in today's health care environment. Mo Med 2010;107(5):324–7.
12. Fakhry SM, Potter C, Crain W, et al. Survey of national usage of trauma response charge codes. An opportunity for enhanced trauma center revenue. J Trauma 2009;67:1352.

13. Champion HR, Mabee MS, Meredith JW. The state of US trauma systems: public perceptions versus reality – implications for US response to terrorism and mass casualty events. J Am Coll Surg 2006;203(6):951–61.
14. Winchell RJ, Ball JW, Cooper GF, et al. As assessment of the impact of trauma systems consultation on the level of trauma system development. J Am Coll Surg 2008;207(5):623–9.
15. Durham R, Pracht E, Orban B, et al. Evaluation of a mature trauma system. Ann Surg 2006;243(6):775–85.
16. US trauma system crisis: lost in the scramble for terror resources. National Foundation for Trauma Care; 2004.
17. Mann NC, Mackenzie E, Teitelbaum SD, et al. Trauma system structure and viability in the current health care environment: a state by state assessment. J Trauma 2005;58(1):136–47.
18. Piontek FA, Coscia R, Marselle CS, et al. Impact of American College of Surgeons verification on trauma outcomes. J Trauma 2003;54(6):1041–7.
19. Maggio PM, Brundage SI, Hernandez-Broussard T, et al. Commitment to COT verification improves patient outcomes and financial performance. J Trauma 2009;67(1):190–5.
20. Norwood S, Cook AD, Berne JD. Level I verification is associated with a decreased mortality rate after major torso vascular injuries. Am Surg 2011;77:32–7.
21. Mackenzie EJ, Weir S, Rivara FP, et al. The value of trauma center care. J Trauma 2010;69(1):1–10.
22. Eastman AB. The Scudder oration: wherever the dart lands: toward the ideal trauma system. J Am Coll Surg 2010;211(2):153–68.
23. Model trauma system planning and evaluation. US Department of Health and Human Services; 2006.
24. Stelfox HT, Bobranska-Artiuch B, Nathens AB, et al. Quality indicators for evaluating trauma care: a scoping review. Arch Surg 2010;145(3):286–95.
25. Stelfox HT, Strauss SE, Nathens AB, et al. Evidence for quality indicators to evaluate adult trauma care: a systematic review. Crit Care Med 2011;39(4):846–59.
26. Brohi K, Cole E, Hoffman K. Improving outcomes in the early phases after major trauma. Curr Opin Crit Care 2011;17:515–9.
27. Lansink KW, Leenen PH. Do designated trauma systems improve outcome? Curr Opin Crit Care 2007;13:686–90.
28. Champion HR, Copes RH, Sacco WJ, et al. The major trauma outcome study: establishing national norms for trauma care. J Trauma 1990;30:1356–65.
29. Celso B, Tepas J, Langland-Orban B, et al. A systematic review and meta-analysis comparing outcomes of severely injured patients treated in trauma centers following the establishment of trauma systems. J Trauma 2006;60(2):371–8.
30. Papa L, Langland-Orban B, Kallenborn C, et al. Assessing effectiveness of a mature trauma system: association of trauma center presence with lower injury mortality rate. J Trauma 2006;61(2):261–7.
31. Moore L, Hanley JA, Turgeon AF, et al. Evaluation of the long-term trend in mortality from injury in a mature inclusive trauma system. World J Surg 2010; 34:2069–75.
32. Twijnstra MJ, Moons KG, Simmermacher KJ, et al. Regional trauma system reduces mortality and changes admission rates: a before and after study. Ann Surg 2010;251(2):339–43.
33. Dutton RP, Stansbury LG, Leone S, et al. Trauma mortality in mature trauma systems: are we doing better? An analysis of trauma mortality patterns 1997-2008. J Trauma 2010;69(3):620–6.

34. Vernberg DK, Rotondo MF. Sustaining an inclusive trauma system in a rural state: the role regional trauma care systems, partnerships, quality of care. J Trauma Nurs 2010;17(3):142–7.

35. Utter GH, Maier RV, Rivara FP, et al. Inclusive trauma systems: do they improve outcomes of the severely injured? J Trauma 2006;60(3):529–35.

36. Sasser SM, Hunt RC, Sullivan EE, et al. Guidelines for field triage of injured patients: recommendations of the national expert panel on field triage. MMWR Recomm Rep 2009;58(No RR-1):1–35.

37. Haas B, Gomez D, Zargosi B, et al. Survival of the fittest: hidden cost of undertriage of major trauma. J Am Coll Surg 2010;211(6):804–11.

38. Faul M, Wald MM, Sullivent EE, et al. Large cost savings realized from the 2006 field triage guidelines: reduction in overtriage to US trauma centers. Prehosp Emerg Care 2012;16(2):222–9.

39. Tiesman H, Young T, Torner JC, et al. Effects of a rural trauma system on traumatic brain injuries. J Neurotrauma 2007;24(7):1189–97.

40. Newgard CD, Nelson MJ, Kampp M, et al. Out-of-hospital decision making and factors influencing the regional distribution of injured patients in a trauma system. J Trauma 2011;70(6):1345–53.

41. Cox S, Smith K, Currell A, et al. Differentiation of confirmed major trauma patients and potential major trauma patients using pre-hospital trauma triage criteria. Injury 2011;42(9):889–95.

42. Holbrook TL, Hoyt DB, Coimbra R, et al. Long-term posttraumatic stress disorder persists after major trauma in adolescents: new data on risk factors and functional outcome. J Trauma 2005;58(4):764–71.

43. Van Beeck EF, Larsen CF, Lyons RA, et al. Guidelines for the conduction of follow-up studies measuring injury related disability. J Trauma 2007;62(2):534–50.

44. Mackenzie EJ, Rivara FP, Nathens A, et al. Impact of trauma center care on functional outcomes following major lower-limb trauma. J Bone Joint Surg Am 2008; 90:101–9.

45. Diggs BS, Mullins RJ, Hedges JR, et al. Proportion of seriously injured patients admitted to hospitals in the US with a high injured patient volume: a metric of regionalized trauma care. J Am Coll Surg 2008;206(2):212–9.

46. Sofer, SCNA edition/journal, Concurrent article.

47. Cisela DJ, Sava JA, Street JH III, et al. Secondary overtriage: a consequence of an immature trauma system. J Am Coll Surg 2008;206(1):131–7.

48. Gupta R, Greer SE, Martin ED. Inefficiencies in a rural trauma system: the burden of repeat imaging in interfacility transfers. J Trauma 2010;69(2):253–5.

49. Rogers FB, Osler T, Lee JC, et al. In a mature trauma system, there is no difference in outcome (survival) between level I and level II trauma centers. J Trauma 2011;70(6):1354–7.

50. Barringer ML, Thomason MH, Kilgo P, et al. Improving outcomes in a regional trauma system: impact of a level III trauma center. Am J Surg 2006;192:686–9.

51. Hemmilla MR, Nathens AB, Shafi S, et al. The trauma quality improvement program: pilot study and initial demonstration of feasibility. J Trauma 2010; 68(2):253–62.

52. Shafi S, Friese R, Gentilello LM. Moving beyond personnel and process: a case for incorporating outcome measures in the trauma center designation process. Arch Surg 2008;143(2):115–9.

53. Cryer HG, Hiatt JR, Eckstein M, et al. Improved trauma system multicasualty incident response: comparison of two train crash disasters. J Trauma 2010;68(4): 783–9.

Trauma System Configurations in Other Countries: The Israeli Model

Dror Soffer, MD[a],*, Joseph M. Klausner, MD[b]

KEYWORDS

- Mass casualty • Trauma • Israel • System • Emergency medical services • Terror

KEY POINTS

- Israel is a small country with a unique trauma system that was developed from the experience gained in peace and in war.
- The state is a full democracy and health care is mandated to all Israeli citizens, without exception.
- The prehospital level is maintained mainly by the emergency medical services, Magen David Adom (MDA, meaning Red Shield of David).
- There are 6 level I trauma centers and 14 level II trauma units in Israel.
- Facing multiple mass casualty incidences, a unique protocol was developed that ensures a fast and effective response to such devastating events.

THE ISRAELI TRAUMA SYSTEM

Israel has a population of around 7 million people. It consists of 20,720 km^2, 423 km from north to south, and between 14.5 and 114 km from east to west. Compared with the United States, with a population of circa 310,000,000, and with an area of some 9,631,365 km^2, Israel is a small country. Only 15.45% of the land is arable, and the rest is made up of urban areas, mountains, and desert. Israel is a full democracy and health care is mandated to all Israeli citizens, without exception. Israel has a Mediterranean climate with long, hot, rainless summers and short, cool winters with some rainfall. The geography is varied, with desert in the southern part and fertile valleys in the north. The coastal plain is flat, and the central part of the country is hilly and crossed by several valleys. The northern part of the central highlands has some mountainous

The authors have no financial disclosures or conflict of interest to disclose.
[a] Division of Surgery, The Yitzhak Rabin Trauma Center, Tel Aviv Medical Center, Sackler Faculty of Medicine, Tel Aviv University, 6 Weizman Street, Tel Aviv 64239, Israel; [b] Division of Surgery, Tel Aviv Medical Center, Sackler Faculty of Medicine, Tel Aviv University, 6 Weizman Street, Tel Aviv 64239, Israel
* Corresponding author.
E-mail address: sofferdror@hotmail.com

terrain (1219 m). The size of the country means that most areas are not remote from one another, although mountainous areas in the north and several gorges are inaccessible to regular vehicles. Most of the population lives in and around the large cities of the nation's capital, Jerusalem, Tel Aviv, Haifa, and Beersheba. There are many other diverse habitats, ranging from the kibbutz to nomadic Bedouin communities.

The development of trauma systems in Israel was initiated by the Ministry of Health in the mid-1990s, according to the recommendations of a designated national committee formed in the early 1990s to improve trauma care.[1] The prehospital level is maintained by 2 organizations: one is the emergency medical services (EMS), Magen David Adom (MDA, Red Shield of David), and the other is the military medical evacuation units. Military evacuation units are used mainly for military operations and are not related to civilian units. Six medical centers are designated as level I trauma centers, and 14 other hospitals are level II trauma centers. A trauma center's level is accredited by a governmental committee assigned by the Ministry of Health, according to designated protocols. Prehospital Trauma Life Support (PHTLS) and the American College of Surgeons Advance Trauma Life Support (ATLS) courses are provided to all paramedics and surgery residents nationwide. The Israeli trauma system is further supported by The Israel National Registry, established in 1995. The trauma registry provides the tools for monitoring and quality assurance, at both the hospital and national levels.[2,3] A national trauma council advises the Ministry of Health on issues related to trauma, such as advances, new technologies, and experience gained by other trauma centers.

According to the National Registry, there are around 36,500 trauma hospitalizations per year nationwide. The trauma rate is 4.7 per 1000 population, and the lifetime risk of injury hospitalization is 1:3. Data collected from the year 2009 showed that 65% of all trauma victims are male. Children in the age range of 0 to 14 years make up the largest group of injured patients (27%), and injuries sustained by motor vehicle accidents (MVAs) comprise 40% of the severe injuries (Injury Severity Score [ISS] ≥15). The main mechanisms of trauma for the year 2009 are detailed in **Fig. 1**. A total of 9.3% of injuries had an ISS greater than 16. The yearly intensive care unit (ICU) trauma-related admission rate for that year was 6.3%, the average ICU stay was 6.7 days, and the average hospital stay was 6.4 days. The mortality among all hospitalized patients with trauma is 1.2% to 2%.[4]

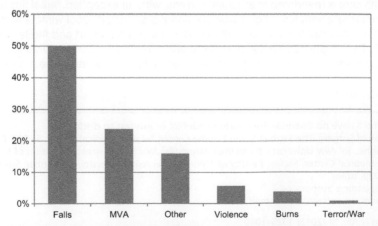

Fig. 1. Mechanisms of injury recorded in the Israeli National Registry trauma database for 2009.

BEFORE HOSPITAL: MDA

MDA was first established in 1930 as a voluntary organization with a single branch in Tel Aviv. After opening branches in Jerusalem and Haifa, it was extended nationwide 5 years later, providing medical support to the public.[5] Its purpose was later defined by law by the Israeli parliament (The Knesset) in 1950, and it consisted of 11 local geographically distinct branches that operated independently. These local centers were eventually united under 1 national EMS management in the early 1980s. MDA funding comes from a variety of sources, the primary source being donations from abroad. Further funding comes from the local municipalities in which MDA operates, and smaller amounts are provided by the national government. Individuals are also expected to pay for ambulance use, for which they can claim reimbursement from their health management organization (HMO).

As the single civilian EMS provider in Israel, MDA is also responsible to national society operations equivalent to the Red Cross in other regions of the world because it is also designated to support the Israeli Defense Forces (IDF) in time of war, as well as any other large-scale national emergency operations. Additional responsibilities are blood collection, blood banking, and blood delivery to hospitals. Centralized management of blood supply on a national level has the advantage of providing blood and blood products in times of mass casualty events and war. EMS in Israel are separate from the fire department and the police, and access to the 11 area dispatch centers is by dialing a free telephone number (101). Approximately 600 ambulances are stationed across the country, and they can be dispatched to any site within minutes. About one-tenth of all ambulances are mobile ICUs.

The MDA medical personnel include emergency medical technicians (EMTs), paramedics, physicians, and volunteers. There are about 600 EMTs who are trained in basic life support skills and can operate automated external defibrillators. Some senior EMTs are trained in manual defibrillation, the preparation of drugs, and in assisting in tracheal intubation.

There are around 450 paramedics employed by MDA. They undergo an 18-month training program during which they take advanced life support (ALS), PHTLS, and pediatric advanced life support (PALS) courses. Some paramedics take academic paramedic courses with university-style programs of 3 to 4 years that provide a degree on completion.

Most of the MDA physicians are hospital-based specialists in emergency medicine and are employed on a part-time basis. In addition to the MDs who staff the mobile ICUs, MDA has a general medical director and a medical director for the paramedic program. The former is in charge of the medical aspects of treatment, including medical protocols, and the latter is in charge of all the training and supervision of MDA paramedics. There are more than 10,000 registered MDA volunteers. They take part in the day-to-day ambulance service, and are also important in multicasualty scenarios. MDA relies heavily on volunteers and provides them with a high level of training, consisting of an 88-hour basic course of study in a generic framework for first aid. As part of its volunteer programs, MDA has a series of on-call first responders who are equipped with medical and communication equipment and operate from home.[6] This pool of volunteers includes doctors as well as off-duty MDA staff,[6] and they can provide emergency care for events that occur close to their residences. When they arrive to the trauma site, they contact the control center and provide essential feedback on the patients' conditions and the required resources. The dispatcher can then decide whether to dispatch a regular or an advanced response unit. The regular unit includes an ordinary ambulance operated by 2 EMTs or by an EMT and a volunteer. These ambulances are equipped to provide basic treatment and life support and transport the injured to the nearest hospital. There are 3 types of advance units (**Table 1**):

- Mobile ICU[7]
- Intensive care ambulance
- Multicasualty response vehicle.[8]

Trauma is responsible for 10% to 15% of MDA's activity. The average response time is 8 minutes. Crews are trained to adopt the save-and-run approach in the trauma setting, and this has led to median times on the scene of only 11 minutes. Save and run was implemented in Israel to contend with mass casualty incidents (MCIs). The protocol is a combination of the scoop-and-run and the stay-and-play doctrines. In the save-and-run protocol, only immediate life-saving interventions are undertaken at the scene, such as oropharyngeal intubation, needle application, and external bleeding control.[9–14]

According to the severity and the type of injury, the on-site MDA team decides to which hospital the patient should be transported. Because the distances between major hospitals are small, trauma victims are usually transported to the nearest level I or II trauma center. In certain situations, the EMS teams might decide to bypass a level II trauma center, even though it may be closer to the trauma site, and transport the patient to the more remote level I trauma center: this could apply, for example, to a patient with an evident severe head injury. MDA teams alert the designated emergency department (ED) when a patient requires immediate attention, and that patient goes directly into the resuscitation bay. Otherwise, the ambulance teams are met at the door of the ED, usually by a senior nurse, and directed to the most appropriate location.

IN HOSPITAL: TRAUMA UNITS

There are 6 level I trauma centers and 14 level II trauma centers in Israel.[15] Level II trauma centers in Israel differ from those in the United States in that, although they all have residency affiliations, they are unable to provide advanced treatment in some medical fields such as neurosurgery or more advanced invasive radiology. All hospital EDs are equipped with appropriate resources for management of complex trauma, and all trauma units are affiliated to the surgical divisions of the respective hospitals. Most heads of trauma units are trauma surgeons who completed their fellowships in trauma and surgical intensive care in one of the university trauma centers in the United States. The rest of the trauma teams are made of general

Table 1		
MDA types of advance units		
Name of Vehicle/Unit	**Operated By**	**Function**
Mobile ICU	Physician, a paramedic, and an EMT/driver	Providing more advanced life support and is usually dispatched when trauma cases are judged by on-site personnel as being severe
Intensive Care Ambulance	One paramedic and 1 EMT	Equipped to respond to conditions that require less advanced life support
Multicasualty Response Vehicle	Change according to the situation	A special stored equipment unit reserved for use during large-scale events that require prolonged operations, such as multiple-casualty incidents

attending surgeons and general surgery residents. Patients with trauma are admitted to surgical departments and treated by attending surgeons and residents supervised by the chief of the trauma unit. Most hospitals do not have a designated trauma ICU, and patients who need ICU care are admitted to either a general or a surgical ICU. In 3 of the level I trauma centers (Tel Aviv Medical Center, Hifa, and Tel Hashomer), there is a dedicated trauma team that cares for these patients. In the remaining centers, patients with trauma are spread across multiple general surgery teams who also care for other surgical conditions.

The Tel Aviv Medical Center is the only level I trauma center hospital in Israel's largest metropolitan area. Since 2001, its trauma unit has functioned according to a unique model, in which all patients with multitrauma are triaged to it. The unit is affiliated to the surgical division, and it is staffed by a multidisciplinary team from various departments of the hospital, including a trauma coordinator, psychologists, physiotherapists, and social workers. Three thousand casualties are admitted annually, of which 89% have blunt injuries and 11% have penetrating injuries. The large population in the hospital's catchment area has led to a considerable variety of urban traumas, mainly pedestrian and road accidents but also criminal and terrorist attacks, and others. During the last decade, there have also been multiple MCIs from terrorist attacks in the city of Tel Aviv and other cities within Israel, to which all of the level I trauma centers have responded at various times.

ISRAELI TRAUMA SYSTEM AND MCIS

MCIs have increased in frequency worldwide in the past few years, and explosions are the main mechanism of injury in those events.[16,17] Because the civilian population is more vulnerable to MCIs than military personnel who have protective gear, armored vehicles, intelligence, and local medical aid, the magnitude of potential and actual injury is formidable. Moreover, such explosions generate a large number of casualties who need urgent medical care. Frykberg and Tepas[18] reported that the mortality in such events reaches 12.6%, and that 30% of the injured are in need of emergent medical aid. Although many of the injured are walking wounded, their numbers contribute to a huge burden on any trauma center. Most of the current MCI protocols were issued by the military, and suit a combat zone. However, Israelis have gained considerable experience in dealing with MCIs over the years, and protocols have evolved over time, some of which are unique and contradict older international protocols.

Between 2000 and 2009, 3786 victims of terror attacks on Israeli civilians were hospitalized. Most victims were evacuated to the level I trauma centers in Jerusalem and Tel Aviv. There have been multiple MCIs nationwide during that period, and those in Tel Aviv are listed in **Table 2**.

Most of the injured were male (82%), and 60% were young (15–29 years of age). The mechanisms of injury were explosion (57%), gunshot wounds (33%), and others (10%). The rate of severely injured patients was 2.5-fold higher than in the normal trauma population (25% vs 10%).[4] The data that were retrospectively collected from the patients' records in the MCI database of the Tel Aviv Medical Center's trauma registry reveal that these victims consume more hospital resources, such as ICU and operating room resources, and have longer hospital stays compared with other patients with trauma. Moreover, many of the injuries occur in multiple body regions (44%), and the mortalities are 3-fold higher than in the general trauma population (5% vs 1.6%). The rates of injuries according to anatomic areas are listed in **Table 3**. The differences in characteristics between terror and trauma victims are described in **Table 4**.

Table 2
Major terrorist attacks in Tel Aviv and its vicinity

Date	Type of Venue	Number of Casualties
June 1, 2001	Suicide bombing inside a night club	191
January 25, 2002	Suicide bombing outside a cafe on a pedestrian mall in Tel Aviv	25
March 5, 2002	Terrorist opened fire on 2 adjacent restaurants	30
March 9, 2002	Guns fired and grenades thrown at cars and pedestrians in the coastal city of Netanya	50
March 20, 2002	Suicide bombing in a bus traveling from Tel Aviv to Nazareth	37
March 27, 2002	Suicide bombing at the Park Hotel in the coastal city of Netanya	140
March 30, 2002	Explosion in a cafe	30
May 8, 2002	Terrorist detonated a suitcase packed with explosives in a crowded gambling and billiards club	73
May 19, 2002	Suicide bombing at an open-air market	50
June 11, 2002	Suicide bomber set off a pipe bomb at a restaurant in the coastal city of Herzliya, north of Tel Aviv	16
July 17, 2002	A double suicide bombing near the old Central Bus Station in Tel Aviv	43
September 19, 2002	Bomb in a bus opposite the Great Synagogue	66
January 5, 2003	Double suicide bombing near the old Central Bus Station in Tel Aviv	144
March 30, 2003	Suicide bombing in the pedestrian mall entrance of a cafe	40
April 30, 2003	Suicide bombing at a beachfront pub in Tel Aviv	63
August 12, 2003	Suicide bombing in a shopping mall in a Tel Aviv suburb	26
December 25, 2003	An explosion near a bus stop at a suburb of Tel Aviv	25
July 11, 2004	Bomb exploded next to a Tel Aviv bus stop	33
November 1, 2004	Suicide bomb exploded in Tel Aviv's busy Carmel market	33
February 25, 2005	Suicide bombing outside a Tel Aviv nightclub	55
July 12, 2005	Suicide bombing outside a shopping mall	95
December 5, 2005	Suicide bombing at the entrance of a shopping mall	55
January 19, 2006	Suicide bombing near the old Central Bus Station in Tel Aviv	30
April 17, 2006	Suicide bombing near the old Central Bus Station in Tel Aviv	49

Table 3	
Injuries by body regions among terror casualties[a]	
Body Region	**%**
Extremities	61.7
Face and neck	30.8
Chest	22.1
Head	20.9
Abdomen	17.3
Pelvis	16.3
Spine	5.7

[a] Some patients had more than 1 injury.

PREHOSPITAL CARE OF CASUALTIES

An MCI was defined by the Israeli Ministry of Health Division for Emergency Services as an event that causes more than 10 casualties or more than 4 severely injured casualties. The activation of any MCI protocol mandates the mobilization of a large number of teams, especially in civilian scenarios. The number of ambulances per event ranges between 24 and 58, which represents 4% to 10% of all MDA ambulances.[11]

The Israeli philosophy is based on the concept that it is more prudent to have a low threshold for activating MCI protocol because surplus manpower that is applied quickly is better than too little manpower that is too late in arrival. It should be expected that the first phase will be chaotic and that it is unrealistic to anticipate order at that stage. The teams should be aware of this and learn to work in chaos, because any attempt to organize the work at the site during the first minutes will lead to unnecessary delays in implementing the EMS structure within the zone of the explosion. That initial phase is usually short-lived and lasts until more teams capable of dealing with large numbers of casualties have been recruited and arrive at the scene. Accumulated data indicate that around 116 medical personnel have been involved in past MCIs, of which 16% were paramedics and only a few were medical doctors. The first ambulances arrived at the scene between 1 and 14 minutes from the time of the explosion. The average time for evacuation of the first victim was 3.9 minutes (5–22 minutes), and the last victim was evacuated no longer than 44 minutes from the time of the explosion.[11]

Care of the injured is decided on by the individual teams, and each team works independently according to basic ATLS protocols. All victims undergo a rapid primary survey that includes opening of an airway (introducing an oropharynx airway when indicated) and external bleeding control (usually by applying tourniquets) (**Fig. 2**).

Table 4		
Differences in characteristics between terror and other trauma victims		
Characteristic	**Terror (%)**	**Other Trauma (%)**
ISS>16	24.8	10.3
ICU	23.6	6.9
OR	57.1	38.7
LOS>14	19.2	7.4

Abbreviations: LOS>14, length of stay longer than 14 days; OR, operating room.

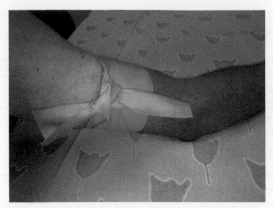

Fig. 2. The Israeli Defense Force tourniquet.

Other interventions are delayed until all the injured have been identified and transported to a safer location.

The medical teams do not usually go into the site until it is declared safe by the security forces. In several events, a second bomb had been concealed and preprogrammed to explode after the rescue team's arrival, causing further damage and injuries among the medical teams as well. Because waiting for clearance by the security forces might cause a major delay in evacuation and treatment, the EMS try to evacuate most of the victims as fast as possible without administering any treatment, apart from simple airway protection and external hemorrhage control.

The first team arriving at the scene does not provide any medical care. Its responsibility is to assess the situation and transmit essential information to the command center. Medical treatment starts only when other medical teams arrive. The first team's assessment should include the type of event (explosion, gunshot, other), the estimated number of injured (few, tens, hundreds), and the severity of the injuries, as well as the location of the event, best routes for arrival and evacuation, and time to the nearest hospital. The first team at the scene cordons off the routes to expedite the arrival of the other teams. When other teams arrive, they spread in the field and take care of injured close to them. The critically wounded who need resuscitation, such as ventilation or cardiac massage, are not treated until enough manpower is in place (discussed later). Colored tags (red, yellow, green) are affixed to the victims according to their estimated urgency to facilitate their evacuation (**Fig. 3**). Only after

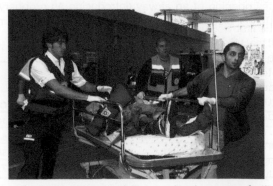

Fig. 3. Multiple-injured trauma patient arriving at a level I trauma facility in Israel.

a local command center has been established are MDA teams divided and they are not assigned to different treatment areas until all the injured have been identified. The establishment of such a front command center is crucial.

The highest-ranking medical authority who arrives first in the field is the Event Commander, and he/she will be replaced by a higher ranking person later on. All EMS personnel are identifiable by special bulletproof vests and headgear, and the Event Commander is easily identified by a yellow cap. These items used for identification should be present in all ambulances.

Triage is one of the cornerstones of prehospital MCI management, and, as such, it is applied to identify the most severely injured patients who require immediate transport to the nearest hospital. The teams should be aware that some victims cannot be saved under MCI conditions, even if they might have had a chance to survive under other circumstances. Therefore, heroic resuscitation efforts must be discouraged. However, overestimation of a patient's injury resulting in overtriage is accepted practice. Although this practice creates a greater burden on the receiving hospitals, it helps to avoid missed injuries.

According to the MDA registry, between 2000 and 2009, the average rate of severely injured (ISS>16) victims was 20%. Only 55% of those injuries were diagnosed as being severe in the hospital setting. Altogether, 10.2% of the injured did not survive to reach the hospital (pronounced dead on arrival), and 34.8% cases considered as being urgent in the field were given an ISS between 9 and 15 (intermediate) in the hospital.[11]

One of the most important aspects in managing an MCI is communication. MDA personnel usually carry designated pagers, beepers, and cell phones, and they can be activated to provide help at any time of the day and anywhere in the country. Much of the current communication is via cell phones. Regular communication networks tend to crash at the beginning of major events.[19] Therefore, steps were take to enable government intervention for shutting down all civilian cell phone communication around the area of an MCI and allow only certain prearranged emergency numbers to function. That intervention allows continuous communication between the teams in the field and the major command center. Communication in the field is kept to a minimum, and the Event Commander uses a battery-operated megaphone (carried by ambulance crews) to give directions. Some wireless communication devices are also used with good results by key personnel in the field and elsewhere. Event Commanders are responsible for the assessment of the number of casualties. They also track the number of crews on scene and the number who have departed for hospitals, and lead search and rescue teams in their areas. The Event Commander reports to the major MDA command center alone and does not deal with other issues such as deflecting the media, or security missions. An MDA liaison situated in each hospital is responsible for the communication between the major command center and the designated hospital. The first victims to be evacuated to the nearest trauma center are the severely injured. If that trauma center is too far away (this has hardly happened in Israel), those patients are transported to the nearest hospital and, after being stabilized, transferred to a major trauma center. Most of the minor injuries are referred to more distant hospitals. The order of evacuation sometimes does not follow the guidelines described earlier because 20% to 30% of the mildly injured evacuate themselves or are assisted by willing bystanders who are welcome to participate in the evacuation process by the teams in the field. An ambulance that is evacuating a severely injured patient may also carry 1 or 2 walking wounded to facilitate evacuation. The Israeli EMS appreciate the value of recruiting willing bystanders and of allowing them to assist in carrying stretchers, in applying local compression for hemostasis, and even in ventilating victims with a bag-valve mask.

IN-HOSPITAL CARE OF CASUALTIES

Reports about an MCI reach the hospital in several ways. All key personnel of the hospital carry dedicated pagers that are connected to the EMS's activating system, which keeps them updated about the developing situation as relayed by the field commanders. It is common for first reports to come from the media, hospital staff, or the unexpected arrival of first victims who self-evacuated from the scene. After the occurrence of an MCI has been verified with the respective authorities (in Israel, they are the police and the MDA dispatch centers), the highest administrative authority of the hospital (the CEO or deputy CEO) is informed. It is their responsibility to declare an MCI, because the activation of MCI protocol is highly resource consuming and requires the shifting of priorities in daily routines on all levels of operation and in all departments. There is a low threshold for the implementation of an MCI protocol in Israel. It is divided into 3 tiers at the Tel Aviv Medical Center: up to 10 casualties, 11 to 50 casualties, and more than 50 casualties. These triaged responses are defined with small numeric differences at each individual hospital. Notification and recruitment of key personnel are via cell phones, beepers, and phone calls that are automatically activated from a central computer. In-hospital personnel are additionally instructed by loudspeakers throughout the buildings.

EDs During MCIs

Most EDs in major downtown hospitals are busy at all times. To cope with a sudden and large influx of MCI victims, all nonurgent patients without trauma must be discharged from the ED and all urgent surgical and medical patients in the ED must be moved to wards without any further work-up. Those patients are taken care of by the physicians and nurses who are left on the wards (usually internal medicine).[20] This process takes only a few minutes and clears the ED within a short period of time. We implement the principle of unidirectional patient flow to ensure that the ED can be set up for the admission of more patients and then for the return to its regular schedule. None of the patients who had been transferred from the ED will return to it. In addition, all attending surgeons and surgical residents who are present in the hospital report to the ED where the senior administrator on call assigns and directs them to one of the sectioned-off areas in the ED. We try to assign at least 1 nurse and physician to each of the most seriously injured patients. The less seriously injured patients are attended to when more help arrives.

The triage officers are the first medical professionals to process the MCI victims in the hospital setting, and their first objectives are to sort patients according to the severity of their injuries. This step is crucial for the proper management of the event. Undertriage at this stage results in failure to identify severely injured patients, whereas overtriage unnecessarily crowds the zone restricted to the severely injured. This responsibility was originally reserved for the most senior ED surgeon at the ED, but experience proved that a less qualified surgeon can handle it just as well. As a result, a surgical chief resident or a young surgical or emergency medicine attending is assigned to triage at the ED's funnel-shaped entrance.

This triage officer directs the flow of victims into 1 of 3 areas. Critically injured victims are assigned to the trauma bay, which is staffed by the most senior surgeons and physicians and headed by the most senior trauma surgeon. Moderately injured victims are assigned to another area to be treated by a smaller number of physicians per patient number and those with less surgical experience. Because the first triage process might miss some severely injured patients, this area is commanded by at least 1 experienced surgical attending. All victims with minor injuries are assigned to the third, more remote area, usually to be taken care of by nonsurgical residents and attendings.

All registration formalities are postponed when there is a large influx of patients. Each patient is tagged by a serial number in the triage station, together with a designated brief record that is put on the bed to be filled in by the medical team on the victim's arrival at the ED. Proper registration (name, identification number, address, and so forth) is postponed until the patient arrives at the ward. Patients who cannot be indentified (unconscious, mutilated, ventilated) are photographed by the hospital photographer and the digital pictures are later shown to families in the information center for identification. Successful MCI management depends on a few key personnel: the medical director(MD), the administrative director(AD), the head nurse(HN),[21] and the emergency medical services coordinator (EMSC).[22] The MD is usually a highly experienced trauma surgeon or a general surgeon equally experienced in trauma. The MD receives all the pertinent information from the triage officer and from the EMSC, such as the location and magnitude of the MCI and the estimated number of victims. The first responsibility of the MD is to establish trauma teams comprising 1 or 2 surgeons and 2 nurses who are assigned to each severely injured patient. The most experienced surgeon in each of these teams is its chief and the only team member who reports directly to the MD. Trauma team members usually do not mix with other teams in the setting of an MCI, where discipline and focus are of the essence to ensure optimal efficacy of operation. Each team is also responsible for its patient until he/she is admitted to the designated ward or operating theater, and beyond if need be. In addition, the MD sends smaller teams to the intermediate injured area and assigns a senior surgeon to supervise that area. The MD guides the teams in implementing the appropriate surgical interventions for stabilizing a given patient and establishes the priorities for further operating room interventions, imaging modalities, and admissions. For example, no patients are transferred to radiology or the computed tomography (CT) scanner without their approval, to avoid overwhelming these facilities with non–critically injured patients and possibly losing track of patients. Laboratory testing is restricted to blood typing. The physician in charge keeps track of all patients who are transferred to the operating room or who are sent to the wards.

The AD alleviates the burden of administrative issues from the MD. We recommend the appointment of the directors of EDs to this position to ensure their vital cooperation. The AD is in charge of all logistics, especially patient transfer, blood bank issues, and coordination of anesthesia experts to different locations and assignments. The AD also handles all communications with the hospital administration. The HN assists the MD by handling all nursing issues. The HN is responsible for directing the large number of recruited nurses from the wards until more ED nurses arrive. The HN is also responsible for collecting patient status and disposition data, and, if special equipment or resources are needed in the ED, the HN arranges for their provision through the central command office. The EMSC updates the triage officer on the expected casualty load, the extent of injuries, the location of the MCI, and the type of explosion. When it becomes apparent that the hospital is overwhelmed with patients and that the system cannot accommodate any more, the transport of new patients is directed to other facilities whenever possible. In such devastating scenarios, the treating hospital might become a triage hospital, and the evacuation of patients to other medical facilities is also accomplished under the direction of the EMSC.

Ancillary Evaluation During MCIs

The special nature and the multitude of injuries encountered during an MCI (eg, the large number of casualties with blast and shrapnel injuries) mandate the use of imaging techniques, but they cannot be made available to all patients at the same time. According to our data, 42% of victims needed some kind of imaging (CT, ultrasound [US], angiography, Doppler US). In addition, 66% of all victims with severe injuries (ISS>16) had advanced imaging, which accounted for 40% of all scans. Because not all imaging techniques are available for all patients, their use needs to be strictly controlled by the decisions of the MD. During MCIs, the need for CT scanning is typically determined according to the routine trauma protocols used in our facility, although, in an MCI, the MD must also consider the number of patients and the availability of the CT scanner.

Rapid evaluation of the victims' conditions as well as rapid hospital resource use is critical to the successful management of an MCI. Because most of the sophisticated diagnostic modalities are not available to all patients in the first minutes/hours of their evaluation during an MCI, a rapidly performed, noninvasive, inexpensive, portable, and easily repeated ultrasound examination for the diagnosis of an abdominal injury is the most logical solution.[23] The incorporation of ultrasonography in the first stages of patient evaluation in an MCI has already been described by us and by others.[24] Considerable experience has been gained in the advantages of the use of sonography for the evaluation of blunt abdominal injury, and its disadvantages in the evaluation of penetrating injuries to the abdomen and torso. A special US team is put into place during an MCI, and it maintains the availability of sonography to all the patients who might need it and restricts unnecessary transport of physicians and patients through the treating area. This team is composed of a radiology resident and an US technician who use a portable US machine and provide the results to the treating on-site physicians/surgeons. Those results are also recorded in the patient's chart by the radiologist.[22]

Previous studies have found that US examination for blunt trauma has a sensitivity of 81% to 88% and a specificity of 97% to 100%,[25] decreasing to 47% to 49% and 82% to 98%, respectively, for penetrating injuries.[21] Because many of the injuries inflicted in terrorist attacks are a combination of both types, it is reasonable to assume that the results are somewhere between the two. Our results showed an overall accuracy of 77%, a sensitivity of 40%, and a specificity of 88%. The positive predictive value (PPV) was 50%, and the negative predictive value (NPV) was 83%. Insofar as a good screening test is characterized by a high sensitivity and specificity, the low sensitivity of US examinations in MCIs indicates that it is not appropriate in that setting. However, its high specificity (88%) might be of value to the MD in helping to determine treatment and diagnostic priorities for other victims.

CT is currently the most important modality for depicting foreign objects and the injury inflicted by them in stable patients. According to Raja and colleagues,[26] close to 90% of injured victims of an MCI in a military setting are scanned. If CT were to be used to identify shrapnel penetrations and trajectories in all patents, the waiting time would be too long to be practical. Therefore, it is essential that patients be prioritized by the MD, who will triage them for CT scans. According to our data, more than 66% of all MCI victims underwent a CT scan, and 40% of them were performed on severely injured patients (ISS>16). With the shifting of CT from selective body area scanning toward a wider field, there has been a similar tendency in the MCI setting: 20% of all CT scans were total body scans (trauma protocol) in 2001, increasing to 80% in 2005.

A rapid evaluation is mandatory for some unstable patients as well as for those who require urgent surgical intervention. If sophisticated imaging modalities are unavailable, we advocate diagnostic peritoneal aspiration (DPA) and diagnostic peritoneal lavage (DPL) to evaluate the abdomen. Our results using this approach indicate that DPL had a sensitivity of 100%, a specificity of 33%, a PPV of 66%, and an NPV of 100%. Our records also show that 10% of the victims who were admitted to hospital underwent a DPL, which was found to be positive in 42%, and 38% of the DPLs were positive in patients who had negative US findings. Most of the injuries to the abdomen were penetrating wounds (this has also been reported by others).

Blood Bank in MCIs

The safe and timely provision of blood products is of crucial importance in the prevention and mitigation of morbidity and mortality resulting from traumatic injuries. The blood bank has a standard operating procedure (SOP) that it follows whenever an MCI is announced. The SOP relates to recruitment and positioning of personnel, reporting on existing supplies and ordering of additional stocks, shifting of work priorities during the event, handling victim samples (and listing them in a designated folder in the computer system), and issuing blood products. **Fig. 4** depicts the flow of events at the blood bank, starting immediately after notification of the occurrence of an MCI. There has not been a shortage of blood in our experience, and the SOP at the Tel Aviv Medical Center enables blood supply in a safe and timely fashion. Following an established SOP allows a smooth flow of work at different sites, including the blood bank, the ED, and the operating rooms. At this point, we use component therapy only, because fresh whole blood is not available in our setup.

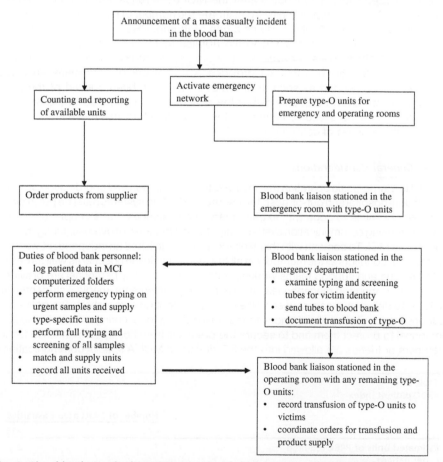

Fig. 4. Blood bank standard operating protocol during a mass casualty incident.

Three processes are triggered simultaneously in the blood bank on the notification of an MCI:

- Counting the available packed red blood cells (PRBCs) and ordering additional units if required
- Notifying the blood bank director and the designated liaison(s) who organize and summon blood bank personnel
- Preparing type-O blood units for transport to the trauma triage room in the ED.

The responsibility of the liaison in the ED is to supervise the collection of the victims' blood samples for typing and screening and transfer to the blood bank, to supply and record each unit of type-O blood transfused to victims.

Our past data indicate that victims admitted to the ED have been resuscitated and transferred to the operating room by approximately 1 hour after the occurrence of an MCI. The liaison from the ED or designated deputy then takes any remaining type-O units to the operating rooms to be dispersed as necessary. At this point, the main activity of the liaison shifts from mostly supervising sample collection to coordinating the requirements of the surgeons and anesthesiologists and the supplies in the blood bank, including the delivery of the blood supplies, where needed. These activities are usually finalized within 1 to 2 hours after the MCI occurrence, and that includes the transfer of PRBCs and type-O units. To estimate the number of blood units for transfer, we devised a simple formula to use as a rule of thumb: PRBC units/patient index, in which 1 PRBC unit per evacuated victim applies to MCIs involving fewer than 25 victims and 2 PRBC units per evacuated victim applies to MCIs involving more than 25 victims (**Table 5**). This formula provides a framework of how many units are expected to be needed as soon as the blood bank has been notified of the MCI. Although it was shown that only half of the evacuated are admitted to the hospital, we prefer to use the evacuated numbers for calculation because these are available earlier in the process of dealing with an MCI.[27]

Other General Considerations

An MCI is a large-scale operation that involves the cooperation and coordination of many essential in-hospital and out-of-hospital resources. Backup systems must be put in place whenever possible to cope with extraordinary circumstances. For example, otherwise smooth-running communication systems might crash because of overuse during the first hours of an MCI. To contend with this likelihood, we established an independent wireless system that connects all the members of all the teams within the hospital as well as designated rescue and support teams working outside its walls. Key personnel are provided with battery-operated megaphones, and runners (eg, volunteers, medical students) are enlisted to deliver messages when voice contact cannot be established. The police are responsible for sealing all entrances to the hospital and for securing access to medical personnel to protect them and to secure the premises from hostile elements. No family members or friends are allowed into the ED during an MCI. A special communications

Table 5 PRBC/patient index		
	Number of Evacuated Casualties	
	<25	≥25
Estimated units of PRBC required per patient	1	2

center staffed by social workers, clergy, and administrators is set up for the victims' families and friends, and a designated staff member functions as a liaison to help relay information to them about the injured. A separate room is assigned for the media, where a hospital public relations representative provides updates and answers questions. Although cameramen are allowed to take pictures outside the ED entrance, at no time are the media allowed in the ED. Access for reporters for the purpose of interviewing consenting victims is permitted only after the MCI is officially declared to be over. Formal debriefing of all key personnel who were involved in the management of the MCI is a crucial aspect,[28] and this takes place as early as possible after the event. This mandatory debriefing is performed according to a standardized tool developed by a consensus group and the Ministry of Health in all hospitals. A designated tertiary survey team composed of an attending surgeon, anesthesiologist, orthopedic surgeon, surgical nurse, trauma coordinator, and social worker reexamines all the admitted patients to confirm that there are no missed injuries and to ensure that the appropriate primary treatment plan has been initiated.

The Israeli model was developed and has proved to be efficient in many real MCIs. It can be easily adopted by any trauma center in any part of the world. The main difference between countries is the prehospital setup. This issue should be addressed by the local authorities, to better control the influx of patients to the different available hospitals and provide more rapid and efficient treatment at the scene.

SUMMARY

The Israeli trauma system uses a well-organized approach that systematically manages the spectrum of trauma care from routine falls and traffic accidents to multicasualty incidents. In the multicasualty incidents, the on-scene commander maintains communication with receiving facilities that also have site commanders from the physician, nursing, and administrative leadership areas. Within this system, years of experience have honed our skills in implementing a system for providing first-class emergency medical services in mass casualty events. Observation of clearly defined and highly regimented protocols helps the teams achieve optimal results by keeping calm in the midst of chaos.

REFERENCES

1. Marganitt B, Rivkind A, Mackenzie EJ. Statewide system approach to the organization of trauma care services–a way to improve the quality of care to the injured. Harefuah 1990;119(1–2):18–23.
2. Michaelson M, Tal-Or E. Trauma registry database. Harefuah 1997;133(12): 656–9.
3. Heruti RJ, Stein M, Barel V, et al. Trauma registry–the concept and its application in Israel. Harefuah 1997;133(3–4):155–9.
4. Peleg K, Mordehai BJ, Givon A, et al. A decade of trauma injuries in Israel 2000-2009. National Report 2011. Available at: http://www.gertnerinst.org.il/e/health_policy_e/trauma/313.htm. Accessed April 12, 2012.
5. Levy N, Michlin A. The beginnings of Magen David Adom. Harefuah 1991;120(3): 157–61.
6. Ellis DY, Sorene E. Magen David Adom–the EMS in Israel. Resuscitation 2008; 76(1):5–10.
7. Peleg K, Pliskin JS. A geographic information system simulation model of EMS: reducing ambulance response time. Am J Emerg Med 2004;22(3):164–70.
8. Avitzour M, Libergal M, Assaf J, et al. A multicasualty event: out-of-hospital and in-hospital organizational aspects. Acad Emerg Med 2004;11(10):1102–4.

9. Cooke MW. How much to do at the accident scene? BMJ 1999;319(7218):1150.

10. Cayten CG, Murphy JG, Stahl WM. Basic life support versus advanced life support for injured patients with an injury severity score of 10 or more. J Trauma 1993;35(3): 460–6.

11. Feigenberg Z. The pre-hospital medical treatment of the victims of multi-casualty incidents caused by explosions of suicide bombers during the Al-Aksa Intifada–April 2001 to December 2004: the activity and experience gained by the teams of Magen David Adom in Israel. Harefuah 2010;149(7):413–7.

12. Pepe PE, Stewart RD. Role of the physician in the prehospital setting. Ann Emerg Med 1986;15(12):1480–3.

13. McCallum AL, Rubes CR. Prehospital interventions. Emerg Med Clin North Am 1996;14(1):1–12.

14. Schuttler J, Schmitz B, Bartsch AC, et al. The efficiency of emergency therapy in patients with head-brain, multiple injury. Quality assurance in emergency medicine. Anaesthesist 1995;44(12):850–8.

15. Peleg K, Aharonson-Daniel L, Stein M, et al. Increased survival among severe trauma patients: the impact of a national trauma system. Arch Surg 2004;139(11): 1231–6.

16. Karmy-Jones R, Kissinger D, Golocovsky M, et al. Bomb-related injuries. Mil Med 1994;159(7):536–9.

17. Stein M, Hirshberg A. Medical consequences of terrorism. The conventional weapon threat. Surg Clin North Am 1999;79(6):1537–52.

18. Frykberg ER, Tepas JJ 3rd. Terrorist bombings. Lessons learned from Belfast to Beirut. Ann Surg 1988;208(5):569–76.

19. Raiter Y, Farfel A, Lehavi O, et al. Mass casualty incident management, triage, injury distribution of casualties and rate of arrival of casualties at the hospitals: lessons from a suicide bomber attack in downtown Tel Aviv. Emerg Med J 2008;25(4): 225–9.

20. Einav S, Aharonson-Daniel L, Weissman C, et al. In-hospital resource utilization during multiple casualty incidents. Ann Surg 2006;243(4):533–40.

21. Soffer D, McKenney MG, Cohn S, et al. A prospective evaluation of ultrasonography for the diagnosis of penetrating torso injury. J Trauma 2004;56(5):953–7 [discussion: 957–9].

22. Kluger Y, Mayo A, Soffer D, et al. Functions and principles in the management of bombing mass casualty incidents: lessons learned at the Tel-Aviv Souraski Medical Center. Eur J Emerg Med 2004;11(6):329–34.

23. Sosna J, Sella T, Shaham D, et al. Facing the new threats of terrorism: radiologists' perspectives based on experience in Israel. Radiology 2005;237(1):28–36.

24. Kluger Y, Kashuk J, Mayo A. Terror bombing-mechanisms, consequences and implications. Scand J Surg 2004;93(1):11–4.

25. Rozycki GS, Ochsner MG, Schmidt JA, et al. A prospective study of surgeon-performed ultrasound as the primary adjuvant modality for injured patient assessment. J Trauma 1995;39(3):492–8 [discussion: 498–500].

26. Raja AS, Propper BW, Vandenberg SL, et al. Imaging utilization during explosive multiple casualty incidents. J Trauma 2010;68(6):1421–4.

27. Soffer D, Klausner J, Bar-Zohar D, et al. Usage of blood products in multiple-casualty incidents: the experience of a level I trauma center in Israel. Arch Surg 2008;143(10):983–9 [discussion: 989].

28. Shapira SC, Shemer J. Medical management of terrorist attacks. Isr Med Assoc J 2002;4(7):489–92.

Research and Analytics in Combat Trauma Care
Converting Data and Experience to Practical Guidelines

Jeremy G. Perkins, MD[a],*, Laura R. Brosch, RN, PhD[b],
Alec C. Beekley, MD[c], Kelly L. Warfield, PhD[d],
Charles E. Wade, PhD[e], John B. Holcomb, MD[e]

KEYWORDS

• Iraq • Afghanistan • Military trauma registry • Research • Clinical practice guidelines
• Human research protection program

KEY POINTS

- The wars in Iraq and Afghanistan have introduced new concepts and understanding, particularly in the field of trauma.
- Efforts to understand patterns of injury and care evolved from case reports/case series into systematic data collection by groups, and ultimately into the first ever formal combat trauma registry within a theater trauma system.
- Research in the deployed environment required appropriate oversight and development of a Human Research Protection Program, and for the first time since Vietnam, dedicated trauma research teams were deployed in theater charged with performing and facilitating research activities.
- Collection of combat casualty data through a trauma registry within a theater trauma system and trauma research provided a framework to develop clinical practice guidelines, and track clinical outcomes after implementation.
- New concepts in medical care introduced during war are often integrated into civilian practice, but need to be validated through prospective research.

Conflict of interest statement: The authors have no conflicts of interest relevant to the subject matter of this article. Dr Wade and Dr Holcomb have received grant support from the US Army and NIH for the conduct of research related to trauma.

The opinions or assertions contained herein are the private views of the authors and are not to be construed as official or as reflecting the views of the Department of the Army or the Department of Defense.

[a] Hematology-Oncology Service, Walter Reed National Military Medical Center, 8901 Wisconsin Avenue, Bethesda, MD 20889, USA; [b] Office of Research Protections, Headquarters, United States Army Medical Research and Materiel Command, 504 Scott Street, Fort Detrick, MD 21702-5012, USA; [c] Department of Surgery, Thomas Jefferson University, 1100 Walnut Street, Philadelphia, PA 19107, USA; [d] Integrated Biotherapeutics, Inc, Department of Vaccine Development, 21 Firstfield Road # 100, Gaithersburg, MD 20878, USA; [e] Center for Translational Injury Research, Department of Surgery, University of Texas Health Science Center, 6410 Fannin Street UPB 1100, Houston, TX 77030, USA
* Corresponding author.
E-mail address: jeremy.perkins1@us.army.mil

Surg Clin N Am 92 (2012) 1041–1054
doi:10.1016/j.suc.2012.04.004
0039-6109/12/$ – see front matter Published by Elsevier Inc.

surgical.theclinics.com

INTRODUCTION

The field army has an opportunity for research that cannot be duplicated by any other organization ... No other institution has an opportunity or responsibility in the field of trauma comparable to that of the Army Medical Service.
—Battle Casualties in Korea, Studies of the Surgical Research Team, 1955, p. 16.

Throughout recorded history wars have resulted in medical advancements, especially in the field of trauma. Such advances have been born out of necessity, concentrated volumes of casualties, and heroic efforts to provide care despite austere conditions and limited resources.[1] The scope of war necessarily brings providers without specific war-trauma care experience into direct contact with large volumes of civilian and military casualties.[2] Fresh sets of eyes, unguided but also unclouded by dogma, observe and strive to understand and solve unfamiliar clinical challenges. This fresh perspective creates an ideal environment to challenge prior understanding, particularly when dogma does not match the on-the-ground reality. The quintessential example is Ambroise Pare, who was a lowly "barber surgeon" but rose to prominence because of his insights into wound care by challenging the dogma of pouring burning oil onto wounds, and his gift for disseminating results.[3] Providers during and after deployment to theaters of war reflect on their experiences, study the impact of their care of patients, publish observations, and often integrate new approaches into their practices. New concepts in medical care introduced during the war can then be studied and validated in the peacetime setting. Twentieth century examples of meticulous record keeping, reflection, analysis, publication, and validation are found in Debakey's landmark article on the treatment of vascular injuries from World War II and Rich's work from the Vietnam Vascular Registry.[4,5] The wars in Afghanistan (Operation Enduring Freedom, OEF) and Iraq (Operation Iraqi Freedom, OIF) have been no exception to identification, analysis, and problem solving of key combat-related clinical issues by providers serving in theaters. This article is intended to describe the evolution of data collection, research, and development of clinical practice guidelines for the wars in Iraq and Afghanistan, and also discusses how to leverage and improve civilian trauma research systems in the United States based on these experiences.

DEVELOPMENT OF THE JOINT THEATER TRAUMA REGISTRY

Deficiencies in combat casualty care had been identified over the course of the shorter, but no less violent conflicts occurring between Vietnam and OIF/OEF, including Somalia and the first Gulf War. During the first Gulf War, it was recognized that there was no system for rapid evacuation for critically injured casualties or system to support medical research.[6] Following the conflict in Somalia, Mabry and colleagues[7] noted the lack of a trauma registry to capture combat casualty data or a trauma system to track outcomes and disseminate lessons learned by providers. Early in OIF/OEF, Holcomb noted the need for better prehospital combat casualty care training, the need for intensive care unit and burn teams, and the need for a unified medical command structure.[8] Such observations and detailed reviews reflected an environment ripe for change over the course of OIF/OEF.

At the beginning of the OEF and OIF conflicts in 2001 and 2003, respectively, systems were in place to record basic data on combat casualties such as demographics, general categories of diagnosis, injury, and basic outcomes (ie, Killed in Action, Wounded in Action, Died of Wounds, and Returned to Duty).[9] While these data are valuable in aggregate for planning military operations, they are less useful for guiding improvements to the medical system of care. Such improvements require analysis of clinically relevant admission, treatment, and outcome data. Individual providers could track this information on patients treated at their particular medical facility, but there was no integrated trauma system or registry in place within the Department of Defense (DOD) to capture such data.

Early efforts to understand patterns of injury and care during these conflicts involved case reports and case series undertaken by individuals or small groups of providers.[10–24] One month after the Iraq invasion in 2003, the US Army Surgeon General sent his consultants for surgery, trauma, orthopedics, and anesthesia into Iraq on a fact-finding mission to "identify what was wrong and fix it." Many recommendations returned from this assignment, one of which was the creation and deployment of a DOD trauma system and trauma registry to parallel civilian approaches in the United States and other countries that had been developed following the medical lessons learned from Vietnam and the first Gulf War. Thus, OIF and OEF represented the first opportunity to implement these systems advances in a protracted, large-scale, armed conflict.[25]

Initial development of a theater trauma system began in May 2004 with the identification of a high-ranking, experienced military trauma surgeon to serve as Trauma System Director.[26] This individual was assigned at the theater's medical command headquarters to introduce the concept and importance of establishing a trauma system in the theater of operations. The Theater Trauma System missions included the following:

- Improve organization and delivery of trauma care
- Develop and implement clinical practice guidelines
- Ensure continuity through improved communication among clinicians in the evacuation chain
- Facilitate morbidity and mortality conferences to promote real-time, data-driven clinical process improvements
- Evaluate and recommend new equipment or medical supplies for use in theater to improve efficiency, reduce cost, and improve outcomes
- Populate a theater trauma registry to evaluate care provided across 3 continents connected with documented outcomes
- Facilitate conduct of formal research.

Independently and at the same time, providers at the busiest combat support hospital in Iraq, the 31st Combat Support Hospital (CSH) colocated in Balad and at the Ibn Sina Hospital in Baghdad, began to collect clinical data into a comprehensive database. The 31st CSH database had the typical limitations of provider-driven clinical databases, namely, there were transcription errors, inexact definitions of data points, and use of terminology with the potential for incorrect interpretation.[27] Regardless, this initiative represented the first OIF/OEF command-supported, organized effort to collect use management and performance improvement data on every combat casualty arriving to the hospital. This database provided an early glimpse of trauma system problems such as hypothermia in casualties arriving at the CSH.[28] Efforts to capture information from casualties managed at far-forward medical treatment facilities close to the point of injury were being developed by the US Navy in 2004 (the Navy and Marine Corps Combat Trauma Registry Expeditionary Medical Encounter Database),[29] and disease-specific databases such as the Balad Vascular Registry were subsequently developed.[30] However, the importance of the 31st CSH database was that it served as a potent catalyst to begin a formal trauma registry to capture data from across the military medical system.

With additional input and resources from the United States Army Institute of Surgical Research (USAISR), trauma registry nurses were deployed to Iraq in November 2004 to CSHs. The trauma registry nurses were tasked to capture data from all casualties requiring surgical care (to include data from casualties treated at Army Forward Surgical Teams and Navy Forward Resuscitative Surgery Systems) using a standard data collection sheet. These nurses then input these data into the Joint Theater Trauma Registry (JTTR).[26] The JTTR captured mechanistic, physiologic, diagnostic, therapeutic, and outcome data on injured patients within a data repository using a dictionary of terms for data entry. Using these data, the Joint Theater Trauma System (JTTS) was able to develop metrics to guide medical practice and medical command decision making with respect to resource allocation, casualty trends, and trauma care outcomes.[31–39]

DEVELOPMENT OF A HUMAN RESEARCH PROTECTION PROGRAM IN A COMBATANT COMMAND

The DOD Directive (DODD) 3216.2 in effect at the beginning of OEF/OIF (updated in 2002 from its original 1983 publication)[40] required that all research involving human subjects conducted or supported by the DOD must comply with 32 CFR 219 (the DOD version of the "Common Rule"), a federal regulation that requires adherence to the 1979 Belmont Report ethical principles of respect for persons, beneficence, and justice. Both the 2002 DODD 3216.2 and the current DOD Instruction (DODI) 3216.02[41] require that human subject research performed at DOD facilities or supported by the DOD is conducted under a DOD Assurance of Compliance (similar to a Federal-Wide Assurance). Each DOD organization seeking an Assurance must demonstrate the presence of an effective system to support the conduct of research by qualified and trained investigators whose research plans are reviewed for scientific validity and ethical/regulatory compliance. These integrated processes are referred to as a Human Research Protection Program (HRPP).

At the beginning of these conflicts, there was no HRPP for oversight of human research in the combat theater. Physicians either collected data under the rubric of quality assurance without approval or attempted to receive approval from various institutional review boards (IRBs) on their return to the United States. In 2004, military health care providers approached the US Army Medical Research and Materiel Command (USAMRMC) Office of Research Protections (ORP) and the Army Medical Department Center and School's Clinical Investigation Regulatory Office to inquire about the appropriate mechanisms for review and approval of research proposed for conduct in theater. Soon thereafter, they received calls regarding mechanisms to approve studies involving retrospective analyses of patient data collected in the combat theater during deployment. In response to these inquires, Army trauma and research oversight leaders set the goal of creating an HRPP to provide a system for scientific review, approval, and compliance oversight for military medical research conducted in the combat area of operations.[42]

The Commander of the USAISR (J.B.H.), who was also the US Army Trauma Consultant to the Surgeon General, contacted the Director, USAMRMC ORP, and requested that a regulatory support mechanism be developed. At this time, deploying providers were also contacting the Chiefs of Departments of Clinical Investigations at Army Medical Centers regarding submission of protocols to their local military IRBs for approval of studies to be conducted in the combat area of operations. Many of these proposals were submitted by investigators at the Brooke Army Medical Center (BAMC), given that BAMC was a Level 1 trauma center and was colocated with the USAISR. A major problem existed, however, in that the assurances held by local military medical facilities did not extend to the conduct of research in a combatant command. This situation was clearly less than optimal.

A coalition of principals from the USAMRMC ORP, BAMC Department of Clinical Investigation, the USAISR, and the Health Policy and Services Directorate of the Office of the US Army Surgeon General worked to develop an innovative HRPP model that would meet the Army's requirements for approval of a DOD Assurance. The Multi-National Corps Iraq (MNC-I) Surgeon, the senior ranking medical officer in Iraq, was identified to serve as the Institutional Official for this new in-theater HRPP. The MNC-I Surgeon possessed both a medical background and high-level authority within the chain of command of medical personnel conducting research in the combat theater. The USAISR provided the scientific review processes and the BAMC IRB performed the ethical/regulatory reviews, approvals, and compliance oversight. The Commanding General of the MNC-I and the US Army Surgeon General signed a Memorandum of Understanding that provided the foundation for the first combat theater HRPP.[43] The first MNC-I DOD Assurance of Compliance for Protection of Humans in Research was approved by the Army Assurance approval authority on 20 July, 2005 (**Fig. 1**).[44] Following the establishment of the Assurance, research protocols were approved following review for scientific merit and compliance with federal, DOD, and Army human subject protection regulatory requirements, conducted with compliance monitoring and continuing IRB review. A second Assurance was implemented for the US Forces—Afghanistan (USFOR-A) in 2007. In 2010, the MNC-I and USFOR-A Assurances were replaced by an overarching US Central Command (USCENTCOM) Assurance that covered the operating areas of Iraq, Kuwait, and Afghanistan. At present, the USCENTCOM Surgeon serves as the Institutional Official, with Human Protection Administrators assigned at USCENTCOM Headquarters in Tampa, Florida, and also in Afghanistan.

LIMITATIONS TO COMBAT-CASUALTY RESEARCH

To date, the vast majority of trauma studies conducted in the combat theaters of operation have been determined by the IRB to present minimal risk to participants, and most have involved descriptive/observational study designs. Many of these studies have sought to describe of the magnitude of various phenomena (eg, face and neck trauma; chest trauma; penetrating injuries to external genitalia; ratios of blood products) or the relationship between clinical interventions administered and patient outcomes (eg, outcomes of patients receiving blood transfusions or the use of tourniquets).

There are clear limitations to the conduct of research in the combat environment. There are no specific regulations prohibiting the conduct of greater than minimal risk research, but there are practical barriers. Of particular importance is the consideration for obtaining informed consent from potential research participants when possible. Most severely injured trauma casualties are unable to give consent, and there are no legal authorized representatives available to serve as surrogates. The DOD's promise to the deploying forces is to provide the highest standard of trauma care available. The use of exceptions from informed consent for emergency care research using Community Consultation raises a variety of ethical concerns when deploying US military forces constitute the "community." One such ethical issue is that military personnel are potentially vulnerable to undue influence from commanders or outranking medical officers. Because of these considerations, combat trauma research has thus far been largely limited to retrospective reviews of existing medical records or prospective observational data collection.[45] Such research presents

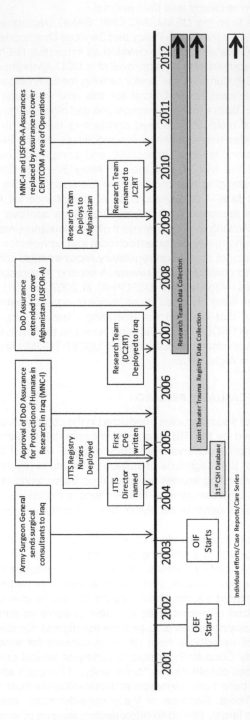

Fig. 1. Timeline of milestones of data collection, trauma system development, oversight, research team deployment, and clinical practice guideline development. CENTCOM, US Central Command; CPG, clinical practice guideline; CSH, combat support hospital; DC2RT, Deployed Combat Casualty Research Team; DoD, Department of Defense; JTTS, Joint Theater Trauma System; MNC-I, Multi-National Corps Iraq; OEF, Operation Enduring Freedom; OIF, Operation Iraqi Freedom; USFOR-A, US Forces—Afghanistan.

minimal risk to participants and, in many instances, qualifies for a waiver of informed consent. A few nontrauma interventional studies have been limited to populations that can provide advance informed consent and who remain available throughout the period of required data collection.

Another unique challenge of combat casualty research relates to the potential involvement of nonmilitary personnel in research. Military facilities in the combat theater actively engage in the care of civilians, security forces, and also detainees, and in many facilities non-US casualties outnumber the US combat casualties. Although data could be collected on civilian noncombatants and security forces, DOD regulations specifically prohibit the conduct of research involving prisoners of war. It was necessary to take special precautions to ensure that information from all detainee personnel were excluded from research databases. The practical application of these concepts evolved over time, and the theater-wide Assurance was critical to ensure ethical and uniform application of these research standards.

DEPLOYMENT OF TRAUMA RESEARCH TEAMS

Dedicated research teams have a long history in US military medicine, with highly productive teams in World War II and Vietnam making major contributions. As OIF and OEF progressed, several approved clinical research protocols merited ongoing collection of data beyond the typical deployment of providers (which varied between 3 and 15 months). Rotating deployments of principal investigators presented special problems for continuity, and ultimately the validity of data and conclusions. In addition, as early information was becoming available, the complexity of clinical and laboratory data collection involved with research trials increased. It became clear that a dedicated research team would greatly facilitate continuity of data collection for such protocols. To address these issues, once again the Commander of the USAISR pressed to establish such a dedicated research team in theater, charged with performing and facilitating research activities across the Iraq theater.

In the fall of 2006, the first team of individuals since the Vietnam War to be dedicated to trauma research was deployed by the USAISR as the Deployed Combat Casualty Research Team (DC2RT), led by one of the authors (J.G.P.). This team consisted of the following members:

- A physician director with demonstrated experience and interest in research
- A deputy director nurse PhD with research, human subject protection, and IRB experience
- Three research nurses with backgrounds in trauma, public health, and/or research
- A senior noncommissioned officer.

The primary role of the research team was to ensure continuous high-quality data collection for approved research studies, despite personnel rotation/turnover. Additional goals of the DC2RT were to integrate into the military hospital by participating directly in the clinical care of patients; serve as principal investigators and conduct research; in concert with the JTTS, implement data-driven changes on near real-time basis; and spread approved research activities to other military treatment facilities within in Iraq, Afghanistan, and Kuwait.

During the deployment of the second Army DC2RT, providers from other military service branches (Navy and Air Force) approached the team seeking IRB oversight for in-theater research initiatives. Because the Army had established an HRPP and DOD Assurance by this point, it made sense to bring all in-theater research under a single umbrella. This action led to the expansion of future research teams assigned at most of the larger surgical hospitals, staffed by a large number of personnel representing all of the US military medical services.

In September of 2009, the DC2RT was renamed the Joint Combat Casualty Research Team. Routine communication with the contiguous United States research leadership and support team ensured the mission stayed on target. Every 6 months the teams rotated and in February 2010, with the addition of a Navy Nurse Anesthetist, the team became tri-service. In the summer of 2010, the USCENTCOM completed a Joint Manning Document and assumed the responsibilities for resourcing future teams. In February 2012, the 12th rotation of JC2RT deployed to Afghanistan to conduct research.

DEVELOPMENT OF CLINICAL PRACTICE GUIDELINES IN THEATER

Collection of combat casualty data through a trauma registry within a theater trauma system and trauma research conducted with appropriate oversight and complemented by research teams provided a framework for critically examining the care of patients, which then permitted the development of clinical practice guidelines (CPGs) in key areas of patient care. A major challenge of trauma care in general is that there is a paucity of Level-I evidence based on randomized controlled clinical trials with which to guide clinical decision making. With notable exceptions, the best available evidence in trauma is often retrospective or based on anecdote and consensus expert opinion. CPGs help to fill the gaps of knowledge and give providers some direction on clinical management, particularly when few or conflicting data exist. CPGs are ideally based on input from a balanced and multidisciplinary group using the highest level of available evidence, and are intended to optimize the care of patients.[46] In civilian trauma care the best examples of these are the Eastern Association for the Surgery of Trauma guidelines.[47] While the civilian trauma guidelines are instructive, for the combat theater CPGs must be written in the context of actual resources and capabilities, and at a level understandable by the general provider. CPGs, however, are not to be blindly followed: it was emphasized and often reiterated that CPGs were not a substitute for clinical judgment.

The early use of blood products with increased ratios of plasma and platelets to red blood cells for patients requiring large-volume resuscitation within the combat theater exemplifies the process of converting data into practice guidelines. The mortality of trauma patients requiring large volumes of blood products is high, and represents a major challenge to providers both clinically and logistically. Efforts to collect transfusion and outcome data on severely injured casualties were initiated in 2004 at the 31st CSH. Although the landmark articles by Borgman and colleagues[48] on blood product ratios and by Perkins and colleagues[49] on platelet use were not published until 2007 and 2009, respectively, these data were available in 2004. Before publication of these data, intense discussions between trauma providers and the blood product supply line ensued, resulting in changed blood bank policies on the availability of thawed plasma and wider deployment of platelets. A Damage Control Resuscitation guideline was written initially at the end of 2004 with the input of clinicians, and based in part on these unpublished data. Both the research team and the JTTS tracked the results of these changes. In 2011, Simmons summarized the impact of all these efforts, describing a 50% decrease in mortality at large surgical hospitals of combat casualties undergoing massive transfusion and laparotomy.[50]

The evolution of prehospital tourniquet use is another example of changing dogma based on theater data. Relatively little modern published data on emergency tourniquet use in military settings had been published before OEF/OIF[51] although research on the optimal tourniquet had been conducted at the USAISR.[52] Tourniquets field tested by Special Operations Forces in 2003 through collaboration with the USAISR provided preliminary real-world feedback. A survey of tourniquet use at the 31st CSH in 2004 demonstrated a relative underutilization of tourniquets in limb injuries and the need to use approved modular tourniquets (eg, Combat Application Tourniquet or CAT-1) over improvised tourniquets.[53] Early prepublication analysis of these data, combined with direct reports from providers in the field and USAISR data on effectiveness of various tourniquet devices, led to the deployment of more than 400,000 tourniquets by 2005. This deployment coincided with the publication of an All Army Action (ALARACT) message in March 2005 entitled "Individual Soldier Tourniquets—Combat Application Tourniquet" and evolution of doctrine to emphasize use of tourniquets as a measure of first resort during care under fire. Subsequent data collection initiated by Kragh and colleagues[54] at the 10th CSH in 2006 and continued by the DC2RT in 2007 demonstrated a substantial increase in their use, and led to the definitive conclusion that tourniquets saved numerous lives on the battlefield. Kragh's work also informed continued refinements on the proper employment of these devices, such as the use of tourniquets in series for continued or refractory hemorrhage.[55,56]

Creation and dissemination of guidelines started in 2004, in parallel with the deployment of the trauma system and trauma registry. Initially these early efforts were coordinated with the Army, Navy, and Air Force trauma consultants and the JTTS Director. In-theater surgeons at each of the large surgical hospitals provided input into the CPGs that were then made available on the USAISR Web site and disseminated as JTTS guidelines. Like the theater itself, this process matured over the ensuing 2 years, and in early 2006 a guideline on how to write and approve a guideline was published. These CPGs are updated routinely, and address issues commonly encountered in theater that deploying providers rarely or never face outside of the deployed environment. These CPGs attempt to incorporate the data generated by recent experience, by the deployed research teams, and by the theater-wide system.[37] The CPGs are living documents, undergoing periodic review, with some documents dating back to the early days of the war (eg, Damage Control Resuscitation). There are currently 34 CPGs (**Table 1**) posted on the Joint Trauma System Web site, which are available via the Web for providers with Internet access (http://www.usaisr.amedd.army.mil/cpgs.html), or by digital or hard copy for providers without computer or Internet access.

One of the areas where improvement can be made is in using these CPGs during the predeployment training phase. The JTTS developed predeployment training to educate providers and familiarize them with common problems involving the care of combat casualties and availability of specific CPGs. However, this predeployment training is considered voluntary, and consequently providers still deploy into theater without knowledge of these hard-won medical lessons.

EVALUATION OF MILITARY GUIDELINES IN THE CIVILIAN ARENA

The process described herein is not unique, and existed in some form during World War II and Vietnam. However, serious errors were made after those wars, with civilians blindly adopting the military guidelines into civilian practice. The classic example after World War II was mandatory colostomy for all colon wounds, which unfortunately resulted in thousands of unnecessary colostomies over the ensuing 50 years. Not until the 1980s, when randomized trials were finally performed, did practice change to a more balanced approach of primary repair for most colon wounds and selective colostomy for the most severe injuries.

Table 1	
2012 Theater trauma system listing of published clinical practice guidelines	
1	01 Clinical practice guideline (CPG) index: 21 Dec 2011
2	02 Central Command Joint Theater Trauma System CPG process: 13 Mar 2010
3	Acoustic trauma and hearing loss: 16 Feb 2010
4	Amputation: 16 Feb 2010
5	Blunt abdominal trauma: 30 Jun 2010
6	Burn care: 21 Nov 2008
7	Canine resuscitation: 18 Apr 2011
8	Catastrophic care: 16 Feb 2010
9	Cervical spine evaluation: 30 Jun 2010
10	Compartment syndrome and fasciotomy: 30 Apr 2009
11	Damage control resuscitation: 10 Aug 2011
12	Emergent resuscitative thoracotomy: 6 May 2009
13	Fresh whole blood transfusion: 30 Mar 2011
14	Frozen blood: 30 Jun 2010
15	High bilateral amputations: 13 Apr 2011
16	Hypothermia prevention: 30 Jun 2010
17	Infection control: 16 Feb 2010
18	Inhalation injury and toxic chemical exposure: 7 Nov 2008
19	Initial care of ocular and adnexal injuries: 16 Feb 2010
20	Intratheater transfer and transport: 19 Nov 2008
21	Management of pain anxiety and delirium: 23 Nov 2010
22	Management of patients with severe head trauma: 30 Jun 2010
23	Management of war wounds: 16 Feb 2010
24	Nutrition: 16 Feb 2010
25	Pelvic fracture care: 30 Jun 2010
26	Postsplenectomy vaccination: 30 Jun 2010
27	Prevention of deep venous thrombosis: 21 Nov 2008
28	Spine injury surgical management and transport: 9 Jul 2010
29	Trauma airway management: 30 Jun 2010
30	Urologic trauma management: 30 Jun 2010
31	Use of electronic documentation: 30 Jun 2010
32	Use of magnetic resonance imaging in management of mild traumatic brain injury in the deployed setting: 4 Aug 2011
33	Use of trauma flow sheets: 1 Dec 2008
34	Vascular injury: 7 Nov 2008
35	Ventilator-associated pneumonia: 16 Feb 2010

Infrastructure and capacity exists for performing prospective, randomized research projects in the civilian arena. With 10% of the United States population injured every year (30 million people) resulting in more than 100,000 deaths, the number of injuries presenting to the 1200 trauma centers across the nation provides a rich research milieu. Adequate funding to fuel such research is crucial. Over the last decade, the DOD and the National Institutes of Health have supported or initiated several collaboratives focused on conducting randomized trials in the civilian trauma population (eg, Resuscitation Outcomes Consortium [http://roc.uwctc.org] and the National Trauma Institute [http://www.nationaltraumainstitute.org]). These efforts have largely focused on resuscitation and hemorrhage control, although large studies on posttraumatic stress disorder, mild traumatic brain injury, and orthopedic injuries are also ongoing. It remains to be seen whether this level of funding will continue after the wars conclude. It is hoped that the exchange of ideas and data-driven practices will remain robust between military and civilian trauma populations.

SUMMARY

At the beginning of the OIF/OEF wars, capture of clinically relevant data across the theater was virtually impossible. Within a relatively short time frame aggregate data collection, analysis, and the rapid turnaround of approved CPGs was a reality. The strength of rapid capture of clinical data lies in the realm where published literature cannot guide clinical decision making. As soon as efforts to collect data had begun, providers sought to examine the aggregate data and to identify trends and opportunities for performance improvement to manage casualties. Providers in theater could give feedback through weekly JTTS teleconferences to identify deficiencies in the CPG or the system itself, and this has led to a data-driven iterative process to review, update, and improve CPGs and clinical care.

The systematic analysis of data from the care of combat casualties is a time-honored tradition and sacred responsibility of military medical personnel. Over the course of the conflicts in Iraq and Afghanistan, the military has developed an effective (and still evolving) theater trauma system to care for casualties on the battlefield. Efforts to integrate the robust performance improvement effort into the clinical milieu are still ongoing. The evolution in data collection and human research protections/research oversight has allowed more effective and efficient techniques to capture and analyze trauma data. Consequently, this has enabled rapid dissemination of data-driven quality improvement measures and CPGs in the midst of war. It is difficult to accurately measure the impact of improved combat medical policies and clinical practice guidelines when the interventions are not randomized and can only be evaluated retrospectively.[57] However, given the constraints inherent on any battlefield, the changes described in this article represent the sum efforts of thousands of dedicated personnel to improve combat casualty care now and in the future.

ACKNOWLEDGMENTS

The authors acknowledge the many dedicated individuals who have devoted countless hours to improve the care of combat casualties. The authors would like to recognize the singular heroic efforts of Ms Annette McClinton, RN, MSN, Chief, Regulatory Compliance and Quality Management, at the USAISR, who tirelessly coordinated the staffing and predeployment training of each the 12 JC2RT teams who have deployed to theater.

REFERENCES

1. Pruitt BA Jr. Combat casualty care and surgical progress. Ann Surg 2006;243(6): 715–29.
2. Medical readiness efforts are underway for DOD training in civilian trauma centers. Washington, DC: General Accounting Office; 1998.

3. Nuland SB. Doctors: the biography of medicine. New York: Vintage Books; 1988. p. 94–119.

4. Debakey ME, Simeone FA. Battle injuries of the arteries in World War II: an analysis of 2,471 cases. Ann Surg 1946;123(4):534–79.

5. Rich NM, Baugh JH, Hughes CW. Acute arterial injuries in Vietnam: 1,000 cases. J Trauma 1970;10(5):359–69.

6. Trunkey DD, Johannigman JA, Holcomb JB. Lessons relearned. Arch Surg 2008; 143(2):112–4.

7. Mabry RL, Holcomb JB, Baker AM, et al. United States Army Rangers in Somalia: an analysis of combat casualties on an urban battlefield. J Trauma 2000;49(3): 515–28 [discussion: 528–9].

8. Holcomb JB. The 2004 Fitts lecture: current perspective on combat casualty care. J Trauma 2005;59(4):990–1002.

9. Holcomb JB, Stansbury LG, Champion HR, et al. Understanding combat casualty care statistics. J Trauma 2006;60(2):397–401.

10. Bilski TR, Baker BC, Grove JR, et al. Battlefield casualties treated at Camp Rhino, Afghanistan: lessons learned. J Trauma 2003;54(5):814–21.

11. Vassallo DJ, Gerlinger T, Maholtz P, et al. Combined UK/US field hospital management of a major incident arising from a Chinook helicopter crash in Afghanistan, 28 Jan 2002. J R Army Med Corps 2003;149(1):47–52.

12. Place RJ, Rush RM Jr, Arrington ED. Forward surgical team (FST) workload in a special operations environment: the 250th FST in Operation Enduring Freedom. Curr Surg 2003;60(4):418–22.

13. Pratt JW, Rush RM Jr. The military surgeon and the war on terrorism: a Zollinger legacy. Am J Surg 2003;186(3):292–5.

14. Lin DL, Kirk KL, Murphy KP, et al. Orthopedic injuries during operation enduring freedom. Mil Med 2004;169(10):807–9.

15. Lin DL, Kirk KL, Murphy KP, et al. Evaluation of orthopaedic injuries in operation enduring freedom. J Orthop Trauma 2004;18(Suppl 8):S48–53.

16. West BC, Bentley R, Place RJ. In-flight transfusion of packed red blood cells on a combat search and rescue mission: a case report from operation enduring freedom. Mil Med 2004;169(3):181–3.

17. Peoples GE, Gerlinger T, Craig R, et al. The 274th forward surgical team experience during operation enduring freedom. Mil Med 2005;170(6):451–9.

18. Peoples GE, Gerlinger T, Craig R, et al. Combat casualties in Afghanistan cared for by a single forward surgical team during the initial phases of operation enduring freedom. Mil Med 2005;170(6):462–8.

19. Rush RM Jr, Stockmaster NR, Stinger HK, et al. Supporting the global war on terror: a tale of two campaigns featuring the 250th forward surgical team (airborne). Am J Surg 2005;189(5):564–70 [discussion: 570].

20. Wedmore IS, Johnson T, Czarnik J, et al. Pain management in the wilderness and operational setting. Emerg Med Clin North Am 2005;23(2):585–601, xi–xii.

21. Acosta JA, Hatzigeorgiou C, Smith LS. Developing a trauma registry in a forward deployed military hospital: preliminary report. J Trauma 2006;61(2):256–60.

22. Beekley AC, Watts DM. Combat trauma experience with the United States Army 102nd forward surgical team in Afghanistan. Am J Surg 2004;187(5):652–4.

23. Beitler AL, Wortmann GW, Hofmann LJ, et al. Operation enduring freedom: the 48th Combat Support Hospital in Afghanistan. Mil Med 2006;171(3):189–93.

24. Craig R, Peoples GE. A novel device developed, tested, and used for warming and maintaining intravenous fluids in a forward surgical team during operation enduring freedom. Mil Med 2006;171(6):500–3.

25. Mullins RJ, Veum-Stone J, Helfand M, et al. Outcome of hospitalized injured patients after institution of a trauma system in an urban area. JAMA 1994;271(24):1919-24.
26. Eastridge BJ, Jenkins D, Flaherty S, et al. Trauma system development in a theater of war: experiences from Operation Iraqi Freedom and Operation Enduring Freedom. J Trauma 2006;61(6):1366-72 [discussion: 1372-3].
27. Klote M, Brosch LR. Respecting our patients by respecting their records. Mil Med 2010;175(3):136-7.
28. Arthurs Z, Cuadrado D, Beekley A, et al. The impact of hypothermia on trauma care at the 31st combat support hospital. Am J Surg 2006;191(5):610-4.
29. Galarneau MR, Hancock WC, Konoske P, et al. The navy-marine corps combat trauma registry. Mil Med 2006;171(8):691-7.
30. Clouse WD, Rasmussen TE, Peck MA, et al. In-theater management of vascular injury: 2 years of the Balad vascular registry. J Am Coll Surg 2007;204(4):625-32.
31. Eastridge BJ, Wade CE, Spott MA, et al. Utilizing a trauma systems approach to benchmark and improve combat casualty care. J Trauma 2010;69(Suppl 1):S5-9.
32. Thomas R, McManus JG, Johnson A, et al. Ocular injury reduction from ocular protection use in current combat operations. J Trauma 2009;66(Suppl 4): S99-103.
33. Ritenour AE, Blackbourne LH, Kelly JF, et al. Incidence of primary blast injury in US military overseas contingency operations: a retrospective study. Ann Surg 2010;251(6):1140-4.
34. Wade CE, Eastridge BJ, Jones JA, et al. Use of recombinant factor VIIa in US military casualties for a five-year period. J Trauma 2010;69(2):353-9.
35. Kragh JF Jr, Wade CE, Baer DG, et al. Fasciotomy rates in Operations Enduring Freedom and Iraqi Freedom: association with injury severity and tourniquet use. J Orthop Trauma 2011;25(3):134-9.
36. Eastridge BJ, Hardin M, Cantrell J, et al. Died of wounds on the battlefield: causation and implications for improving combat casualty care. J Trauma 2011; 71(Suppl 1):S4-8.
37. Ennis JL, Chung KK, Renz EM, et al. Joint Theater Trauma System implementation of burn resuscitation guidelines improves outcomes in severely burned military casualties. J Trauma 2008;64(Suppl 2):S146-51 [discussion: S151-42].
38. Stansbury LG, Lalliss SJ, Branstetter JG, et al. Amputations in U.S. military personnel in the current conflicts in Afghanistan and Iraq. J Orthop Trauma 2008;22(1):43-6.
39. Kelly JF, Ritenour AE, McLaughlin DF, et al. Injury severity and causes of death from operation iraqi freedom and operation enduring freedom: 2003-2004 versus 2006. J Trauma 2008;64(Suppl 2):S21-6 [discussion S26-7].
40. Department of Defense Directive (DODD) 3216.2: protection of human subjects and adherence to ethical standards in DoD-Supported Research, 2002. Available at: http://www.med.navy.mil/sites/nmrc/documents/hspp_dod3216_2.pdf. Accessed April 21, 2012.
41. Department of Defense Instruction (DODI) 3216.02: protection of human subjects and adherence to ethical standards in DOD-supported research, 2011. Available at: http://www.dtic.mil/whs/directives/corres/pdf/321602p.pdf. Accessed April 21, 2012.
42. Brosch LR, Holcomb JB, Thompson JC, et al. Establishing a human research protection program in a combatant command. J Trauma 2008;64(2 Suppl): S9-12 [discussion: S12-3].
43. Memorandum of Understanding between the United States Surgeon General and the Commander, Multi-National Corps, Iraq; SUBJECT: the conduct of human

subjects research in army medical treatment facilities in the multi-national corps, Iraq area of operations, signed 16 and 19 March 2005.

44. DOD Multiple Project Assurance (MPA) of compliance for the protection of human research subjects. Multi-National Corps Iraq; 2005.

45. Beekley AC, Martin MJ, Nelson T, et al. Continuous noninvasive tissue oximetry in the early evaluation of the combat casualty: a prospective study. J Trauma 2010; 69(Suppl 1):S14–25.

46. Clinical Practice Guidelines we can trust: Institute of Medicine of the National Academies. 2011.

47. Eastern Association for the Surgery of Trauma Guidelines. Available at: http://www. east.org/research/treatment-guidelines/category/trauma. Accessed April 21, 2012.

48. Borgman MA, Spinella PC, Perkins JG, et al. The ratio of blood products transfused affects mortality in patients receiving massive transfusions at a combat support hospital. J Trauma 2007;63(4):805–13.

49. Perkins JG, Cap AP, Spinella PC, et al. An evaluation of the impact of apheresis platelets used in the setting of massively transfused trauma patients. J Trauma 2009;66(Suppl 4):S77–84 [discussion: S84–5].

50. Simmons JW, White CE, Eastridge BJ, et al. Impact of improved combat casualty care on combat wounded undergoing exploratory laparotomy and massive transfusion. J Trauma 2011;71(Suppl 1):S82–6.

51. Lakstein D, Blumenfeld A, Sokolov T, et al. Tourniquets for hemorrhage control on the battlefield: a 4-year accumulated experience. J Trauma 2003;54(Suppl 5): S221–5.

52. Walters TJ, Wenke JC, Kauvar DS, et al. Effectiveness of self-applied tourniquets in human volunteers. Prehosp Emerg Care 2005;9(4):416–22.

53. Beekley AC, Sebesta JA, Blackbourne LH, et al. Prehospital tourniquet use in operation Iraqi freedom: effect on hemorrhage control and outcomes. J Trauma 2008;64(Suppl 2):S28–37 [discussion: S37].

54. Kragh JF Jr, Walters TJ, Baer DG, et al. Survival with emergency tourniquet use to stop bleeding in major limb trauma. Ann Surg 2009;249(1):1–7.

55. Kragh JF Jr, Walters TJ, Baer DG, et al. Practical use of emergency tourniquets to stop bleeding in major limb trauma. J Trauma 2008;64(Suppl 2):S38–49 [discussion: S49–50].

56. Kragh JF Jr, O'Neill ML, Walters TJ, et al. The military emergency tourniquet program's lessons learned with devices and designs. Mil Med 2011;176(10): 1144–52.

57. Simmons JW, White CE, Eastridge BJ, et al. Impact of policy change on US Army combat transfusion practices. J Trauma 2010;69(Suppl 1):S75–80.

Graduate Medical Education in Trauma/Critical Care and Acute Care Surgery
Defining Goals for a New Workforce

Edward Kelly, MD*, Selwyn O. Rogers Jr, MD, MPH

KEYWORDS

- Trauma • Emergency surgery • Critical care • Graduate medical education
- Acute care surgery • Fellowship

KEY POINTS

- Advances is surgical technology have resulted in ever more technically complex operations for acutely ill patients.
- Superspecialization has led to diminishing numbers of surgeons qualified in emergency general surgery.
- Demand for emergency general surgery services is higher than ever, and increasing.
- A new specialty in general surgery has been developed to meet the public health need and enhance training: Acute Care Surgery.

INTRODUCTION

In the evolving field of general surgery, change has been constant. Technical advances such as minimally invasive surgery, an aging patient population, and an ever expanding demand to respond to urgent surgical conditions has catalyzed change in the definition of general surgery. General surgery has traditionally included a significant component of emergency surgery over a wide variety of anatomic sites, in response to traumatic injury and nontraumatic causes (eg, peptic ulcer disease, cancer, infections), which naturally included critical care medicine in the perioperative setting. With the growing trend toward specialization, surgical training has evolved in

The authors have nothing to disclose.
Division of Burn, Trauma, and Surgical Critical Care, Harvard Medical School, Brigham and Women's Hospital, 75 Francis Street, Boston, MA 02115, USA
* Corresponding author.
E-mail address: Ekelly1@partners.org

Surg Clin N Am 92 (2012) 1055–1064
doi:10.1016/j.suc.2012.04.006
0039-6109/12/$ – see front matter © 2012 Elsevier Inc. All rights reserved.

surgical.theclinics.com

response to demands from within and without the discipline of surgery to provide efficient, effective training in ever more complex and urgent surgical problems. This review demonstrates how general surgery has changed to meet these new needs, which has led to the new specialty of acute care surgery (ACS).

CHANGES IN SURGICAL NEED

Surgical practice is in constant flux. With the development of new techniques and technologies, the modern surgeon is constantly improving his or her repertoire of skills. The surgical resident in training must master an ever expanding set of learning objectives. By way of example, the advancement of laparoscopic techniques for cholecystectomy has led to a decline in the number of open cholecystectomies while increasing the total number of cholecystectomies performed.[1] Furthermore, common bile duct (CBD) explorations, once common, are now exceedingly rare with the wide availability of endoscopic retrograde cholangiopancreatography for the management of CBD stones. The newer and often better technology has nearly supplanted many of the open approaches to common surgical conditions, such as the management of biliary disease, morbid obesity, and gastric reflux.

To maintain a viable practice, surgeons have had to learn the new techniques and were often rewarded with more cases once they had mastered the new approach. In trauma surgery there have been analogous examples, including the widespread adoption of damage-control surgery,[2] hypotensive resuscitation,[3] damage-control resuscitation,[4] advanced hemostatic dressings,[5] and video-assisted surgery for chest injury.[6] The practice of trauma and ACS continues to evolve, leading to more effective care and improved outcomes, while at the same time demanding that practicing surgeons and trainees acquire and maintain an ever increasing and ever more technical body of knowledge.

Even as technical advances are changing surgical practice, the surgical patients are changing as well. With modern, effective, and less invasive treatments, patients are living longer and better with chronic diseases[7] but are now subject to diseases of survivorship. These patients can present with traditional surgical problems, which are harder to diagnose and manage because of the multiple comorbidities. For example, cystic fibrosis, a once fatal disease in childhood, is now a disease that complicates surgery in adults. Adults with cystic fibrosis are known to have a higher incidence of gastrointestinal tract malignancy.[8] Thus, a higher index of suspicion for cancer is indicated in the setting of acute digestive complaints in these patients. Furthermore, with the aging of the American population, there is an ever expanding pool of baby boomers in need of urgent and emergent surgical care. The patients seen by the trauma and acute care surgeons of today have significant active medical issues that greatly affect their surgical management.

While the need for emergency surgical care is changing, the demand for skilled surgeons to service that need is higher than ever. With advancing surgical technology and the expanding knowledge base required in all surgical disciplines, fellowship training and subspecialization is becoming the norm among United States surgical residents,[9] leading to a deficit of skilled providers in general surgery. As many subspecialty surgeons are unwilling to practice outside of their area of focus, there is a growing gap in coverage for emergency surgical care.[10]

NEW MANDATES IN SURGICAL TRAINING

Parallel to the advances in technology in surgical treatment, there has been significant advancement in surgical training. For much of the last century, surgical training had followed an apprenticeship model, whereby the trainees (residents or fellows) would spend long hours in the hospital, learning by example, without an organized curriculum or a standard for progress in technical or cognitive skills. The residents were often in competition with each other to maintain their positions in so-called pyramidal programs. The apprenticeship model began to show its age in the early 1980s, when interest in general surgery residency among US Medical School seniors began a decades-long decline.[11] Lifestyle was cited by medical students as the primary reason for not pursuing a career in general surgery. Concerns were voiced both about the lifestyle in training and the lifestyle of the attending surgeon. The decline in interest led to a decrease in the number of applicants to surgical programs and unfilled residency positions, leading some to asked the question, were we still training the best and the brightest?[12]

Other influences were acting concurrently to change the face of surgical residency training. Concerns about patient safety were raised in response to recognition of resident fatigue in working long shifts and long working weeks, resulting in the 80-hour work-week mandate. Medicare, Medicaid, and private health care payors have increased the requirement for attending involvement in teaching cases, greatly restricting the role of the senior resident as a teacher.

Simultaneously with the changes in resident work hours, effective nonoperative treatments emerged for treating traumatic injuries. As a result, the operative experience in trauma surgery decreased dramatically in all but the busiest trauma centers. By 2003, a survey conducted by Fakhry and colleagues[13] showed that at more than 80 major trauma centers, residents would perform 15 or fewer laparotomies for injury. This figure was not considered adequate to prepare trainees for clinical practice. In a survey of 300 General Surgery Program directors, Bell and colleagues[14] found that the mean number of operative cases for major abdominal, vascular, and bladder injury was less than zero, and for liver and neck exploration the figure was less than 2 per resident. These investigators also concluded that this was insufficient experience to prepare the residents for clinical practice.

THE NEW GENERAL SURGEON/ACUTE CARE SURGEON IN PRACTICE

These evolving trends in surgical need and surgical technology combined with new mandates in surgical training have shaped the development of the new specialty of ACS. Surgical patients are more complicated than ever before, yet continue to have urgent surgical needs. The acute care surgeon, like the trauma surgeon of old, needs to be able to provide excellent surgical care with limited time to prepare. The acute care surgeon needs a wide base of knowledge to be able to diagnose and treat the medically complex surgical patient; thus, critical care is a core competency of the acute care surgeon. In addition, the acute care surgeon needs to be adept in the use of modern surgical technology, and having an active, if limited, practice in elective surgery can provide the clinical material to refine technical skill. ACS is more accurately defined by the mastery of a wide body of knowledge than by expertise in a narrow set of technical skills. General surgeons who concentrate their practice on emergency care have always been known by different names in the past, often determined by their area of greatest interest: critical care surgeon, emergency general surgeon, trauma surgeon, among others. The modern definition of ACS integrates all of these functions.[15] ACS involves a much wider scope of practice than more technically oriented surgical specialties and overlaps with many of them. This scenario is clearly illustrated in the table of contents of the first textbook of ACS, published in 2007, which contains chapters on management of vascular, colorectal, infectious, and pancreatic conditions, among many others.[16]

Within the wide scope of practice, ACS does require collaboration with experts in the other surgical disciplines, referring physicians (ie, primary care providers and emergency room physicians), and the prehospital community. ACS fills the void for emergency surgical services around the clock and around the calendar. An ACS specialist must work in collaboration with partners, associates, and consultants for close comanagement of patients, for seamless coverage, and coordinated care. ACS requires a multidisciplinary approach to patient care and requires team-building and team-leading skills. The net effect will be to bring the ACS specialist to the center of integrated urgent care, much like the "service-line" approach used with cardiovascular care.[17] The opportunities for professional and academic development in this integrated service line are vast and will be very attractive for residents and medical students. In fact, there is evidence of growing interest in ACS among medical students exposed to this specialty.[18]

THE ACUTE CARE SURGEON IN TRAINING

To meet the challenges of training surgeons in the evolving field of acute care surgery, the American Association for the Surgery of Trauma (AAST), representing senior trauma surgeons in the field, drafted and published a set of guidelines that defined the Fellowship in ACS.[19] The stated goals for setting these guidelines were to develop a comprehensive 2-year curriculum, which embraced clinical trauma, emergency general surgery, and surgical critical care. The goals were outlined to foster a match program for these fellowships, to work with the American Board of Surgery (ABS) to redefine the core training in general surgery residency, and to promote a collaborative relationship among clinicians currently in practice in the 3 component disciplines. The AAST asserted that ACS encompassed a clear body of medical knowledge distinct from the core of general surgery, and that mastery of this field required completion of general surgery residency before eligibility for Fellowship training. The guidelines included completion of an ABS-accredited surgical critical care Fellowship with added training in related surgical fields[20] and significant exposure to emergency surgery (**Table 1**). The guidelines also required a minimum of 12 months of trauma call responsibility. This curriculum addressed the decline in operative experience in trauma by United States general surgery residents and solidified the link between urgent surgical care and surgical critical care. To further demonstrate their commitment to ACS as a specialty, in 2010 the AAST added "Clinical Congress of Acute Care Surgery" to the name of their annual meeting. Similarly, the primary journal for trauma surgery, the *Journal of Trauma, Injury, Infection, and Critical Care*, has recently been renamed the *Journal of Trauma and Acute Care Surgery*.

Table 1 AAST surgery curriculum rotations	
Acute care surgery	4–6 mo
Thoracic	1–3 mo
Transplant/hepatobiliary/pancreatic	1–3 mo
Vascular/interventional radiology	1–3 mo
Orthopedic surgery	1 mo
Neurologic surgery	1 mo
Electives	1–3 mo
(Burn surgery and pediatric surgery recommended; others could include endoscopy, imaging, plastic surgery, and so forth)	
Total	15 mo

SETTING UP AN ACUTE CARE SURGERY FELLOWSHIP

The AAST guidelines have been adopted by many surgical training programs throughout the country. Seven Fellowship programs have been reviewed and formally approved by the AAST (**Box 1**). This represents a very rapid adoption of the curriculum, as the process for review and accreditation only began in 2008. All of these 7 had an accredited surgical critical care program before establishing ACS Fellowship, and all are Level I trauma centers. As expected, the programs with established infrastructure and senior leadership in trauma and critical care were able to move swiftly through development and accreditation. Now, several years later, programs without previously established surgical critical care Fellowships are building the ACS Fellowship from scratch.

Surgical critical care training is regulated by both the Accreditation Council for Graduate Medical Education (ACGME) and the ABS. Both of these governing bodies require a 12-month fellowship period, of which no more than 3 months may be spent in operative experience. The ACGME mandates that the Program Director (PD) must be certified by the ABS in surgical critical care, approved by the sponsoring institution's Graduate Medical Education Committee (GMEC), and ensure a Fellow to patient ratio of at least 1:5. In addition, Faculty supervising clinical Fellows must be ABS certified, the didactic program must comply with ACGME standards (**Box 2**), and the Fellows must be reviewed regularly in their progress in the ACGME competencies (**Box 3**).[21] The Residency Review Committee—Surgery approves the number of Surgical Critical Care Fellows. ACGME limits work-hours to an average of 80 per week (including moonlighting), limits work shifts to no more than 24 hours, and limits in-house call to no more than every third night.

The ABS administers the Certifying Examination for Added Qualifications in Surgical Critical Care, which is a written test[22] with defined content (**Table 2**). Applicants for the examination must have passed the Qualifying Examination for General Surgery, have an unrestricted license to practice medicine, have completed an ACGME-approved Fellowship, must have critical care privileges in clinical practice, and must submit a case log of 50 patients treated during Fellowship, including all deaths (up to 25). Residents who complete critical care Fellowship before completing surgical residency may sit for the examination but do not receive certificates until successful completion of residency and passing the Qualifying and Certifying Examinations in General Surgery.

Once the ACGME and ABS surgical critical care requirements are met, the program must seek approval from the sponsoring institution's GMEC for adding the AAST 1-year curriculum. To secure approval, the PD must be able to demonstrate

---

Box 1
AAST-approved ACS programs

University of California, San Francisco—Fresno, Fresno, California

University of Colorado School of Medicine, Denver, Colorado

University of Maryland/R. Adams Cowley Shock Trauma Center, Baltimore, Maryland

University of Nevada School of Medicine, Las Vegas, Nevada

University of Pittsburgh Medical Center, Pittsburgh, Pennsylvania

Massachusetts General Hospital, Boston, Massachusetts

University of Texas Health Science Center, Houston, Texas

Box 2
ACGME standards for medical knowledge in critical care fellowship

Cardiorespiratory resuscitation

Physiology, pathophysiology, diagnosis, and treatment of disorders of the cardiovascular, respiratory, gastrointestinal, genitourinary, neurologic, endocrine, musculoskeletal, and immune systems, as well as of infectious diseases

Metabolic, nutritional, and endocrine effects of critical illness

Hematologic and coagulation disorders

Critical obstetric and gynecologic disorders

Trauma, thermal, electrical, and radiation injuries

Inhalation and immersion injuries

Monitoring and medical instrumentation

Critical pediatric surgical conditions

Pharmacokinetics and dynamics of drugs

Metabolism and excretion in critical illness

Ethical and legal aspects of surgical critical care

Principles and techniques of administration and management

Biostatistics and experimental design

---

that the Fellowship will not take away valuable teaching cases for existing residencies, that the Fellows will have ample learning opportunities and supervision, and that the PD and Faculty meets the standards as set by the AAST.

The PD must be a faculty member of the sponsoring institution, certified in general surgery and surgical critical care, and be a member of the AAST. The PD gathers and communicates the program's vital statistics to the AAST on an annual basis. The faculty must have ABS certification in general surgery or other certification approved by the AAST, and must be active staff at the sponsoring or participating institutions. The sponsoring institution must provide the majority of the clinical experience, but participating institutions may be employed for specific rotations. Fellows must log their operative experiences in a case log, and are encouraged to use the online case log run by the AAST.

The AAST requires documentation of Fellows' progress in the ACGME competencies, and restricts duty hours to 80 per week (inclusive of all in-house activities) and mandates 1 full day completely off from clinical or scholarly activities per week, on average. Duty shifts may not exceed 24 hours, and in-house call may not exceed every third night. Moonlighting is not forbidden but must be included in the work-hours limitations. Fellows must receive regular updates on their progress, and Faculty evaluations and must have a final evaluation from the PD as part of their permanent record. Similarly, every accreditation cycle Faculty must be evaluated by Fellows and peers.

Once all of the requirements are in place and the PD has submitted the Program Information Form, the application is reviewed by the AAST site surveyors. If the application meets all standards, a site visit is arranged. Two surveyors review the program in person. If the program is approved, the AAST accredits the Fellowship for a period of 5 years. If there are minor deficiencies, the Fellowship may be granted provisional accreditation for 1 year, during which time the deficiencies must be corrected. A focused repeat site visit can then grant full accreditation.

Box 3
ACGME core competencies

Patient care

Evaluated through: direct observation, clinical outcomes, patient presentations, bedside rounds

Medical knowledge (biomedical, clinical, cognate sciences, and their application)

Evaluated through: annual otolaryngology examination scores, direct observation, direct questioning during clinical care and teaching experiences, journal club and conference discussions (for cognate sciences), patient presentations, scores on self examinations

Practice-based learning and improvement (investigation and evaluation, appraisal, and assimilation of evidence)

Evaluated through: progressive, graded improvement in clinical care and surgical technique, the use of evidence-based medicine, and the evaluation of the best-available evidence in routine clinical care

Interpersonal and communication skills (effective information exchange, teaming with patients and families)

Evaluated through: direct observation of communications with other residents, consulting and attending physicians, nonphysician clinical staff, nonphysician nonclinical staff, and patients and their families, as well as reviews of pertinent sections of regular evaluations

Professionalism (performing professional responsibilities, ethics, sensitivity)

Evaluated through: responsibility in performing their professional duties (continuity, responsiveness, availability, and self-sacrifice), following ethical principles, and sensitivity to diverse patient populations

Systems-based practice (awareness and responsiveness to larger context and system of health care, use of system resources)

Evaluated through: use of the entire health care system in patient care, and teamwork; direct observation in patient care and at the Morning Report meeting

There is no formal match currently set up for ACS Fellowship; therefore, it is unclear how many ACS Fellowships are operating or are in early stages of development. The Eastern Association for the Surgery of Trauma Web site (www.east.org) hosts an extensive Fellowship listing for trauma, critical care, and acute care surgery positions. The Web site advertised 11 non–AAST-approved programs in 2011. As the AAST is an organization of senior surgical leadership and not an accrediting body like the ACGME, Fellowship programs can operate without AAST approval but will be in competition with approved sites for the best candidates.

THE FUTURE

Significant challenges still exist for fellowship training in ACS. While there is no doubt that there is an extreme need for surgeons in acute care, Fellowship-trained ACS surgeons will have little difficulty finding work in academic, community, or rural settings.[23] It is too early to tell whether ACS Fellowships as currently constructed provide the proper training for all settings, or if programs should be tailored for specific aspects of ACS more appropriate to each setting (eg, academic, community, and rural). Furthermore, funding for Fellowship training is in question not only for ACS but for all surgical specialties. Federal funds subsidize postgraduate medical education through the Centers for Medicare and Medicaid Services for programs accredited by the ACGME, for up to 5 years of clinical training. As ACS involves training after the

Table 2 ABS certifying examination content	
Topic	Weight (%)
I. Initial Resuscitation	6
II. Cardiovascular Physiology, Pathophysiology, and Therapy	10
III. Respiratory Physiology, Pathophysiology, and Therapy	9
IV. Fluid and Electrolyte, Pathophysiology, and Therapy	11
V. Neurologic Physiology, Pathophysiology, and Therapy	5
VI. Metabolic, Endocrinologic, and Nutritional Effects of Surgical Illness	5
VII. Infectious Disease, Pathophysiology, and Therapy	10
VIII. Hematologic Disorders Secondary to Acute Illness/Blood Transfusion	2
IX. Acute Gastrointestinal, Genitourinary, and Obstetric-Gynecologic Disorders	10
X. Trauma	10
XI. Thermal Injury	4
XII. Monitoring, Bioengineering, and Biostatistics	6
XIII. Life-Threatening Pediatric Conditions	2
XIV. Principles and Techniques of Administration	3
XV. Pharmacology, Pharmacokinetics, and Drug Metabolism in Critical Illness	2
XVI. Ethical and Legal Aspects in Surgical Critical Care Medicine	2
XVII. Immunology, Transplantation, and Cell Biology	4

fifth year, no Fellowship Program qualifies for the subsidy, leaving the Programs to seek financial support from clinical revenues, hospital subsidies, and industry. In addition, industrial support has been significantly curtailed by ACGME rules changes in 2009, in response to public concern over conflicts of interest.[24,25]

With more than 80% of current surgical residents planning on seeking Fellowship training and diminishing funding from federal and industry sources, many Fellowship programs, including ACS, are turning to clinical revenues to provide support for Fellows' salaries, leading to conflicting financial and educational mandates. On the one hand, all ACS Fellows are ABS certified or eligible to practice general surgery, and may have hospital privileges and bill for their services. Thus, each Fellow is capable of generating clinical revenue for his or her own salary. On the other hand, ACGME guidelines do not allow Fellows to practice and bill within the specialty of their fellowship, and ACS programs that depend on these clinical revenues would not be ACGME compliant. At present, the ACGME does not accredit ACS Fellowship, so ACS Fellows can bill without concern about the Program being cited. However, if ACS is to develop into a specialty recognized by the ABS, with a certifying examination, ACGME compliance may ultimately be necessary, or a new pathway independent of ACGME will need to be validated.

The ABS has recognized this conflict and has tried to identify ways to improve federal support of Fellowship training. One method under consideration is the "Integrated Fellowship" approach already in place for cardiothoracic surgery and plastic surgery, which combines residency and Fellowship into a single 5- or 6-year program, with the first years given over to more traditional general surgery and the final 2 years spent in the subspecialty. The graduate of the Integrated pathway is eligible only for Board certification within the specialty but not general surgery. To implement an

Integrated Program for Acute Care, a new Board examination would need to be structured to ensure competence in all 3 of the key components of ACS: emergency general surgery, trauma, and surgical critical care. Until there is more experience with the current model of Fellowship training, integrated training is probably not viable.

SUMMARY

Emergency surgical needs have changed dramatically in the past 20 years, but there is more need for urgent surgical care than ever before. While the surgical need continues to expand, the pool of surgeons capable and willing to provide emergency care has diminished, due to professional and market forces encouraging superspecialization. At the same time, experience in emergency surgical care among surgical trainees has been curtailed by increasing effectiveness in nonoperative management, decreased exposure to surgical emergencies due to limitation of working hours, and increasingly earlier pressure toward specialization. The gap in trained surgeons to provide emergency care has become a crisis in some areas, and a new generation of surgeons is needed to fill it. The goal of ACS training is to fill the gap with energetic young surgeons who are skilled in advanced techniques; trained in the management of acutely ill and moribund patients; experienced in complex, rapid decision making; and able to lead a diverse team of other health care specialists. Training programs to produce these surgeons are being developed in a multidisciplinary fashion, with collaboration by senior surgical leadership in trauma, surgical critical care, and general surgery. Despite the significant challenges, new programs have already begun training Fellows in ACS, and the number of programs is rapidly increasing. Fellowship-trained acute care surgeons should outnumber non–acute care surgeons who manage emergency surgery patients within 10 years.

REFERENCES

1. Steiner CA, Bass EB, Talamini MA, et al. Surgical rates and operative mortality for open and laparoscopic cholecystectomy in Maryland. N Engl J Med 1994;330(6): 403–8.
2. Rotondo MF, Schwab CW, McGonigal MD, et al. 'Damage control': an approach for improved survival in exsanguinating penetrating abdominal injury. J Trauma 1993;35(3):375–82 [discussion: 382–3].
3. Bickell WH, Wall MJ Jr, Pepe PE, et al. Immediate versus delayed fluid resuscitation for hypotensive patients with penetrating torso injuries. N Engl J Med 1994; 331(17):1105–9.
4. Borgman MA, Spinella PC, Perkins JG, et al. The ratio of blood products transfused affects mortality in patients receiving massive transfusions at a combat support hospital. J Trauma 2007;63(4):805–13.
5. Rhee P, Brown C, Martin M, et al. QuikClot use in trauma for hemorrhage control: case series of 103 documented uses. J Trauma 2008;64(4):1093–9.
6. Abolhoda A, Livingston DH, Donahoo JS, et al. Diagnostic and therapeutic video assisted thoracic surgery (VATS) following chest trauma. Eur J Cardiothorac Surg 1997;12(3):356–60.
7. Federal Interagency Forum on Aging-Related Statistics. Older Americans 2010: Key Indicators of Well-Being. Federal Interagency Forum on Aging-Related Statistics. Washington, DC: U.S. Government Printing Office; 2010.
8. Neglia JP, FitzSimmons SC, Maisonneuve P, et al. The risk of cancer among patients with cystic fibrosis. Cystic Fibrosis and Cancer Study Group. N Engl J Med 1995;332(8):494–9.

9. Borman KR, Vick LR, Biester TW, et al. Changing demographics of residents choosing fellowships: long-term data from the American Board of Surgery. J Am Coll Surg 2008;206(5):782–8.

10. Committee on the Future of Emergency Care in the United States Health System. Hospital-based emergency care: at the breaking point. Washington, DC: Institute of Medicine of the National Academies; 2006.

11. Bland KI, Isaacs G. Contemporary trends in student selection of medical specialties: the potential impact on general surgery. Arch Surg 2002;137(3):259–67.

12. Zinner MJ. Surgical residencies: are we still attracting the best and the brightest? Bull Am Coll Surg 2002;87(3):20–5.

13. Fakhry SM, Watts DD, Michetti C, et al. The resident experience on trauma: declining surgical opportunities and career incentives? Analysis of data from a large multi-institutional study. J Trauma 2003;54(1):1–7 [discussion: 7–8].

14. Bell RH Jr, Biester TW, Tabuenca A, et al. Operative experience of residents in US general surgery programs: a gap between expectation and experience. Ann Surg 2009;249(5):719–24.

15. Velmahos G, Jurkovich G. The concept of acute care surgery: a vision for the not-so-distant future. Surgery 2007;141(3):3.

16. Britt LD, editor. Acute care surgery: principles and practice. New York (NY): Springer; 2007.

17. Cohn L. The times they are a-changin'. J Thorac Cardiovasc Surg 2010;140:2.

18. Moore HB, Moore PK, Grant AR, et al. Future of acute care surgery: a perspective from the next generation. J Trauma 2012;72(1):6.

19. Committee to Develop the Reorganized Specialty of Trauma SCC, and Emergency Surgery. Acute care surgery: trauma, critical care, and emergency surgery. J Trauma 2005;58(3):614–6.

20. Committee on Acute Care Surgery American Association for the Surgery of Trauma. The acute care surgery curriculum. J Trauma 2007;62(3):553–6.

21. ACGME program requirements for graduate medical education in surgical critical care. Available at: http://www.acgme.org/acWebsite/downloads/RRC_progReq/442_critical_care_surgery_01012009.pdf. Accessed May 24, 2012.

22. Surgical critical care: content outline for the certifying and recertification examinations. Available at: http://www.absurgery.org/xfer/SCC-CE-RECERT.pdf. Accessed May 24, 2012.

23. Sheldon G. The surgeon shortage: constructive participation during health reform. J Am Coll Surg 2010;210(6):8.

24. Industry funding of medical education—report of an AAMC task force. Washington, DC: Association of American Medical Colleges; 2008.

25. Field MJ, Lo B, editors. Conflict of interest in medical research, education, and practice. Washington, DC: Institute of Medicine of the National Academies; 2009.

Index

Note: Page numbers of article titles are in **boldface** type.

A

Abdomen
    NCTH control in, 851
Acute care surgery
    fellowship for
        setting up, 1059–1061
    graduate medical education in, **1055–1064**
        changes in surgical need effects on, 1056
        future directions in, 1061–1063
        new mandates in surgical training, 1056–1057
        new surgeon in practice, 1057–1058
        new surgeon in training, 1058
Acute traumatic coagulopathy (ATC)
    hemostatic resuscitation with, 886–887
    new understandings in, 880–883
AE system. *See* Aeromedical evacuation (AE) system
Aeromedical evacuation (AE) system
    history of, 926–927
Afghanistan
    war in, 1042
Airway control
    in prehospital emergency trauma care and management, 824–826
Amputation
    in complex extremity injury management, 991–992, 998–1003
        complications of, 1000–1001
        described, 998–999
        level of amputation, 999–1000
        prosthetics after, 1001–1003
        rehabilitation after, 1001–1003
Antibiotics
    topical
        in burn patients, 972–973
Anxiety
    in burn patients
        during ICU care
            management of, 968
ATC. *See* Acute traumatic coagulopathy (ATC)

B

Bleeding control
    in prehospital emergency trauma care and management, 826–829

Surg Clin N Am 92 (2012) 1065–1076
http://dx.doi.org/10.1016/S0039-6109(12)00121-1
0039-6109/12/$ – see front matter © 2012 Elsevier Inc. All rights reserved.

surgical.theclinics.com

Printed and bound by CPI Group (UK) Ltd, Croydon, CR0 4YY

03/10/2024

01040440-0006